TREATING SELF-INJURY

Treating Self-Injury
A Practical Guide

BARENT W. WALSH

THE GUILFORD PRESS
New York   London

Paperback edition 2008

Last digit is print number: 9 8 7 6 5 4 3

Library of Congress Cataloging-in-Publication Data

Walsh, Barent W.
    Treating self-injury : a practical guide / Barent W. Walsh.
      p. cm.   Includes bibliographical references and index.
    ISBN 978-1-59385-216-0 (hardcover : alk. paper)
    ISBN 978-1-59385-981-7 (paperback : alk. paper)
    1. Self-mutilation—Treatment.   I. Title.
    [DNLM: 1. Self-Injurious Behavior—therapy.   WM 165 W223t 2006]
RC552.S4W36 2006
616.85′82—dc22
                                                  2005020983

For Virginia Walsh and Valerie Wedge,
the most generous spirits

About the Author

Barent W. Walsh, PhD, has worked with self-injuring persons since the late 1970s. He is the long-time Executive Director of The Bridge of Central Massachusetts, headquartered in Worcester, Massachusetts. The Bridge consists of over 35 programs serving emotionally disturbed, mentally ill, or developmentally delayed children, adolescents, or adults. These programs emphasize the implementation of evidence-based practice models, including dialetical behavior therapy, illness management and recovery, assertive community treatment, integrated dual disorder treatment, and wraparound services in public sector settings. Dr. Walsh has conducted research, written extensively, and presented internationally on self-injury. He has consulted on this topic at numerous schools, universities, outpatient clinics, group homes, special education programs, psychiatric hospitals, and correctional facilities. He previously taught in the Graduate School of Social Work at both Simmons College and Boston College.

Preface

At first glance, Steve and Brandy appear to have nothing in common. Steve, age 25, has a long history of being troubled and in trouble. He was first hospitalized for self-destructive behavior at age 15. Over the years, he has received a variety of psychiatric diagnoses, including bipolar, borderline personality, and posttraumatic stress disorders. Steve comes from a chaotic family history of divorce, violence, and alcohol abuse. Even worse, he was sexually abused by an uncle from age 8 to 12. After numerous false starts and failures in the community, Steve is now part of the adult mental health system. He lives in a supported housing program, is striving for stability, and is able to work part-time.

Brandy's profile is entirely different. At age 16, her major life frustrations to date have been modest—at least in contrast to Steve's. She comes from an intact family. Her parents are consistently caring and involved. She has no history of trauma, carries no psychiatric diagnoses, and has many strengths. A junior in high school, Brandy is a fine student who receives A's and B's. She has several close friends with whom she spends time almost every weekend, and she is also the star pitcher on her high school softball team.

So where do the paths of Steve and Brandy intersect? Although they have never met and are unlikely to, they share an ongoing, alarming dilemma. Both Steve and Brandy cut themselves several times a week, usually on their forearms or legs, and burn themselves episodically several times a year.

And this is not all that they have in common. Both frequently experience intense emotional distress, are baffled as to how to manage it, and turn to self-injury as their last, best solution. Both have come into treatment hoping for some answers to their problems, not the least of which are the scars on their bodies that seem to keep multiplying beyond their control.

I wrote this book to assist professionals who work with people like Steve and Brandy. It is intended for a broad range of mental health clinicians, school personnel, and other professionals who work with self-injuring persons. The goal of the book is to provide a series of practical suggestions for understanding, managing, and treating the behavior. This book addresses common forms of self-injury as well as atypical and even severe examples. It does not, however, discuss self-injury in individuals with autism, mental retardation, and other forms of developmental disabilities.

Common examples of self-injury include scratching and cutting of the wrists, arms, and legs; self-inflicted burns; excoriation of wounds; self-hitting; and self-biting (although there are many other forms). Unfortunately, self-injury is presently an increasingly common behavior found in a wide range of settings, including middle and high schools, colleges, outpatient clinics, and private practices. Self-injury has long been found and continues to be a problem in programs serving more challenged individuals, such as those in special education schools, group homes, day treatment programs, inpatient psychiatric hospitals, and correctional facilities.

My background for writing this book is my work as a therapist with self-injurers since the late 1970s. I have conducted a number of empirical studies with a focus on adolescent and adult self-injurers, and I have also presented hundreds of workshops on the topic internationally. In addition to my own experience, this book draws heavily on the voluminous literature pertaining to self-injury and emphasizes treatment strategies that are current and evidence based.

This book is divided into three parts. Part I defines self-injury, distinguishes the behavior from suicide, places self-injury within the broader context of other forms of self-harm, identifies groups in which self-injury occurs, and differentiates self-injury from body modification, such as tattoos and body piercing.

Part II is the heart of the book. Assessment and treatment are discussed at length with numerous illustrative case examples. This book employs a biopsychosocial model to explain self-injury. Consistent with this perspective, the assessment and treatment techniques recommended include psychopharmacological and cognitive-behavioral forms of intervention. The discussion of psychological treatment moves from the most basic to the most complex. I begin with a discussion of using a low-key, dispassionate, interpersonal style in first responding to self-injury. Next, I discuss assessment with an emphasis on the myriad details that are important in coming to know a client and his or her patterns of self-harm. The presentation of more formal treatment interventions starts with a review of contingency management and continues with chapters devoted to replacement skills training, cognitive therapy, body image work, and exposure treatment. The discussion also includes a review of family therapy approaches and a chapter on the psychopharmacological treatment of self-injury written by Gordon Harper, MD. Finally, a chapter is provided on managing the negative reactions of therapists and other caregivers that frequently emerge in response to self-injurious behavior.

The third and final section of the book focuses on several specialized topics. The first of these is the challenging problem of contagion or epidemic self-injury. Usually found in groups of adolescents, contagion is addressed by reviewing the empirical literature pertaining to the concept and by discussing several examples of contagion episodes. Following this chapter is a presentation of a protocol used in public schools to prevent contagion and manage self-injury effectively. The principles used in this protocol can also be applied to other group settings, such as group homes, residential schools, and inpatient units. Finally, I discuss how to understand, prevent, and treat "major self-injury," including acts that involve extensive tissue damage and/or injury to the eyes, face, or genitals. Such behavior is usually associated with severe psychopathology, extensive trauma, or other extreme circumstances.

In closing, I express my hope that this book will benefit two categories of professionals: those who treat self-injurers who have major mental health challenges (such as Steve) and those who work with the new generation of healthier self-injurers (such as Brandy). Both types of clients deserve respectful, compassionate, and effective care. My intent in this book has been to make a contribution toward this important psychotherapeutic goal.

Acknowledgments

Writing a book involves sacrifice for the author and those around him. My profound thanks to my wife, Valerie, and my children, Ben and Anna, who did without my presence for many hours as I sat sequestered, tapping out words on the computer.

My thanks also to my longtime colleagues at The Bridge of Central Massachusetts. They patiently endured my being preoccupied with this effort and took up the slack, running over 30 programs for emotionally disturbed, mentally ill, or developmentally disabled individuals. Specifically, I wish to thank my very committed management team of Steve Murphy, Fred Battersby, Milt Bornstein, Donna Bradley, Tina Wingate, Doug Watts, and Nancy Bishop; my very talented division directors, including Carol Tripp-Tebo, Christy Clark, Jen Eaton, Jodie Rapping, Margaret Crowley, Laura Winton, June David-Fors, and Erica Robert; and the Board of Trustees, including Board President J. Christopher Collins.

I also wish to thank the major funders of The Bridge, who are supportive in so many ways. These include Elaine Hill, Sue Sciaraffa, Ted Kirousis, Babs Fenby, Jack Rowe, and Richard Breault from the Massachusetts Department of Mental Health; Terry O'Hare from the Department of Mental Retardation; and Marty Cohen from the Metrowest Community Health Care Foundation.

Beyond those directly involved in my day-to-day professional work, there are many others who had an impact on this project. I wish to thank colleagues in the field of self-injury for their scholarship and wisdom. These include authors Paul Rosen, Wendy Lader, Karen Conterio, Tracy Alderman, Jane Hyman, Caroline Kettlewell, Daphne Simeon, Armando Favazza, Kate Comtois, Milton Brown, Kim Gratz, Sarah Shaw, Efrosini Kokaliari, and Jan Sutton.

I also wish to thank those who have assisted me in learning mindful-ness, including Marsha Linehan, Charlie Swenson, Zindel Segal, and the late Cindy Sanderson. I am particularly indebted to my meditation teach-ers, Soto Zen priest, Issho Fujita, and the venerable Lobsang Phuntsok, Tibetan monk.

My greatest inspiration in writing on the topic of self-destructive behavior has been the intellectual giant, suicidologist, Ed Shneidman. As the saying goes, he has forgotten more than I will ever know about the topic of self-harm. I also want to thank Lanny Berman, Executive Director of the American Association of Suicidology, for enabling me to present on self-injury for many years at the Association's annual conference.

Finally, I want to acknowledge those who have taught me the most about self-injury: self-injurers themselves. The secret to understanding and treating self-injury is first and foremost developing an ability to really lis-ten. Approaching self-injurers nonjudgmentally, respectfully, and compas-sionately puts one is a position to learn from them. Based on that learning, the therapist can facilitate growth, problem solving, and healing. The role of the therapist with these individuals is primarily one of intermediary. Self-injurers are some of the most inspiring people I have known. Many of them have worked so hard to overcome so much in order to move to a better, stronger place. I appreciate the learning they have sent my way and hereby pass it on.

Contents

PART III. SPECIALIZED TOPICS

TREATING SELF-INJURY

PART I

Definition and Contexts

CHAPTER 1

Definition, Differentiation from Suicide, and Classification

The most important point should be stated at the outset: Self-injury is separate and distinct from suicide. Self-injury is not about ending life but about reducing psychological distress. Self-injury is often a strangely effective coping behavior, albeit a self-destructive one.

TERMINOLOGY

Since the mid-1990s, the language used to refer to behaviors such as self-inflicted cutting, scratching, burning, hitting, and excoriation of wounds has changed. Previously referred to as "self-mutilation," the more common and popular term has become "self-injury." Both self-injuring people and those who treat them have advocated that "self-mutilation" is too extreme and pejorative a term (e.g., Hyman, 1999; Connors, 2000; Simeon & Favazza, 2001). These advocates have argued that most people who self-injure employ the behavior as a coping mechanism to deal with psychological distress; therefore, the behavior has adaptive features. Moreover, they have correctly stated that the large majority of self-inflicted wounds involves only modest physical damage that leaves little, if any, long-term scarring. The wounds do not result in a "mutilation" of the body. The *Merriam-Webster Dictionary* defines "mutilate" as, "to cut up or alter radically so as to make imperfect" and "to maim, cripple" (1995, p. 342). I accept the contention that the term "self-mutilation" is derogatory, even sensationalistic, in referring to the behavior (Simeon & Favazza, 2001), and therefore use the term "self-injury" in this text.

3

FORMAL DEFINITION

In this book, self-injury is defined in the following way:

> *Self-injury* is intentional, self-effected, low-lethality bodily harm of a socially unacceptable nature, performed to reduce psychological distress.

The components of this definition require some explication. As explained above, the term "self-injury" is descriptive and nonpejorative. It is also nonexaggerative. The word "intentional" specifies that self-injury is deliberate; it is not accidental or ambiguous as to intent. Self-injury is also "self-effected." This term is chosen rather than "self-inflicted" because many individuals self-injure with the assistance of others. Not uncommonly—especially with adolescents—two or more people may take turns or simultaneously hurt each other. For quite a few people, self-injury is an interpersonal experience. The next term in the definition is "low lethality." Self-injury, by definition, involves those forms of self-harm that do modest physical damage to the body and pose little, or no, risk to life. The distinction of self-injury from suicide is explicit and fundamental, as is discussed in detail later in this chapter.

Self-injury is primarily about "bodily harm." The behavior alarms others because of the tissue damage. A person may present with talk or planning about self-injury, but until he or she crosses the line into actively damaging the body, there is no self-injury.

The phrase "of a socially unacceptable nature" is included in the definition to emphasize social context. Favazza (1996) has written extensively about the multifarious body modifications that occur around the world. In most cultures, body modification is symbolically meaningful and culturally endorsed. It may have profound religious significance and be part of a complex rite of passage. That is not the case for common self-injury, which, although it may have many meanings for its perpetrators, is not endorsed by the prevailing culture. Granted, self-injury can often seem to be part of an adolescent expression of angst and alienation. Among teens there may be considerable social reinforcement for the behavior. However, there are no organized, culturally endorsed rituals that surround it. Self-injury is not connected to any socially sanctioned rite of passage.

The final phrase in the definition is "performed to reduce psychological distress." Self-injury is enacted because of its ability to modify and reduce psychological discomfort. It is usually immediately and substantially effective and therefore is often repeated. The behavior is not suicidal, but it is psychologically motivated. Self-injury is a behavior that cannot be explained via biological mechanisms alone. Rather, it is a self-conscious, self-intentioned, distress-reduction behavior.

DIFFERENTIATING SELF-INJURY FROM SUICIDE

The above section has emphasized that self-injury should be considered separate and distinct from suicide. The remainder of this chapter discusses nine points of distinction between self-injury and suicide. These points are provided to justify the contention that self-injury and suicide should be understood, managed and treated differentially. All too often self-injury is inappropriately labeled "suicidal," resulting in poorly designed interventions. The nine points of distinction presented here provide a practical roadmap for determining whether a self-destructive behavior is suicidal or self-injurious. This distinction has major implications for all the assessment and treatment that follow. A concise summary of the nine points is provided in Table 1.1.

Intent

A fundamental place to start in differentiating suicide from self-injury is with the topic of intent. Clinicians need to know what the person is intending to accomplish via the behavior. What are his or her goals in acting self-destructively? Some people are quite insightful and articulate in explaining the intent of their self-harming behavior. They provide clinicians with explanations of their behavior that are clear and concise. For example, some self-injuring people say, "I cut myself to feel better. I don't want to die. I just want to get the anger out." In a similar vein, some suicidal individuals make their motives quite evident. They may say, "If I don't have this relationship in my life, it's not worth living. My life is over. That's why I took the overdose." In both examples, intent could not be more clear.

However, more frequently than not, clinicians find it difficult to elicit a clear articulation of intent. Self-destructive persons are emotionally overwhelmed and often very confused about their own behavior. When asked why they acted self-destructively, many individuals provide ambiguous responses, such as, "I'm not sure why I took the overdose; it just seemed like the thing to do." Others speak with considerable vagueness, such as, "I wouldn't cut myself now, but I had to do it then" and refuse, or are unable, to say more.

Some individuals seem to be disconnected from conscious thought processes when they hurt themselves, such as the individual who said, "At one point, I looked down at my arms, saw a lot of blood and had no idea

TABLE 1.1. Differentiating Suicide Attempts from Self-Injurious Behavior

Assessment focus	Suicide attempt (Shneidman, 1985)	Self-injury (Walsh & Rosen, 1988)
1. What was the expressed and unexpressed intent of the act?	To escape pain; terminate consciousness	Relief from unpleasant affect (tension, anger, emptiness, deadness)
2. What was the level of physical damage and potential lethality?	Serious physical damage; lethal means of self-harm	Little physical damage; nonlethal means used
3. Is there a chronic, repetitive pattern of self-injurious acts?	Rarely a chronic repetition; some overdose repeatedly	Frequently a chronic, high-rate pattern
4. Have multiple methods of self-injury been used over time?	Usually one method	Usually more than one method over time
5. What is the level of psychological pain?	Unendurable, persistent	Uncomfortable, intermittent
6. Is there constriction of cognition?	Extreme constriction; suicide as the only way out; tunnel vision; seeking a final solution	Little or no constriction; choices available; seeking a temporary solution
7. Are there feelings of hopelessness and helplessness?	Hopelessness and helplessness are central	Periods of optimism and some sense of control
8. Was there a decrease in discomfort following the act?	No immediate improvement; treatment required for improvement	Rapid improvement; rapid return to usual cognition and affect; successful "alteration of consciousness"
9. What is the core problem?	Depression, rage about inescapable, unendurable pain	Body alienation; exceptionally poor body image in clinical populations

how it happened." Another variation is the all-too-common encounter with adolescents who, when asked why they performed some self-destructive act, reply with that classic roadblock to psychological progress, "I don't know."

Intent can be successfully elicited from both suicidal and self-injuring persons, but the process often requires a combination of profound compassion and investigative persistence. Our discussion of differentiating suicide from self-injury begins with key points of distinction pertaining to intent.

Suicidal Intent

In his classic work *Definition of Suicide* (1985), Shneidman identified a number of salient points that differentiate suicide from self-injury. The first of these is intent. Shneidman states that the intent of the suicidal person is generally not so much to kill the body; rather, the intent is to "terminate consciousness." The suicidal person wants to stop the psychological pain, to escape the "psychache," as Shneidman calls it (Shneidman, 1993). The suicidal person will do whatever it takes to make the pain go away *permanently*.

Self-Injurious Intent

In contrast, the intent of the self-injuring person is not to *terminate* consciousness, but to *modify* it. The overwhelming majority of self-injurers report that they harm themselves in order to relieve painful feelings. The type of emotional distress they want to relieve falls into two basic categories. The majority of those who self-injure report hurting themselves in order to relieve *too much* emotion (Favazza, 1987; Walsh & Rosen, 1988; Alderman, 1997; Conterio & Lader, 1998; Brown, 1998, 2002; Brown, Comtois, & Linehan, 2002). The minority report harming themselves in order to relieve *too little* emotion or states of dissociation (e.g., Conterio & Lader, 1998; Shapiro & Dominiak, 1992; Simeon & Hollander, 2001). Those who report feeling too much emotional distress identify such feelings as:

- Anger
- Shame
- Anxiety, tension, or panic
- Sadness
- Frustration
- Contempt

Studies differ regarding the order of uncomfortable emotions cited by self-injurers. (See Brown, 2002, for a thorough review of studies on emotions that precede self-injury.)

A smaller proportion of self-injurers report feeling too little emotion. They state that they feel empty, "zombie-like," dead, or "like a robot." These individuals self-injure to alleviate this absence of feeling. As a young adult female once told me, "When I cut myself and see the blood, it's very reassuring, because I can see for myself that I'm still alive." Many of these individuals may be experiencing states of dissociation immediately prior to self-injuring.

The key point regarding intent is that the suicidal person wants to eliminate consciousness permanently; the self-injurer wants to modify consciousness, to reduce distress, in order to live another day.

Level of Physical Damage and Potential Lethality

Given the difficulty of eliciting clearly articulated intent from clients, clinicians often have to focus on the acts of self-harm in order to perform an accurate assessment. Fortunately, the chosen method of self-harm often communicates a great deal about the intent of the self-destructive person. Certain behaviors convey suicidal intent; others suggest self-injurious motivation.

Suicide Methods

Research has shown repeatedly that people who die by suicide use a rather short list of high-lethality methods. For example, recent statistics from the Centers for Disease Control and Prevention identify death by suicide as occurring via seven basic methods (cdc.gov website, 2002; see Table 1.2). Note that the primary methods that people use to end their lives are shooting themselves, hanging, pill or poison ingestion, and jumping from a height. Note also that the most common form of self-injury (cutting) is reported to result in death for only 1.4% of those who die by suicide. That is to say, the 98.6% of individuals who die by suicide in the United States use methods other than cutting. It should be emphasized that the type of cutting that is likely to result in death is severing the carotid artery or jugular veins in the neck. It is not cutting of the arms or legs, the most common bodily locations for self-injury.

Moreover, if the statistics for cause of death by suicide are reviewed for the age group of 15–24 years, the percentage of those dying by cutting becomes even lower. This is the age group in which self-injury is most common (see Table 1.3). Note that for the younger age group the same methods of self-harm result in death: self-inflicted gunshot, hanging, overdose and

TABLE 1.2. Deaths by Suicide in the United States, 1999; All Ages, All Races, Both Sexes

Cause of death	Number of deaths	Percentage of deaths
1. Firearm	16,599	56.8
2. Suffocation (e.g., hanging)	5,427	18.6
3. Poisoning (e.g., overdose, carbon monoxide)	4,893	16.8
4. Fall (e.g., jumping from a height)	693	2.4
5. Cut/pierce	404	1.4
6. Drowning	311	1.1
7. Other (many different types, such as self-immolation or transportation related)	872	3.0

Note. Total deaths = 29,199.

self-poisoning, and jumping from a height. Note also that the proportion of 15- to 24-year-olds who die by cutting/piercing drops to 0.4%. *Thus, 99.6% of youth who die by suicide use methods other than cutting.* Once again, those youth who die by cutting generally do so by cutting the carotid artery or jugular vein in the neck, not arms or legs.

Self-Injury Methods

There are no comparable data from large samples regarding the methods of self-injury. The largest sample reported in the literature to date is Favazza

TABLE 1.3. Deaths by Suicide in the United States, 1999, Ages 15–24, All Races, Both Sexes

Cause of death	Number of deaths	Percentage of deaths
1. Firearm	2,315	59.3
2. Suffocation	966	24.8
3. Poisoning	328	6.4
4. Fall	112	2.9
5. Other	97	2.5
6. Drowning	31	0.8
7. Fire/burn	18	0.5
8. Transportation related	18	0.5
9. Cut/pierce	16	0.4

Note. Total deaths = 3,901.

and Conterio's study (1988). Their study employed a convenience sample that responded to a Phil Donahue television show devoted to self-injury. Responding to a request to complete a mail-in questionnaire, 250 people, 96% of whom were female, did so. The results indicated that respondents used the following methods: cutting (72%), burning (35%), self-hitting (30%), interference with wound healing (22%), hair pulling (trichotillomania; 10%), and bone breaking (8%).

Some additional data regarding types of self-injury are available from a small sample study I conducted in the late 1990s (Walsh & Frost, 2005). The study sample consisted of 70 adolescents who were receiving intensive treatment in either special education or residential programs. Of the 70 adolescents, 34 were identified as poly-self-destructive, meaning they had histories of suicide attempts and recurrent self-injury and multiple forms of indirect self-harm, including risk taking, substance abuse, and eating disorders. Of these 34 youth, 23 were female and 11 were male. These youth reported that their self-injury took the following forms: cutting (82.4%), body carving (64.7%), head banging (64.7%), picking at scabs (61.8%), scratching (50%), burning (58.8%), self-hitting (58.8%), and self-piercing (52.9%). Other less common forms of self-injury for these youth were self-inflicted tattoos (47.1%), self-biting (44.1%), and hair pulling (38.2%). Although many of these behaviors were alarming, it is important to emphasize that none was life threatening. Note also that when the categories of cutting, scratching, and carving are combined, body incising (91.2%) was by far the most popular method of self-injury for this sample.

Across the literature on self-injury (e.g., Favazza, 1987; Walsh & Rosen, 1988; Alderman, 1997; Conterio & Lader, 1998; Brown, 1998; Simeon & Hollander, 2001), the most common methods of self-injury reported consist of the following:

- Cutting, scratching, and carving
- Excoriation of wounds
- Self-hitting
- Self-burning
- Head banging
- Self-inflicted tattoos
- Other (e.g., self-biting, abrading, ingesting scrap, inserting objects, self-inflicted piercing, hair pulling)

These are presented in the general order of frequency, although the exact order varies from study to study. Cutting is almost always the most common form reported.

It is important to emphasize that none of these behaviors is likely to result in death, except in the most extreme circumstances (e.g., self-burning that takes the form of self-immolation, an exceedingly rare behavior). If cutting behaviors are unlikely to result in death, particularly the most common forms of cutting arms, wrists, and legs, it is quite reasonable to conclude that the behavior is generally about something other than suicide. If cutting is generally not about trying to end one's life, then what is it about? This is the question I attempt to address in the rest of this book.

Chapter 2 discusses the broad category of direct self-harm, which can be divided into two groups: suicide and self-injury. When clients discuss plans to use (or actually employ) any of the top four behaviors listed in Tables 1.2 and 1.3 (i.e., shooting, hanging, self-poisoning, jumping from a height), it is appropriate to conclude that their intent is suicidal. These are high-lethality behaviors that frequently result in death. In contrast, if clients discuss, or actually perform, acts of cutting, excoriation, self-hitting, self-burning, or self-biting, it is appropriate generally to view the behaviors as self-injurious rather than suicidal.

Frequency of the Behavior

Another point of distinction between suicide and self-injury is the frequency with which the behaviors occur. In general, self-injury occurs at much higher rates than suicide attempts. The large majority of people who attempt suicide do not do so recurrently or frequently. The most common pattern is that people attempt suicide once or twice when they are in a particularly stressful period in their lives. For most persons this type of crisis period passes and they move on with their lives. Most individuals are resilient and/or obtain professional help and are unlikely to attempt suicide again.

However, there are others—those in the minority—who attempt suicide recurrently over extended periods of time, years, even decades. These are usually persons who have a serious and persistent mental illness (e.g., a major depression, bipolar illness, borderline personality disorder). Most frequently, it appears that recurrent suicide attempters employ pill overdose as their methods. These individuals appear to know how much prescribed or over-the-counter medications they can ingest and still survive. Or they may take serious, even lethal dosages, but quickly disclose their actions to others, resulting in protective intervention. However, even for these recurrent suicide attempters, the rates of their attempts pale in comparison to rates of self-injury in many persons.

Many, probably the majority, of self-injuring persons perform the behavior frequently. A commonly reported frequency by self-injuring clients is 20–100 times over a multiple-year period (Walsh & Rosen, 1988). Even adolescents who are in their early teens describe a several-year course of self-injury, with as many as 20–30 episodes per year. Sometimes the frequency of self-injury can be hard even to count for some clients. For example:

Eloise's favorite form of self-injury was to cut many finely executed parallel lines on her left forearm. She would begin near her wrist and cut progressively up her forearm until she reached the inside of her elbow. On one occasion, as part of a behavioral assessment, we attempted to count the exact number of separate and distinct cuts executed during a single episode. The count was about 78. Also, several days after inflicting such self-injury, Eloise would tend to reopen the wounds by scraping a razor blade "across the grain" repeatedly. This type of self-harm defied any attempts at counting.

Many persons self-injure many, even hundreds of, times. Almost no one attempts suicide at such rates.

Multiple Methods

Another point of distinction between suicide and self-injury is whether the perpetrators use multiple methods. As noted above, persons who attempt suicide repeatedly are relatively rare and tend to use the method of overdosing on prescribed or over-the-counter medication. Although there are no precise statistics on these suicide repeaters, clinical experience suggests that most suicide repeaters employ one method over time, that being overdose. In contrast, most self-injuring persons use more than one method. Note that in the small sample study of adolescents mentioned above, over 70% employed more than one method. In the Favazza and Conterio (1988) study cited above, 78% of 250 responders had used multiple methods.

The use of more than one method may be related to at least two factors: preference and circumstances. Many self-injuring persons state that they use different methods of self-injury because they prefer to do so. For example, some self-injuring people say that they cut when they are anxious and burn when they are enraged. Others say that they cut when dissociating but hit themselves when angry. The range of links between types of affective distress and forms of self-injury is almost infinite. An important detail in the assessment and treatment of self-injury is determining whether or not an individual uses more than one method and how he or she decides on a specific method at any one point in time.

Sometimes the decision on method of self-harm is more related to circumstance than personal preference. For example, adolescents placed in a group home or an inpatient unit may have difficulty obtaining a razor to cut because of close staff supervision. Although cutting may be their preferred method, they may have to resort to self-hitting or self-biting due to the unavailability of the preferred tool.

Level of Psychological Pain

Shneidman (1985) emphasized that "unendurable, persistent pain" drives the suicidal crisis. The "psychache" of the suicidal person is so profound, deep, and excruciating that it is intolerable, unlivable. Moreover, the pain is persistent, wearing down the person and producing profound psychic fatigue. Given the phenomenological experience of this pain, it is no wonder that the suicidal person contemplates a permanent escape. For the large majority of suicidal persons this experience of intense pain is fraught with significant cognitive and emotional distortions. Nonetheless, within the mindset of suicidal persons is a certain logic that compels them in the direction of suicide in order to escape.

In contrast, a different type of psychic distress characterizes self-injury. The pain of the self-injuring person is intense and uncomfortable, but it does not reach the level of a suicidal crisis. The psychological anguish of the self-injurer is interruptible and intermittent, rather than permanent and unalterable. One reason for the difference is that the self-injury itself offers a method to interrupt and reduce the pain, rendering it temporary and partial.

Constriction of Cognition

Another key feature of the suicidal crisis is cognitive constriction. Shneidman (1985) has used several terms to explain this mindset including "constriction," "tunnel vision," and "dichotomous thinking." They all mean essentially the same thing. In the suicidal person, life is channeled down to an all-or-nothing option. The suicidal person thinks in a radically narrow or constricted way. A particularly common example is the belief "I must have this relationship with this person or I will die," but there are many other scenarios. Other examples encountered in clinical practice include:

> "If I lose my fortune, I will kill myself."
> "If this disease is incurable, I will end it all."
> "I can't tolerate getting a bad grade. If I get a mere B, I'll overdose."
> "If I can't get this job back, I'll kill my boss and myself."
> "If I can't have custody of my children, no one will."

(Note that the last two are murder–suicide scenarios.) However diverse the content, all these examples have constricted thinking in common. The basic formula is "X must happen or I will kill myself."

Self-injury is not characterized by dichotomous thinking. More frequently than not, the thought process of self-injurers is disorganized rather
than constricted. They do not reduce their lives to an all-or-nothing predicament. Rather, they still perceive themselves to have choices in their lives
and options from which to select. One of these options—and not the best
one—is to self-injure. For self-injuring persons the option to cut or burn is
oddly reassuring.

Helplessness and Hopelessness

Suicide research has long identified both hopelessness and helplessness as
important components of depression and suicidal behavior (Beck, Rush,
Shaw, & Emery, 1979; Seligman, 1992; Milnes, Owens, & Blenkiron, 2002).
Helplessness refers to a loss of controllability (Seligman, 1992). People who
feel helpless believe that they have no real influence or control over their
situations. They are convinced there is nothing they can do to impact or
improve their lives. Such cognitive pessimism is very conducive to the "giving up" that suicide entails.

Hopelessness is the counterpart to helplessness. When people feel
hopeless, they believe their pain is endless, permanent; they have no
future. Persons in a suicidal crisis feel unendurable pain that seems infinite
and over which they believe they have no control. Within such a bleakly
pessimistic mindset, it is no wonder that people consider suicide as the
remaining option.

Another way to describe the helpless and hopeless world view of the
suicidal person is in terms of the "cognitive negative triad of depression"
(Beck et al., 1979). Within this perspective, suicidal people think, "I'm no
good [self], everything around me is terrible [world], and nothing will ever
change [future]."

In contrast, helplessness and hopelessness do not characterize the self-
injury scenario. Self-injuring persons generally do not feel they have no
control over their psychological pain. In fact, the option of self-injury provides a key sense of control. Most self-injuring people find it reassuring
that cutting, burning, or some other form of self-harm is available whenever
they may need it to reduce distress. The control that self-injury offers is
antithetical to hopelessness. The future is not one of endless inescapable
pain because self-injury often works as a tension-reduction mechanism.
Granted, self-injuring persons may be episodically pessimistic and despair
that their lives include so much discomfort. But their distress lacks the
sense of inescapability and permanency that is fundamental to the suicidal
crisis.

Psychological Aftermath of the Self-Harm Incident

The aftermath of suicidal and self-injury behaviors also differs. Most people who survive suicide report feeling no better following the attempt. Instead, they often report feeling even worse. They may make bitterly self-critical comments, such as, "I even screwed this up—I'm such a loser" or "I didn't even kill myself right." Other statements include: "I didn't have the guts to do it, but next time I will" or "Now I feel even worse than I did before I took the pills." These are people who, despite the attempt at suicide, have in no way diminished their psychological pain and their intent to kill themselves. One case vignette conveys the tone and content of the suicidal aftermath quite well:

Erin was a 17-year-old with a history of depression and recurrent suicide attempts by overdose. Recently released from a psychiatric unit where she was deemed to be safe, Erin became enraged and despondent when her mother was critical of her. Erin walked to a nearby bridge and jumped from a 30-foot height into frigid winter water. She survived only because an off-duty policeman saw the incident and pulled her out. Once medically cleared, Erin was immediately placed on a locked psychiatric unit.

Interviewed the next day on the ward, Erin was asked if she was feeling any better. In a bitter, sarcastic tone, she spat out her reply, "My only regret is that I didn't jump off something higher onto something harder!"

This vignette points to the common features of suicide aftermath. Persons often show persistent, intense psychological pain and high-lethality intent even after the attempt.

The aftermath of self-injury behavior is often the *direct opposite* of the suicide attempt. The "draw" of the self-injury episode is its effectiveness in reducing emotional distress. Moreover, the relief obtained is *immediate.* Self-injuring persons emphasize the importance of the relief obtained and the accessibility of the effect. They make such comments as:

"As soon as I cut, it was like all the anger was let out and I felt so much better."
"After cutting my arms or legs, all the tension leaves my body and I can go to sleep."
"Once I burn myself, I can see my rage on the outside, so I don't have to feel it inside anymore."

Clinicians should be especially alert when clients report that their self-injury is no longer producing the desired effect. When self-injury fails to provide its usual "therapeutic" effect, persons who rely on it for relief begin to feel hopeless and helpless and may start to panic, feeling that the pain is inescapable. This loss of escape can catapult self-injurers into a suicidal crisis. The pain is no longer manageable and within their control. As the pain escalates and they are unable to reduce it, the conditions for a suicidal crisis may emerge and protective intervention may be necessary.

The Core Problem

The core problem for the suicidal person is usually some combination of depression, sadness, and rage about his or her primary source of unendurable pain. Maltsberger (1986) has emphasized that the despair that drives the suicidal crisis is not only about sadness, loneliness, and isolation but also includes elements of "murderous hate." This hatred provides much of the energy for the suicidal behavior and is often directed both at the self and at others.

The challenge in assisting suicidal individuals is therefore to identify the primary source of unendurable pain and to reduce it. Shneidman (1985) stresses that if the professional can add a third term to the dichotomous thinking of the suicidal person, then suicide risk will be reduced. For example, if the constricted thinking of an individual is "I must have this relationship or I will die," adding a third term might mean introducing the option of counseling with a focus on the relationship. The dichotomous scenario of "This must happen or I will die" is expanded (and lethality simultaneously diffused) by adding a third term, "This must happen or I will die *or* I will address the relationship in counseling."

Finding the *specific* source of the unendurable, inescapable pain is the primary focus in working with suicidal persons. The more precisely defined the source, the more effective the work is likely to be. Moving from the global (e.g., "All of my life is terrible") to the idiosyncratic (e.g., "I'm tired of being humiliated by my boss at work") is at the heart of the therapeutic work.

In contrast, the core problem for many self-injuring persons often involves their body image. Not surprisingly, many people who hurt themselves repeatedly often have especially negative attitudes toward their bodies (Walsh & Rosen, 1988; Alderman, 1997, Hyman, 1999). For many, a profound sense of body alienation or body hatred drives them to self-injure. Key questions that become central foci in the treatment of self-injury are "Why do you repeatedly inflict harm on your body?" and "What are the origins of this relationship with your body?" The relationship between body alienation and self-injury is discussed at length in Chapter 11.

However, one emerging group of self-injuring persons does not appear to have significant body image problems. This group appears to comprise the healthier individuals who surfaced only since the late 1990s as a self-injury phenomenon. The core problem for these individuals appears to be a combination of intense stress, inadequate self-soothing skills, and peer influences that endorse self-injury. The challenges that drive these individuals to self-injure are reviewed in Chapter 3.

CLASSIFYING SELF-INJURY

Over the years a number of ways of classifying self-injury have been proposed (e.g., Menninger, 1938/1966; Ross & Mckay, 1979; Walsh & Rosen, 1988). The most widely accepted has come from Favazza, who has presented a series of classification schemes that have been evolving since 1987 (Favazza, 1987; Favazza & Rosenthal, 1990; Favazza, 1996; Favazza, 1998; Simeon & Favazza, 2001). The most recent of these, and the one with which Favazza is most satisfied (personal communication, 2002), is presented in Simeon and Favazza (2001).

The classification scheme presented by Simeon and Favazza (2001) is an important advance in the study of self-injury that should be reviewed. They propose that self-injurious behavior be organized in terms of four categories: stereotypic, major, compulsive, and impulsive. Within these categories they discuss the types of self-injury included, the associated tissue damage, the biological correlates, the rates and patterns of behavior, and the diagnostic categories associated with the behavior.

In this book, I have chosen to use some aspects of Simeon and Favazza's classification scheme, but not others. The first category presented by Simeon and Favazza is "stereotypic self-injury," which refers to behaviors such as head banging, self-hitting, biting, picking, and scratching as enacted by individuals with mental retardation, developmental disability, autism, and other conditions. Simeon and Favazza state that this behavior is different from self-injury in other populations in that it can occur at extremely high rates (e.g., thousands of times per day) and is "fixed, contentless, and driven" (Simeon & Favazza, 2001, p. 5). Although I suspect that stereotypic self-injury in the developmentally disabled has more psychological content than is generally recognized, I otherwise accept the Simeon and Favazza conceptualization. The topic of stereotypic self-injury is not covered in this book. Excellent books already exist that are devoted exclusively to the assessment and treatment of it (e.g., Gardner & Sovner, 1994; Schroeder, Oster-Granite, & Thompson, 2002). Stein and Neihaus (2001) also provide a fine brief review of the topic.

The second category presented by Simeon and Favazza (2001) is the concept of "major self-injury," which includes acts of self-harm that are often associated with psychosis and which cause considerable damage. Major self-injury can be medium- to high-lethality in nature. Examples of major self-injury cited by Simeon and Favazza are self-enucleation, auto-castration, and self-amputation. I accept the concept of major self-injury as described by Simeon and Favazza and discuss it at length in Chapter 18.

The major departure in this book concerns the two categories of compulsive and impulsive self-injury presented by Simeon and Favazza. Compulsive self-injury refers to behaviors such as hair pulling, skin picking, and nail biting. Simeon and Favazza (2001) state that this category is associated with disorders such a trichotillomania and stereotypic movement disorder. The behavior tends to appear as part of a compulsive behavior pattern, sometimes with elaborate rituals. These behaviors often occur several times per day and can occur "automatically, without any conscious urge, or with a complex variety of associated thoughts and affects" (Simeon & Favazza, 2001, p. 9, citing Christenson et al., 1993). They also note that this category of behavior appears to have a strong association with the diagnoses of obsessive–compulsive disorder (OCD) and OCD-related disorders (see Christenson, MacKenzie, & Mitchell, 1991).

Simeon and Favazza (2001) group self-inflicted skin cutting, burning, and hitting under the rubric of impulsive self-injury. They note that these behaviors are associated with borderline personality disorder, antisocial personality disorder, posttraumatic stress disorder (PTSD), and eating disorders. They indicate that this category can be subdivided into episodic and repetitive self-injury, stating:

> In the repetitive type, self-injury may become an organizing and predominant preoccupation, with a seemingly addictive quality, that is incorporated into the individual's sense of identity. The self-injury may become almost an automatic response to various disturbing internal and external stimuli, typically beginning in adolescence and persisting for decades. (2001, p. 15)

Although Simeon and Favazza do not discuss the episodic type at length, Favazza has done so elsewhere (1995). He stated:

> The term episodic refers to behavior that occurs every so often. Episodic self-mutilators do not brood about this behavior, nor do they have a self-identity as a "cutter" or "burner." They deliberately harm themselves to feel better, to get rapid respite from distressing thoughts and emotions, and to regain a sense of control. (1996, p. 234)

The episodic subcategory includes the same types of behavior (cutting, burning, and picking) as the repetitive, but the behaviors occur less frequently and are less of a central preoccupation for the individuals.

Simeon and Favazza's (2001) formulation of compulsive versus impulsive self-injury is problematic in that too many examples of self-injurious behavior do not fit it. They acknowledge the limitations of their own categories, saying, "the distinction between compulsive and impulsive repetitive may not always be sharp and clear. Impulsive repetitive self-injury can, at times, become so habitual as to occur on a daily or weekly basis and with clearly identifiable precipitating external events or affective states, as though it were a compulsion" (Simeon & Favazza, 2001, p. 16).

Self-injuring persons are often quite fluid in how they harm themselves. Sometimes they self-injure episodically, such as every few weeks or months, and they do not seem preoccupied with or controlled by the behavior. When their stress level rises, they may self-injure much more frequently and begin to resemble the repetitive, impulsive self-injurer described by Simeon and Favazza. However, they may also go through periods when the behavior becomes very high rate, almost automatic, that is to say, compulsive in nature.

Moreover, I have worked with a number of clients who present with *both* compulsive and impulsive self-injurious behaviors *at the same time.* The following example describes such a situation.

Hilda had many self-destructive behaviors in her repertoire. Her hair pulling had produced multiple bald spots on her head. She stated that she pulled out her hair every day, often without awareness, when she was on the phone or using her computer. She collected some baseline data as part of her treatment and reported that her rate of hair removal ranged from 0 to over 230 hairs per day over a 3-week period. During the same time period, Hilda cut herself repeatedly. On several occasions she did this in an impulsive rage, cutting jagged wounds into her forearm that caused damage just short of needing medical attention. At other times, she would methodically lay out her blades and execute small, precise cuts on a single area of her wrist during an episode that took several hours.

In this example, the client presents with all three types of behavior in combination: compulsive (hair pulling), impulsive–repetitive (frequent, rageful cutting), and impulsive–episodic (occasional methodical cutting). This convergence of diverse behaviors within single individuals suggests that the associations between the impulsive and compulsive categories and separate and distinct psychiatric diagnoses may not be very strong.

Simeon and Favazza's attempt at classification is the best proposed to date, even though it has problems yet to be resolved. Their work and that of their colleagues (Simeon & Hollander, 2001) on attempting to identify biological correlates to the different types of self-injury is particularly important. Such research has considerable potential for the development of more targeted psychopharmacological interventions in the future.

In this book I use a much simpler classification scheme, that of common self-injury versus major self-injury. This way of categorizing the behaviors can be easily grasped and employed by clinicians in the field. Classification models such as Simeon and Favazza's (2001) are important for research purposes but are unlikely to be used by caregivers in fast-paced environments such as schools, outpatient clinics, group homes, and hospitals. Staff persons in these settings need "quick and dirty" ways to conceptualize the behavior that can be directly linked to assessment and treatment.

CHAPTER 2

An Overview of Direct
and Indirect Self-Harm

Comprehensive assessment of self-destructive behavior considers *all* forms of self-harm. A clinician assessing for self-injury should seek not only to differentiate it from suicide (as discussed in the previous chapter), but also to evaluate for other self-destructive behaviors such as substance abuse, eating disorder, risk taking, and medication discontinuance.

A CLASSIFICATION SCHEME FOR DIRECT
AND INDIRECT SELF-HARM

Farberow (1980) provided a classic formulation of self-destructive behaviors that is still relevant today. In his discussion of the entire spectrum of self-destructive acts, he made the distinction between *direct* and *indirect* self-harm. Pattison and Kahan (1983) elaborated on this distinction and proposed a classification scheme that remains the best of its kind. In this framework the concept of direct versus indirect self-harm is combined with the dimensions of lethality and number of episodes. I have employed a modified version of the Pattison and Kahan classification scheme because it provides an excellent framework for organizing information regarding the entire spectrum of self-destructive behavior (see Figure 2.1). The schema shown in Figure 2.1 is one that can be easily used in conducting an assessment of self-destructive behavior, regardless of client or setting. A checklist based on this conceptual model is provided at the end of this chapter in Figure 2.2.

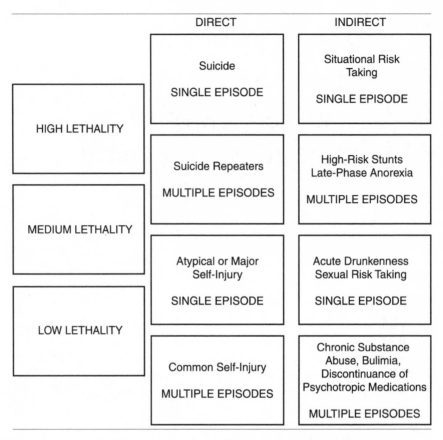

FIGURE 2.1. Differential classification of self-damaging behavior. After Pattison and Kahan (1983).

Direct Self-Harm

The first dimension in the schema is the distinction between *direct* and *indirect* self-harm. Direct self-harm refers to behavior that involves immediate tissue damage and for which intent is generally unambiguous. The category of direct self-harm applies to people who deliberately and concretely hurt themselves, and the damage inflicted is immediate. As shown in Figure 2.1, the main types of direct self-harm are suicidal behavior, major self-injury, and common self-injury. These range from high-lethality behaviors (suicide) to medium-lethality (recurrent suicide attempts and atypical or major self-injury) to low-lethality (self-injury) behaviors. As shown in Figure 2.1, the behaviors can involve either single or multiple episodes.

Indirect Self-Harm

Substance Abuse and Eating Disorders

Indirect self-harm refers to behavior in which the damage is generally accumulative (and/or deferred) rather than immediate. In addition, with indirect self-harm, intent is often very ambiguous. Common examples of indirect self-harm are patterns of substance abuse and eating disorder that damage physical health. For both types of behavior, the physical harm is usually accumulative rather than immediate in nature (acute alcohol or drug overdoses are exceptions). In addition, individuals who abuse substances or are eating disordered tend to deny self-destructive intent. Substance abusers may justify their behavior by saying they "just like to get high" or "live to party." Eating-disordered individuals may explain their behavior by stating they are "too fat" or "out of shape."

The following excerpt is an excellent example of indirect self-harm. The person described is an eating-disordered client whose anorexia had reached life-threatening proportions, yet she adamantly denied any self-destructive intent:

Alyssa had struggled throughout her teen years with anorexia nervosa. She was hospitalized multiple times on specialized eating disorder units due to dangerously low body weights, unstable vital signs, and other related health problems. Appearing to have made progress by the time she reached age 18, Alyssa left home to attend college in a nearby state. At the time she left for school, she had a marginally acceptable body weight of 90 pounds (at a height of 5 feet 2 inches).

Three weeks later Alyssa returned for a therapy meeting utterly transformed. When she walked into the therapist's office, her appearance resembled that of a concentration camp victim. The skin on her face was stretched tightly across her skull, giving her a skeletal appearance. The skin on her hands and limbs was tautly stretched across the bones. Shocked by Alyssa's appearance, the therapist insisted that the client go to an emergency room immediately. The hospital found her vital signs to be extremely unstable and her weight to be 72 pounds. She was admitted directly to an intensive care unit.

Several days later, the therapist interviewed Alyssa at the hospital. When the therapist asked her quite directly why she was trying to kill herself, Alyssa replied indignantly, "I'm not trying to kill myself! I'm too fat!"

Alyssa's dilemma is a classic example of indirect self-harm. It took years for her anorexia to become life threatening. When Alyssa went to college, she was unsupervised by family or professionals for the first time.

Without oversight from others, Alyssa's anorexia quickly careened out of control. Yet when she was asked about the potential lethality of her eating disorder, she vehemently denied self-destructive intent. Her eating disorder met both conditions of indirect self-harm: the damage was accumulative rather than immediate in nature and the intent was very ambiguous.

Substance abuse also can result in serious health risks. Use of street drugs may result in death via overdose or the contraction of the HIV/AIDS virus. The deleterious effects of chronic alcoholism are well known, ranging from damage to the liver, heart, and other organs to Korsakoff's syndrome with its related memory loss and dementia. Yet it is a rare substance abuser who acknowledges that his or her behavior has self-destructive motivations.

Risk Taking

Risk-taking behavior is another major type of indirect self-harm. There are three main types of risk-taking behavior: situational, physical, and sexual. Situational risk taking refers to behaviors that are not risky, in and of themselves. The behavior becomes potentially harmful only in relation to a particular context. For example, taking a walk is not a dangerous activity per se; however, choosing to walk alone at night in a high crime area of a city is potentially quite dangerous. Some people are prone to putting themselves in harm's way due to poor judgment and/or minimal investment in life (Orbach et al., 1991; Orbach, Lotem-Peleg, & Kedem, 1995). Consider the following as a representative example of situational risk taking:

Tiku was a seriously self-destructive individual who not only frequently cut herself, but also had the habit of going off with strangers. On one occasion she was walking alone in a city late at night when a car occupied by four young men pulled up. They showed her a supply of beer they had in the car and asked if she'd like to "party with them." She thought, "This sounds like fun!" so she jumped into the car. Later that evening, after some heavy drinking, she was gang-raped by the four men. After the sexual assaults were over, the four men drove off with her clothes, leaving her to fend for herself naked.

Tiku's poor judgment and failure to take normal precautions in dealing with strangers is an example of situational risk taking. It is important to emphasize that labeling a behavior as risk taking is not tantamount to blaming a victim. In Tiku's case, the rapists were reprehensible and responsible for their assaults. Nonetheless, the young woman's failure to protect herself played a role in the outcome. Moreover, her tendency to take such risks repeatedly represented a self-destructive pattern.

Physical risk taking is a second type of the behavior. Many self-injuring youth and adults are notorious physical risk takers (Lightfoot, 1997; Ponton, 1997). They may walk in high-speed traffic, sit on the edge of a roof of a multistory building, or straddle an open stairway at a high elevation. Here the risk is not situational but concrete. A slight miscalculation could result in serious injury or even death. Many youth report feeling exhilarated when they take physical risks. As one adolescent once told me, "I feel most alive when I flirt with death. It so cool!"

Sexual risk-taking behavior comes in many forms. Some forms involve having multiple partners within a short period of time or unprotected sex with strangers. Others entail having sex with intravenous drug users or with individuals known to have sexually transmitted diseases. Still others include having sex while intoxicated and being unaware of one's activities. Unprotected oral, vaginal, and anal sex can represent serious risks, particularly when the partner's sexual history is not well known. A person's sexual behaviors can be so impulsive and erratic that they assume self-destructive proportions. Granted, the actual extent of physical risk is often ambiguous at the time of the act. It is generally impossible to know if a particular sexual encounter will lead to genital herpes, gonorrhea, syphilis, chlamydia, or HIV/AIDS. However, some individuals have so many random or impulsive sexual encounters that they markedly increase their risk of disease and even death.

Few individuals deliberately attempt to get HIV/AIDS or other sexually transmitted diseases. Nonetheless, when individuals fail to protect themselves repeatedly, such behavior should be viewed as sexual risk taking that is potentially self-destructive in nature. The self-destructive intent of the individual may be more of omission than commission, but the results are the same. The following anecdote is an example of sexual behavior that has self-destructive motivations:

Early in treatment, Jim described himself as "wild and crazy." One of his favorite weekend activities was to drink heavily at a gay bar and have sex with several partners. Jim's pattern was to give oral sex and receive anal sex, usually in a restroom stall. He took precautions only when a partner demanded it. Jim complained that, "Using condoms takes the spontaneity out of it. Besides I lose them most of the time."

Over time in treatment, Jim admitted to being depressed about being thrown out of his parent's house for being gay. He also said that he didn't really care if he lived or died, so the "sexual precaution stuff is irrelevant." This minimal investment in life reflected Jim's depression and hopelessness.

After Jim had been in treatment for several months, he began to acknowledge that his drinking and unprotected sexual behaviors were both self-demeaning and self-destructive in nature. He identified that his real goal was to have an ongoing stable relationship. He also discussed his pain related to his family's rejection and came to accept that reconciliation was unrealistic for the time being, due to his family's homophobia.

ASSESSING FOR RISK-TAKING BEHAVIORS

A thorough assessment of self-destructiveness explores all three types of risk-taking behaviors. This can be accomplished by asking a few very basic questions, as outlined below:

Situational risk taking	*Physical risk taking*	*Sexual risk taking*
"Do you ever walk in a dangerous area of a city alone at night?"	"Do you ever take physical risks, such as walking in high-speed traffic or standing on the edge of a roof?"	"Have you ever had sex with people you barely know?"
"Have you ever gotten into a car with strangers?"	"Have you done risky things, such as walk on train tracks in a tunnel?"	"Have you had sex while very intoxicated and had little or no memory of the experience afterward?"
"Do you ever hitchhike alone?"	"Do you find physically risky activities thrilling?"	"Have you ever had unprotected anal sex?"
"Do you place yourself in risky situations?"		"How many sexual partners have you had in the last year?"
		"Do you think of your sexual behavior as risky?"

Some individuals respond quite enthusiastically to questions about risk taking, indicating that they relish such activities. Motivations are complex in those who report high rates of risk taking (Lightfoot, 1997; Ponton, 1997). For many the payoff appears to be some combination of enjoying the adrenaline rush associated with the risk taking, while simultaneously indulging a desire to demean or destroy the self. A recurrent pattern of situational, physical, and/or sexual risk taking should be viewed as potentially life threatening as high-lethality suicidal behavior.

Asking a series of questions about risk-taking behaviors should be done with great care and compassion. A therapeutic alliance usually has to be well established before reliable information can be obtained, especially about sexual behaviors. Inquiring about these risk-taking behaviors should be done in a supportive, nonjudgmental manner. Clients should not feel that they are being subjected to an evaluation of their morality. The goal is to assess the person's self-destructiveness in all its manifestations. The presence of these major forms of indirect self-harm points to the client being in significant distress and lacking important coping skills. Both should be targeted in treatment.

Medication Discontinuance or Abuse

Yet another form of indirect self-harm is the unauthorized discontinuance or abuse of prescribed medications. It is well known that many people do not comply with medication regimens completely. For example, significant percentages of people who are prescribed an antibiotic for a bacterial infection fail to complete the entire course. This is *not* the type of medication discontinuance deemed to be self-destructive here.

Many self-injuring people are on psychotropic medications, be they antidepressants, antianxiety agents, antipsychotics, or mood stabilizers. Unfortunately, many clients episodically discontinue or abuse these medications. The noncompliance with prescribed regimens is part of a recurrent self-destructive pattern for some individuals. For example:

In the course of treatment, Erika identified a number of key steps that preceded her self-injuring behavior. She found that some sort of relationship disappointment generally triggered the downward spiral. Once this had occurred, she began drinking or smoking pot heavily. Before long, Erika would abruptly stop taking her antipsychotic medication without telling her doctor. This decision quickly led to paranoid thinking and increased anxiety. As her cognitive and affective distress increased, she became more and more focused on "the only solution." This was to cut herself on her forearms and legs, after which she felt calm for several days.

In the course of treatment, Erika recognized that it was important for her to stay on her medication. Her impulse to discontinue was part of a self-destructive pattern that culminated in cutting behavior. She decided that if she were to give up cutting, she needed to remain on her medication and to avoid heavy drinking and pot smoking. She also had to work on her relationship skills in order to reduce the frequency of her disappointments.

Erika was involved in multiple forms of indirect self-harm, including alcohol and marijuana use and discontinuance of prescribed medications. All three behaviors were part of a web of self-harm that led to cutting. Untangling this web enabled her to reduce her cutting behavior while she also worked on acquiring new skills.

COMORBIDITY OF INDIRECT SELF-HARM WITH SELF-INJURY

Thoroughness is one reason to assess for all forms of direct and indirect self-harm. Another is because the various forms of direct and indirect self-harm have frequently been found to co-occur. The relationships have been reported both within and across the categories of direct and indirect self-harm. More specifically, self-injury has frequently been found to be associated with suicidal behavior (e.g., Walsh, 1987; Linehan, 1993a; Favazza, 1996). As mentioned in Chapter 7, persons who frequently self-injure may turn to suicide when their self-injury stops working as an effective affect management technique.

Self-injury has also frequently been found to be associated with the major forms of indirect self-harm. Walsh (1987) reported that the number one predictor of self-injury in his study of 52 adolescent self-injurers was the presence of an eating disorder. Favazza et al. (1989) described a sample of 65 self-injuring clients in which 50% reported having a past or present eating disorder. Within the Favazza sample, 15% identified their eating disorder as anorexia, 22% as bulimia, and 13% as both (Favazza et al., 1989). Paul, Schroeter, Dahme, and Nutzinger (2002) reported that in a sample of 376 inpatient women being treated for eating disorder, 34.4% had self-injured at some point in their lifetimes.

In an unpublished study I conducted in the 1990s (Walsh & Frost, 2005), over 60% of a sample of 34 poly-self-destructive adolescents reported having vomited in order to lose weight. Favarro and Santonastaso (1998), Parkin and Eagles (1993), and Mitchell, Boutacoff, and Hatsukami (1986) have also reported an association between eating disorder and self-injury.

Another important relationship has been reported between self-injury and substance abuse. In the unpublished study cited above (Walsh & Frost, 2005), a sample of 34 poly-self-destructive adolescents reported having major problems with substance abuse; 77% reported sniffing glue, 53% stated that they drank alcohol frequently, 85% reported having used marijuana, 32% cocaine, and 42% LSD. Clearly, this sample of self-injuring and suicidal adolescents was also abusing several substances.

Other publications have pointed to the comorbidity of self-injury and substance abuse. Simeon and Hollander (2001) reviewed studies of skin picking, hair pulling (trichotillomania), and nail biting and reported associations with substance abuse. Greilsheimer and Groves (1979) reviewed reports of male genital self-mutilation and cited acute intoxication as a precipitant in a number of cases. Alderman (1997), Hyman (1999), Connors (2000), and Linehan (1993a) have also linked substance abuse with self-injurious behaviors.

For many individuals the affect-modulating effects of substances may complement the tension reduction capabilities of self-injury. Emotionally dysregulated people tend to seek relief from their distress in multiple directions. Sometimes they may self-injure to deal with anxiety, anger, sadness, or shame; at other times they may drink or use drugs to deal with the same or different feelings. Relatively few individuals report self-injuring while they are under the influence of a substance. For example, Linehan and colleagues reported that 13.4% percent of a sample of 119 self-injuring persons had used alcohol shortly before the act. An example of this atypical scenario is described below:

Sarah had been self-injuring a few times a year for about a 3-year period. She stated that she only cut herself when she was high on marijuana or alcohol. She explained that she "really didn't like doing it." She added that it hurt when she cut, and because of that, she was scared to do it. However, sometimes "the pressure just got to be too much" and she "just had to." Being high helped her "to build up the courage."

Yet another relationship exists between self-injury and risk-taking behaviors. In the Walsh and Frost (2005) study, 94% of the sample of 34 poly-self-destructive adolescents reported physical risk-taking activities and 85% situational risk taking. In addition, 41% reported having had sex with strangers; 15%, anal sex without a condom; 18%, sex with no memory afterward due to intoxication; and 32%, who averaged 15.81 years of age had had eight or more sexual partners, suggesting another area of sexual risk taking.

CONCLUSION

This chapter has reviewed the spectrum of self-destructive behaviors in relation to the categories of direct and indirect self-harm. The interrelationships between various self-destructive behaviors have also been discussed. A checklist (Figure 2.2) is provided at the end of the chapter that includes the major types of direct and indirect self-harm. Although reasonably inclusive, the checklist does not pretend to be exhaustive. Unfortunately, self-destructive people are creative and often come up with new forms of self-harm. One example of this creativity is the frequent emergence of new designer drugs. Another is the development of new methods to disfigure or mar the body. Therefore, an "other" category is provided in several places within the checklist.

Clinicians who use the checklist will find that it can be quickly memorized and employed informally while interviewing clients. Inquiring about all of the items on the checklist should provide a reasonable degree of confidence that a thorough inventory of self-destructive behavior has been obtained.

Check those that the client reports having done at any time.

Direct Self-Harm

____ Suicide attempts (e.g., overdose, hanging, jumping from a height, use of a gun)

____ Major self-injury (e.g., self-enucleation, autocastration)

____ Atypical self-injury (mutilation of the face, eyes, genitals, breasts, or damage involving multiple sutures)

____ Common forms of self-injury (e.g., wrist, arm, and leg cutting, self-burning, self-hitting, excoriation)

Indirect Self-Harm

Substance abuse
____ alcohol abuse
____ marijuana use
____ cocaine use
____ inhalant use (e.g., glue, gasoline)
____ hallucinogens, ecstasy, etc.
____ IV drug use
____ other; specify:

Eating-disordered behavior
____ anorexia nervosa
____ bulimia
____ obesity
____ use of laxatives
____ other; specify:

____ Physical risk taking (e.g., walking on a high-pitched roof or in high-speed traffic)

____ Situational risk taking (e.g., getting into a car with strangers, walking alone in a dangerous area)

____ Sexual risk taking (e.g., having sex with strangers, unprotected anal intercourse)

____ Unauthorized discontinuance of psychotropic medications

____ Misuse/abuse of prescribed psychotropic medications

____ Other forms of indirect self-harm; specify:

FIGURE 2.2. Checklist for direct and indirect self-harm behaviors.

CHAPTER 3

Major Groups in Which Self-Injury Occurs

The prevalence of self-injury in the United States appears to be growing markedly. In the early 1980s, Pattison and Kahan (1983) estimated the rate of deliberate self-harm to be 400 per 100,000 in population. By the late 1980s this estimate had grown to 750 per 100,000 (Favazza & Conterio, 1988), and as of the late 1990s, it had advanced to 1,000 per 100,000 in population (Favazza, 1998). If these estimates are correct, the rate of self-injury has grown by 150% over a 20-year period. An alternative explanation is that self-injury is more in the public eye now, recognized as an important public health problem, and, as a result, the reporting may be more accurate. Or both may be true: The rate of self-injury may have increased, *and* the reporting may be more precise. Regardless of the explanation, it should be emphasized that the prevalence numbers of self-injury are approximations only. One of the frustrations for those who desire to understand self-injury is that there are no large nationwide epidemiological studies of the behavior to date. An interesting finding that points to the scope of the problem comes from the Youth Risk Behavior Survey data in Massachusetts for 2003 (Massachusetts Department of Education, 2004): 18% of Massachusetts high school students reported having self-injured during the past year (2003). Thus, at least for one state, the behavior has become a significant public health problem.

It may be instructive to compare the rate of self-injury to other forms of direct and indirect self-harm. The suicide rate in the United States is approximately 11 per 100,000 (Miller & Hemenway, 2001), and the rate of alcohol abuse is estimated to be about 5,600 per 100,000 (Grant et al., 1994). Thus, using Favazza's most recent estimate, individuals are about 90 times more likely to self-injure than to commit suicide, and are about 5½ times less likely to self-injure than to abuse alcohol.

What accounts for the increasing rate of self-injury nationally? One explanation is that the behaviors are now occurring in broader segments of the population. In the past, self-injury was reported in the following groups of people:

- Outpatients with serious emotional disturbance or mental illness (Linehan, 1993a; Alderman, 1997; Deiter, Nicholls, & Pearlman, 2000).
- Persons presenting at psychiatric emergency rooms (Clendenin & Murphy, 1971; Weissman, 1975).
- Seriously and persistently mentally ill persons in day treatment or partial hospitalization programs (Deiter et al., 2000).
- Seriously and persistently mentally ill adults living in community-based residential or supported housing programs.
- Patients in short- and long-term psychiatric and forensic units (Offer & Barglow, 1960; Phillips & Alkan, 1961; Pao, 1969; Podvoll, 1969; Kroll, 1978; Darche, 1990; Langbehn & Pfohl, 1993; Himber, 1994; Conterio & Lader, 1998; Gough & Hawkins, 2000; Paul et al., 2002).
- Youth in special education schools, residential treatment, or juvenile detention facilities (Ross & McKay, 1979; Cullen, 1985; Walsh & Rosen, 1985; Rosen & Walsh, 1989; Chowanec, Josephson, Coleman, & Davis, 1991; Boiko & Lester, 2000; Heinsz, 2000).
- Prison inmates (Virkunnen, 1976; Haines & Williams, 1997; Howard League for Penal Reform, 1999; Ireland, 2000; Motz, 2001).

These groups, of course, are not mutually exclusive. For example, individuals can be discharged from total institutions such as hospitals or prisons and become clients in residential or outpatient settings, or vice versa.

Not surprisingly, people being treated in the above settings have tended to acquire major psychiatric diagnoses. These include, first and foremost, borderline personality disorder (Gardner & Cowdry, 1985; Linehan, Armstrong, Suarez, Allmon, & Heard, 1991; Linehan, 1993a; Dulit, Fyer, Leon, Brodsky, & Frances, 1994; Zweig-Frank, Paris, & Guzder, 1994; Bohus et al., 2000), followed (in no particular order) by PTSD (van der Kolk, McFarlane, & Wiesaeth, 1996; Briere & Gil, 1998; Simeon & Hollander, 2001), dissociative disorders (Briere & Gil, 1998), anorexia nervosa and/or bulimia (Walsh & Rosen, 1988; Favazza & Conterio, 1988; Warren, Dolan, & Norton, 1998; Favaro & Santonastaso, 2000; Rodriguez-Srednicki, 2001; Paul et al., 2002), depression (Ross & Heath, 2002), anxiety (Ross & Heath, 2002), obsessive–compulsive disorder (Gardner & Gardner,

1975; Favaro & Santonastaso, 2000; McKay, Kulchycky, & Danyko, 2000; Simeon & Hollander, 2001), antisocial personality disorder (Mckerracher, Loughnane, & Watson, 1968; Virkkunen, 1976), and a variety of psychoses (Menninger, 1938/1966; Green, 1968; Rosen & Hoffman, 1972; Greilsheimer & Groves, 1979; Favazza, 1987; Walsh & Rosen, 1988).

During the period from the 1960s through the 1980s, the assumption (correct or not) was that a person who self-injured was probably seriously disturbed and suffering from considerable functional impairment, including compromised social functioning and a diminished ability to deal with the demands of school and/or work.

This level of impairment was often linked to aversive childhood experiences. Self-injuring persons were described as having experienced major family dysfunction such as sexual abuse (Walsh & Rosen, 1988; Darche, 1990; Shapiro & Dominiak, 1992; Miller, 1994; van der Kolk et al., 1996; Alderman, 1997; Favazza, 1998; Briere & Gil, 1998; Turell & Armsworth, 2000; Rodriquez-Srednicki, 2001; Paul et al., 2002), physical abuse (van der Kolk, Perry, & Herman, 1991; van der Kolk et al., 1996; Briere & Gil, 1998; Low, Jones, MacLeod, Power, & Duggan, 2000), loss and divorce, exposure to family violence, family alcoholism, or family mental illness and suicidality (Walsh & Rosen, 1988; Turell & Armsworth, 2000). In other words, until recently, self-injuring persons were deemed to be seriously disturbed, to be functionally impaired, and to have come from seriously dysfunctional family backgrounds. Moreover, consistent with these profiles, these persons were seen as requiring intensive and expensive long-term treatment.

SELF-INJURY IN THE GENERAL POPULATION

Somewhat astonishingly, this pattern changed in the late 1990s when self-injury began to appear in ever-greater numbers in people who did not fit the above profiles. This is not to say that self-injury declined in the usual populations thought to be associated with the behavior. Persons with major psychiatric diagnoses continued to have high rates of self-injury. But at the same time a new generation of self-injuring persons was emerging from the general population rather than clinical settings. Although generalizations not based on data are risky, it can be stated that the new population of self-injurers appears to be of diverse age, less psychologically challenged, and less functionally impaired in the areas of social relationships and school and/or work. Also important is that many of these self-injuring persons may have experienced far less in the way of trauma.

This new, emerging group of self-injurers includes:

- Youth in middle and high schools serving regular education students
- Adolescents and young adults in colleges and universities
- Adults in the general population

Writings on this new group of self-injurers are scarce, and large-sample empirical studies are almost nonexistent. Next, the three groups identified above are considered in order of chronological age.

SELF-INJURERS IN MIDDLE AND HIGH SCHOOLS

Until recently the only discussions about middle and high school students who self-injure were case reports by such authors as Orenstein (1994), Pipher (1994), and Levenkron (1998). An important recent contribution is an empirical study of self-injuring high school students conducted by Ross and Heath (2002), who studied a sample of 440 youth from urban and suburban high schools in Canada. They found that 61 (or 13.9%) of the students reported having self-injured. Of these, 39 (or 64%) were girls and 22 (or 36%) were boys. These 61 students were compared with non-self-injuring students and were found to have significantly higher scores for depression and anxiety (using the Beck Depression Inventory and the Beck Anxiety Inventory).

Because the Ross and Heath study is one of the only to employ a community sample, their descriptive information regarding the self-injury of these youth is worth reviewing. Of the 61 high school students who self-injured, only 10 (or 16.4%) reported using more than one method. This is quite different from the clinical sample reported by Walsh and Rosen (1988) in which 50% used more than one method, and from Favazza and Conterio's clinical sample (1988) in which 78% used more than one method. The types of self-injury reported in the Ross and Heath study were skin cutting (41%), followed by self-hitting (32.8%), pinching (6.5%), biting (5%), and burning (3.3%). In addition, 18% of the sample reported hitting walls (which may or may not be self-injurious). These methods appear to be similar to those reported in previous clinical studies.

The raw frequency of self-injury reported by Ross and Heath (2002) was startling in that 13.1% of the sample stated they self-injured at least *once a day*. If accurate, this is clearly a very high rate that would seem to compete with, or even exceed, the rates in many clinical samples. In addition, 27.9% of the high school self-injurers stated they self-injured a couple of times a week, and 19.6%, a couple of times a month. Another 19.6% reported self-injuring episodically. However, one problem with the Ross and Heath sample is that 18% reported having self-injured only once, which raises questions as to whether they should have been included in the sample. Empirical studies have generally required more of an established pattern of self-injury for inclusion in a study sample. How the Ross and Heath (2002) study results would have been affected if the single-time self-injurers had been excluded is not known.

Also important from the Ross and Heath (2002) report is age of onset: 59% of the sample reported starting in seventh or eighth grade and 11.5% in ninth grade. Particularly striking is that 24.6% stated they had started in sixth grade or earlier. This means that a quarter of the sample had started engaging in self-injuring behavior by age 12 or earlier—which is very early, indeed. On the far more encouraging side, of the 61 self-injurers studied, 64% of the sample reported no longer self-injuring. If this rate is accurate (i.e., not distorted by an adolescent sense of time or unwarranted optimism), the rate of recovery would appear to be quite high. It is not known how many of these youth had received psychological treatment. Ross and Heath also did not report a follow-up component to the study. It would be very useful if they were to conduct a follow-up and collect data regarding continuance/discontinuance of self-injury.

In that the Ross and Heath (2002) study and the Massachusetts Department of Education (2004) report are the only community samples of adolescents to date, we are forced to rely on anecdotal information for additional insights. I ask the reader's indulgence here to share some clinical impressions of the new group of self-injuring youth from middle and high schools. Over the past 10 years, I have treated or consulted to schools regarding approximately 120 self-injuring youth from the community. Although my experiences may be idiosyncratic, that is not my sense from talking to professionals and self-injurers around the country. My clinical impressions are that this new generation of self-injuring youth is comprised of both genders, with females outnumbering males roughly 2 to 1, who come from a wide range of ethnic, racial, and economic backgrounds. Often they have started self-injuring as early as age 11 or 12. Many have considerable strengths and are doing well in school or at least adequately. Most have never been identified as needing special education services, and many are not disciplinary problems. Few have had previous psychological treatment.

Two brief case examples may be representative of the self-injurers encountered in middle and high school settings:

Amy is a 13-year-old seventh grader who attends a small private school for girls. She is a B+ student, a fine artist, and she plays the cello in her school orchestra. Amy is articulate and personable. She is slightly underweight and can be episodically bulimic, especially when her peers make an offhand remark about her size. Amy has close friends whom she sees every weekend.

She poses no disciplinary problems with her mother, who is a single parent. Recently it came to light through friends at school that Amy has been cutting herself once or twice a week for about 6 months. She tends to cut when exam pressures mount or she has an upcoming cello performance. She reports that the cutting relaxes her and is "no big deal." Amy usually inflicts the cuts on her left forearm with a razor blade. The cuts draw blood but do not require sutures and do not appear to be leaving permanent scars.

Sean is a 17-year-old junior in a large urban public high school. He is a C student and member of the football team. Most of Sean's friends are team members. Sean lifts weights on a daily basis as part of his training for football. He is an attractive young man who is meticulous about his appearance. He is not talkative in therapy, but he is cooperative and responsive when asked direct questions.

Sean lives with his parents and a younger brother. His self-injury started about a year ago. He has carved designs into his upper arms with a razor and has burned his forearms and legs with cigarettes (although he does not smoke). Sean's self-injury appears to be linked to intense anger. He resents parental curfews and is frequently infuriated by the dictatorial style of his football coach. Sean reports that cutting or burning himself helps him "not to hit people." He states that if he were to get into a physical altercation with his parents or coach, he "would have too much to lose," so he "handles it in his own way." Sean says he can't wait to get to college, where he will run his own life.

Many of these youth have a substantial circle of friends. In some cases their friends may self-injure as well. An example of this type of peer interaction and influence is described in the following anecdote.

The principal of a middle school in a middle-class suburb was alarmed to discover that her students were experiencing an epidemic of self-injury. All the more surprising were the specific students involved in the self-harm. None of the students had been in trouble in school and most were doing well academically. The primary self-injurers were eight females in the seventh grade. All eight knew each other, but only about half were close friends. The principal learned that the two more influential leaders in the group had been cutting themselves for about 9 months, sometimes alone, sometimes together. The others had begun to cut more recently, within the last 6 weeks. Asked about the family lives of these girls, the principal replied that the large majority of the students had concerned and involved parents. The principal said that when the parents learned of the cutting, they were horrified and

sprang into action, looking for professional services. The response from the
parents was everything the principal could have hoped for.

It should be emphasized that although this new group of self-injuring
adolescents often has major strengths, the students are nonetheless experiencing serious distress. Self-injury in middle and high school students
should not be minimized or dismissed as "attention seeking" or "just a fad."
When people take the radical step of harming their bodies, they should be
taken seriously and the sources of their stress addressed.

Usually a friend has introduced these youth to self-injury (although
most adolescents will deny imitating others). Once they have tried self-
injuring, they may quickly come to rely on it as a preferred way of managing and reducing emotional pain. Almost always these youth lack the
healthy coping skills necessary to acknowledge and reduce emotional distress.

Another interesting feature regarding this new generation of self-
injurers is what is *not* wrong with them. In the past I have argued that body
alienation is central to understanding self-injury (Walsh, 1987; Walsh &
Rosen, 1988; Walsh, 2001; see also Chapter 11). Time and again, when
encouraged to tell their stories, self-harming persons from the 1970s and
1980s disclosed histories of trauma, especially sexual and/or physical abuse.
Very consistently, those who had been abused reported a profound sense of
bodily hatred or alienation derived from the trauma. These persons had suffered greatly at the hands and organs of others and had come to view their
bodies as contaminated, dirty, and broken. Moreover, they often blamed
themselves (irrationally) in some way for the abuse and seemed to condemn
the body as the culprit or co-conspirator in the trauma history.

Many of the new group of self-injuring persons deny any history of
sexual or physical abuse and do so convincingly. Moreover, when they are
asked detailed questions about body image, they present with normal attitudes. Many are not body alienated; they do not loathe their bodies and do
not report experiences of dissociation derived from trauma. One line of
demarcation between the old and new groups of self-injurers may be
whether or not they present with negative attitudes regarding the body (see
Chapter 11 for an extended discussion and some empirical data regarding
this topic).

Not surprisingly, given that many of these youth are psychologically
healthier and have strengths in the areas of family, peers, and school, they
also tend to give up the behavior more quickly. Unlike individuals from
clinical populations who may self-injure for years, many of these youth
cease after 6 months to 2 years. Treatment often has a role in helping these
individuals stop self-injuring. In therapy, these clients can be very respon-

sive, cooperative, and motivated. They often are quite receptive to learning new self-soothing skills, which they may practice quite diligently.

Peer influences are often crucially important as well. If a small circle of friends stops self-injuring, an individual may give it up with or without treatment. Mutual support among peers can also be quite helpful in assisting self-injurers to stop. These considerable peer factors do not imply that these adolescents are not in real distress. They are in intense pain and need assistance until they mature and can handle their emotional distress more effectively through other means.

Another way to understand the world of this new group of adolescent self-injurers is to read Kettlewell's *Skin Game* (1999), the first book-length autobiographical memoir of a "cutter's journey." Ms. Kettlewell grew up living on the campus of a Virginia prep school where her father was an administrator. She lived in an intact family and was not subjected to abuse. She first cut in the seventh grade. She received little in the way of professional treatment until she was in her 20s, and that pertained more to relationship issues than cutting. Throughout her youth, despite her emotional turmoil and persistent cutting, she was an exceptional student, as evidenced by her attending and graduating from Williams College, one of the more academically competitive colleges in the country. After majoring in English at Williams, she subsequently obtained her master's in writing from George Mason University. Ms. Kettlewell is an exceptional writer, perhaps the most incisive and poignant voice ever to describe the act of self-injuring. An example of her ability to articulate the experience of self-injury is provided below:

> I intended to kill something *in* me, this awful feeling like worms tunneling along my nerves. So when I discovered the razor blade, cutting, if you'll believe me, was my gesture of hope. That first time, when I was twelve, was like some kind of miracle, a revelation. The blade slipped easily, painlessly through my skin, like a hot knife through butter. As swift and pure as a stroke of lightning, it wrought an absolute and pristine division between before and after. All the chaos, the sound and fury, the uncertainty and confusion and despair—all of it evaporated in an instant, and I was for that moment grounded, coherent, whole. *Here is the irreducible self.* I drew the line in the sand, marked my body as mine, its flesh and its blood under my command. (Kettlewell, 1999, p. 57)

Ms. Kettlewell is a key spokesperson regarding self-injury, particularly for that new group of self-injurers who are so capable and accomplished. Ms. Kettlewell now lives in Virginia with her husband and son. Although she no longer self-injures, she has an ability to describe and share the anguish of the self-injuring experience like no one else.

SELF-INJURERS IN COLLEGES AND UNIVERSITIES

Youth from middle and high schools who self-injure eventually grow up and leave home. Some enter the general population as workers; others go to college. Youth who have harmed themselves during adolescence may continue or resume self-injuring in adulthood. Those who attend college may be more likely to come to the attention of professionals, because they often are referred to, or appear at, university health services. In one study, Favazza and Rosenthal (1990) reported that 12% of a college-age sample claimed to have self-injured.

Shaw (2002) described a group of college-age self-injurers in a recent qualitative study. In her report, she discussed a sample of six women in college who had extensive histories of self-injury. These women ranged in age from 18 to 21 years old. They had self-injured from 1 to 5 years. The level of physical damage associated with their self-harm ranged from very modest self-injury to extensive self-mutilation. The number of episodes of self-injury for these woman was from about 10 to over 50. Their involvement in treatment differed greatly. One had been hospitalized repeatedly and three others had had extensive outpatient treatment; however, two of the six had received no treatment whatsoever.

The women in Shaw's study appear to be good examples of the new type of self-injurer. All six were functioning quite adequately in their college settings. Some were excelling academically. Most were engaged is serious relationships. Moreover, of particular interest is that all six had *ceased* self-injuring. These women were experiencing considerable distress in their lives and had repeatedly used self-injury in the past to manage emotional pain. Nonetheless, they had considerable strengths and were able to discontinue self-injury through the use of treatment and/or their own internal resources and naturally occurring external supports.

An example of a college-age self-injuring person from my own experience echoes Shaw's (2002) findings.

Shauna was a 20-year-old college junior who had been self-injuring on and off since about age 16. She denied a history of physical or sexual abuse, but complained bitterly about her autocratic, hypercritical father. "There's no pleasing this guy," said Shauna, yet she tried desperately to do so.

Shauna stated that she tended to self-injure when academic deadlines approached or when a relationship began to get serious. She elaborated that when she had dated someone for very long and it began to get physically more intimate, inevitably she felt compelled to break it off. Shortly thereafter she would find herself feeling lonely and angry that she had "bungled another relationship." This self-deprecation would lead to cutting, which in turn would relieve her despair. Shauna stated that she wanted to be able to have a relationship but felt too frightened. She said she deserved to cut herself because she "made such a mess of things and hurt other people."

On the positive side, Shauna responded very well to short-term treatment. She found mindful breathing exercises and visualization techniques to be good alternatives to cutting. She also reconceptualized her dating problems and was able to give herself permission to go slowly with physical intimacy. She became much more skilled at communicating her need for patience to a partner. She also came to recognize that she needed to do some additional work regarding her relationship with her father.

ADULT SELF-INJURERS
IN THE GENERAL POPULATION

For decades, self-injury was described as a type of behavior found in adolescents and young adults. Clinicians were aware of only a few relatively rare, self-injuring persons who persisted harming themselves into middle age. These tended to be people with serious and persistent mental illness who were part of an adult mental health system of care.

In an important study, Briere and Gil (1998) employed a national sampling service to generate "a stratified, random sample of the U.S., based on geographical location of registered owners of automobiles and individuals with listed telephones" (p. 611). The resulting sample consisted of 927 adults, with equal gender representation. The authors founds that 33 (or 4%) of the sample reported having self-injured at least occasionally, and 3 (or 0.3%) reported *often* engaging in the behavior. The self-injurers had a mean age of 35 years, clearly indicating the adult nature of the sample. Also of note is that there was no significant gender difference for the 33 self-injuring subjects, with 4% of the females and 3% of the males reporting self-harm. Based on their findings, Briere and Gil concluded that self-injury is "relatively rare in the general population" (p. 612), given the rate of 4% obtained in their sample.

Although 4% of any group may not seem like a large amount, we can reach a different conclusion when considering national census data. The U.S. Census for 2000 reported that there were 104,004,252 persons between the ages of 20 and 44 in the country (factfinder.census.gov/servlet). (I selected this age range for adults as the one in which self-injury is more likely to occur. The age range may, in fact, be too narrow in discussing self-injury in the general population of adults, but it was used here in order to be conservative.) Using Briere and Gil's prevalence rate, 4% of the 20- to 44-year-old population in the United States equals 4,160,170 persons. Thus, based on the Briere and Gil (1998) study, we can estimate that there may be more than 4 million adults in the general population who have self-injured. If we consider only those who stated that they self-injured "often" in the Briere and Gil report, then the rate drops to 0.3% of the sample. This percentage (0.3%) yields an estimate of approximately 312,013 persons in the United States between the ages of 20 and 44 who have *often* self-injured. The results from the Briere and Gil study begin to point to the scope of the problem of self-injury in the general adult population.

One way to approach the problem of self-injury in adults is via epidemiological statistical analysis; another is through qualitative research. Hyman's book (1999) is an innovative and informative qualitative study of self-injury in adults. Her work focused on 15 women who had self-injured for years and were willing to tell their stories in detail. The women ranged in age from 26 to 51, with a mean of 36.9 years. Thus, the ages of Hyman's group further dispel the notion that self-injury is solely an adolescent and young adult problem.

The women that Hyman came to know and wrote about had not had easy lives. All 15 had been sexually abused as children; all but one had been repeatedly sexually abused by a parent or stepparent. The trauma continued to be a focal point of their lives and a key antecedent in their long histories of self-injury. What is particularly instructive (and inspirational) about the lives of these women is their resilience and related level of functioning. At the beginning of her book, Hyman (1999) identified each woman in terms of a pseudonym, age, and profession. This list bears repeating because it is inherently revealing:

Edith, 51, physical therapist
Karen, 49, human services worker
Elizabeth, 25, typist
Jane, 39, treasurer
Erica, 43, editor and writer
Peggy, 34, human services worker
Mary, 47, technology manager for communications company
Esther, 40, central security station operator and store sales associate
Jessica, 46, part-time social worker, in graduate school for social work
Rosa, 30, drafter for engineering and architectural firm
Meredith, 26, part-time social worker, in graduate school for social
    work

Caroline, 30, office staff worker and student in music school
Helena, 28, freelance proofreader and copyeditor
Sarah, 27, part-time worker, in graduate school for pharmacy

Hyman's list dispels another myth about self-injury: that persons who self-harm well into adulthood must be seriously disturbed and suffering from considerable functional impairment. The 15 women in Hyman's book display an impressive level of accomplishment in the workplace. In addition, most are engaged in ongoing relationships and have meaningful social networks. Although the stories of Hyman's informants are fraught with anguish and psychic pain, they nonetheless convey a crucially important message of hope and recovery. Toward the end of *Women Living with Self-Injury*, Hyman described her follow-up contact with 9 of the 15 women. Her conversations or correspondence with the women occurred 1½–5 years after the initial interviews.

> I often heard tales of improvement and recovery from voices that sounded full and cheerful, contrasting with the sometimes audible shame, anxiety, and distress of the original interviews. Two of my informants have decreased self-injury, five have stopped self-injury altogether, and four of these five have also stopped feeling the need to self-injure. (Hyman, 1999, p. 177)

EXPLANATIONS REGARDING THE INCREASED PREVALENCE OF SELF-INJURY

Why is there such a marked increase of self-injury in our society? Why is the behavior surfacing in healthier segments of the population of the United States, Europe, Japan, and Taiwan? To address questions such as these, we must inevitably go beyond the individualistic approach of psychology and talk about sociocultural factors. Favazza (1996) has written about self-injury from a transcultural perspective. He has reviewed the practice of self-induced body modification around the world and linked it to such themes as religious transformation, pubertal rites of passage, shamanistic magic, and the mythologies of garnering power over the natural and spiritual worlds. He writes:

> Because of their persistence and the "deep" meanings attributed to them by societies, self-mutilative rituals inform us about basic elements of social life. Examination of the rituals . . . reveals that they serve an elemental purpose, namely, the correction or prevention of a destabilizing condition that threatens

the community. A few examples of destabilizing conditions are diseases; angry gods, spirits or ancestors; failure of boys and girls to accept adult responsibilities when they mature; conflicts of all sorts, for example, male–female, intergenerational, interclass, intertribal; loosening of clear social role distinctions; loss of group identity and distinctiveness; immoral or sinful behaviors; ecological disaster.

Self-mutilative rituals (and some practices) serve to prevent the onset of these conditions and to correct or "cure" them should they occur. The rituals work by promoting healing, spirituality, and social order. (1996, p. 226)

It is not difficult to cull from Favazza's discussion of worldwide phenomena many aspects that fit our own situation. These include the challenging problems of disease (e.g., HIV/AIDS and the impact on youthful sexuality); conflict between the sexes, generations, and classes; loss of cohesiveness in the social order; confusion regarding the moral order; and widespread ecological disaster. Moreover, using Favazza's (1996) three dimensions, it can be said that the contemporary version of self-injury entails aspects of *healing* (ironically, via hurting the body), *spirituality* (or at least an alteration of consciousness), and the *promotion of the social order* (by provoking a response in the social network). Thus, the self-injury of today may not be so far removed from the culturally endorsed body modifications of the past.

Feminist writers have advanced other explanations for self-injury. Shaw (2002) has provided an excellent summary of feminist formulations of self-injurious behavior. She emphasizes the link between self-injury and the cultural standards of "feminine beauty" that are imposed on, and used to exploit, women. Shaw writes:

Women voluntarily undergo culturally sanctioned procedures which are painful and physically destructive for the sake of Western beauty ideals. Such behavior is not interpreted as pathological or deviant. Women pluck, cinch, inject toxic substances, and have cellulite vacuumed out of their thighs. As Dworkin asserts, "not one part of a woman's body is left untouched, unaltered. No feature or extremity is spared the art, or pain of improvement" (1974, p. 113). "Pain is an essential part of the grooming process . . . no price is too great, no process too repulsive, no operation too painful for the woman who would be beautiful" (Dworkin, 1974, p. 115). (2002, p. 32)

Through the feminist lens, self-injury can even be viewed as an act of empowerment and body reclamation. As Shaw states:

Self-injury is uniquely distressing because it reflects back to the culture what has been done to girls and women. Whether or not it is a conscious process, by refusing to remain silent, by literally carving, cutting, and burning their experiences of violation and silencing in their arms and legs, girls and women claim ownership of their bodies and their subjectivity. They refuse to relinquish what they experience as true. This is a radical and threatening act because part of what holds patriarchy in place is girls' and women's silence. (2002, p. 35)

One problem with feminist formulations such as Shaw's is that they provide little in the way of explanation regarding *male* self-injury. Given that self-injury is increasing for both genders, a feminist articulation explicates only about half the problem. Interestingly, the perspective of Fakir Musafar closely matches the feminist view, despite the gender difference. Musafar is an originator, perhaps *the* originator, of the "Modern Primitive Movement" of body modification. He has pierced, tattooed, corseted, suspended, cinched, and winched virtually every part of his body. He is featured in the publication *Modern Primitives* (Vale & Juno, 1989) that served as a prototype for much of the popularity of piercing and tattoos that emerged in the late 1980s and early 1990s. Musafar reports that these various forms of body modification and stimulation produce not pain and torture but "a state of grace" in him and others (Musafar, cited in Favazza, 1996, p. 325). Musafar writes about his and his colleagues' commitment to body modification:

We had rejected the Western cultural biases about ownership and use of the body. We believed our body belonged to us. We had rejected the strong Judeo-Christian body programming and emotional conditioning to which we had all been subjected. Our bodies did *not* belong to . . . a father, mother, or spouse; or to the state or its monarch, ruler, or dictator; or to social institutions of the military, educational, correctional, or medical establishment. And the kind of language used to describe our behavior ("self-mutilation"), was in itself a negative and prejudicial form of control. (cited in Favazza, 1996, p. 326)

Although I find the feminist and "Musafarian" formulations regarding self-injury to be intriguing and insightful, my own view comes from a more "experience-near" psychotherapeutic perspective. As a clinician I am not so much concerned with broad cultural influences (over which I have little influence) as with the day-to-day forces directly affecting my clients' lives. I believe there are many factors that play a role in their decisions to self-injure. A list of these elements falls into four broad categories of (1) environmental influences, (2) direct media influences, (3) peer-group dimensions, and (4) internal psychological elements. This list particularly pertains to adolescents and young adults, for whom self-injury appears to be growing most rapidly. I concede that this list is no more than a set of speculations or hypotheses.

Environmental Influences

- School and work environments are fraught with high stress.
- Multitasking lifestyles are conducive to persistent low-level stress and anxiety.
- Heavy emphasis on competition in schools and the workplace is conducive to isolation and distrust.
- The media heavily market a reliance on over-the-counter and prescription medications to alter mood, achieve desired feeling states, induce sleep, etc.
- Modification of consciousness is viewed as something that can be achieved quickly and affordably via use of alcohol or street drugs.
- Many adolescents and adults believe that celebration requires intoxication.
- Families, schools, and peers rarely teach healthy self-soothing skills.
- The culture emphasizes acquisition of material goods over quality of life.
- With both parents working, children are left alone for substantial portions of each day. When parents are home they are often exhausted and psychologically unavailable. Children are left with little soothing time with either parent.
- The divorce rate of 50% stresses not only children, but single parents, day care personnel, teachers, and beyond.
- There is an overall diminished sense of community and social supports to assist those in distress.
- The prevailing culture overemphasizes physical appearance and sets impossible standards of beauty for its youth in terms of weight, breast size, muscular configuration, etc. That which is unattainable can easily become a negative self-attribution.

Direct Media Influences

- Popular television shows and movies portray self-injurers (e.g., *Girl, Interrupted, Thirteen*).
- Music videos frequently portray self-injurious acts.
- People prominent in the media have reported self-injuring (e.g., actress Angelina Jolie, Princess Diana).
- Most television talk shows have featured self-injury as a topic.
- Many chat rooms are dedicated to the topic of self-injury.
- Many websites focus on self-injury; all too many of these provide extensive examples of poetry, artwork, and even photographs

describing or depicting self-injury acts, wounds, or scars. (See Appendix C for an annotated list of self-injury websites.)

Adolescent Peer-Group Dimensions

- Adolescents routinely experience powerful emotions and lack the coping skills to manage them.
- Adolescent peer groups view extensive substance use as a normative rite of passage.
- Substance use often begins at early ages, in middle and even grammar school.
- Substance use forestalls normative problem solving and the development of healthy self-soothing skills.
- Adolescents place high value on being viewed as "outrageous outsiders" by peers and adults.
- Peer-group cohesion is enhanced by behaviors that adults condemn or fear.
- Youth are action-oriented; self-injury is dramatic, visible, and produces immediate results.
- Adolescents are desensitized to self-injury because of the peer group's endorsement of body piercings, tattoos, brandings, and scarifications.
- Self-injury is viewed as "not much different" from these popular forms of body art or modification.

Internal Psychological Elements

- Self-injury works; it (temporarily) reduces tension and restores a sense of psychological equilibrium.
- Self-injury has powerful communication aspects.
- Self-injury provides a sense of control and empowerment.

There are, of course, many more internal psychological factors than those listed above. These additional factors are discussed at length in the second and third sections of this book. Let us now turn to the topic of when body modification should be considered self-injurious.

CHAPTER 4

Body Piercing, Tattooing, Branding, Scarification, and Other Forms of Body Modification

Since the late 1980s, a remarkable cultural phenomenon has emerged in the United States in the form of the increased popularity of body piercings, professional tattoos, scarifications, brandings, and other forms of body modification. Clinicians often ask if these forms of "body art," as they are sometimes called, should be considered self-injurious. There is no simple answer to this question. One way to address the issue is to refer to the definition of self-injury provided in Chapter 1.

Body piercings, professional tattoos, scarifications, and brandings may, at first glance, seem to meet some of the elements of self-injury. Tattoos and piercings, for example, are acquired intentionally and are self-effected, in that they are deliberately obtained by going to a professional. These forms of body modification are also very low in lethality if normal sterile procedures are employed.

Whether tattoos, body piercings, and other body modifications meet the definition of self-injury becomes a more complex determination for the remainder of the definition. Should tattoos and piercings be considered a form of "bodily harm" (and therefore self-injury)? This judgment is in the eye of the beholder. Most people who select and acquire professional tattoos consider them to be attractive and a decided improvement to their appearance. Certainly, many professional tattoo artists are very skilled and produce exceptional body art. As for body piercings, it seems unlikely that these should be considered disfiguring in that the large majority of the perforations created for body jewelry fully heal, and fill in, if left unadorned over time. Brandings and patterned scarifications are another matter in that the designs are permanent. However, those who obtain them often do so because they wish to proclaim affiliation to some group (e.g., football players to a team or fraternity, or youth to a gang). In these latter cases, the body modification is symbolically meaningful and endorsed by an influential social group.

SOCIAL CONTEXT AND BODY MODIFICATION

In the international culture of the early 21st century, tattoos and piercings (and to a lesser extent, brandings and scarifications) have widespread acceptance in diverse social contexts. In the late 1980s when I showed slides of elaborate tattoos and body piercings to professional audiences and asked if they considered them to be examples of self-injury, 80–90% said yes. In the mid-2000s, when similar audiences are shown the very same slides, the yes response drops to 5–10%. Clearly there has been a major shift in the acceptance of body modification as normative, even socially desirable, behavior. Therefore, it seems inappropriate to consider such body modification to be self-injurious because of the social endorsement. Body art is distinguishable from self-harming behavior in many instances because the tissue damage is viewed as either symbolically meaningful or beauty enhancing, or both.

INTENT AND BODY MODIFICATION

Very few individuals would state that they acquire tattoos or piercings to reduce psychological distress. Some talk of an "addiction to ink" or piercings, but they seem to be speaking figuratively rather than literally. Therefore, if the behaviors are not pursued to manage psychological distress or crisis, then it would appear that body modification can clearly be distinguished from self-injury. And that would appear to be the end of the story.

Of course, it turns out to be not quite that simple. There is also the matter of *self-inflicted* tattoos, piercings, scars, and brands. These are behaviors that almost always lack the aesthetic accomplishment of the professional versions. Moreover, in some cases, the behaviors are linked to distress management. Two examples from clinical practice make the point.

Naomi is a 16-year-old living in a group home. She was referred due to recurrent suicide attempts via overdose and multiple episodes of self-injury (wrist cutting). In addition, on one occasion, Naomi had mutilated her genitals. In the group home Naomi was working hard to learn new skills to deal with her depression and rage. She was especially motivated to earn weekend passes to visit her friends and her mother. One of the conditions for these passes was that she have no incidents of self-harm during the previous week.

During one time period, Naomi seemed especially agitated and restless. Staff learned from Naomi's roommate that she may have pierced her body. Subsequently, a staff nurse discovered that Naomi had pierced one of her nipples using a sewing needle. On examination the wound appeared to be in the early stages of infection. Naomi argued that there should be no consequences for the self-inflicted piercing because "everyone is doing it these days." Staff denied Naomi's request for a weekend pass, saying that professional piercings acquired under sterile conditions are different from self-inflicted piercings using nonsterile methods. Staff continued to work with Naomi regarding alternative ways to deal with agitation and restlessness.

In Naomi's case, the staff correctly viewed the behavior to be self-injury rather than body modification. Naomi's piercing was clearly related to psychological distress and was also unsafe medically. Naomi was astute enough to try to exploit the current climate of acceptance regarding body modification, but staff did not accept her line of reasoning because of the details of her piercing behavior.

Ian, an 18-year-old living with his parents, stated that his goal in life was to become the most famous tattoo artist of all time. He said he intended to top the great names of Don Ed Hardy, Lyle Tuttle, and Hanky Panky. No one in Ian's family had a problem with his goal, but they had serious reservations about his plan to achieve it. Ian said he was "an innately gifted artist" and was quite capable of being "self-taught" as a tattooist. He was adamant that he needed no training in the technical art of tattooing, claiming that he could learn everything he needed on the Internet or in books. Trouble was, Ian started out on his own body, using third-hand equipment, and the results weren't promising. Ian discovered that what he could do on paper turned out differently on skin. He became enraged and depressed at the unsightly mess he had made of his arms.

Despairing that he had failed at his life's goal, Ian agreed begrudgingly to see a family therapist with his parents. In treatment, no one challenged Ian's overall plan—even though it involved dropping out of junior college. Through a process of negotiation, the family worked with Ian to find a way to move him closer to his goal. Eventually, Ian agreed to apprentice at a well-known tattoo shop. Once he started work, Ian was relieved to learn that the owner could cover the mistakes on his arms with attractive professional tattoos.

In Ian's case the problem wasn't so much psychological distress as poor planning and impulsivity. Some family ingenuity turned behavior that resembled self-injury into a vocational plan with some promise.

BODY MODIFICATON AND MENTAL HEALTH STATUS

Favazza (1998) has suggested that heavily pierced and tattooed individuals may have more psychopathology than the general public. Not much in the way of data are available to support or disconfirm this hypothesis, but one study suggests that tattoos may have both advantages *and* disadvantages. Drews, Allison, and Probst (2000) studied differences between tattooed and nontattooed college students. In a sample of 235 they found that the tattooed students rated themselves as more adventurous, creative, and artistic than the nontattooed students. The students with tattoos also viewed themselves as more likely to take risks.

Drews and colleagues also analyzed their results by gender. They found that the tattooed males viewed themselves as more attractive and reported having more sexual partners. These males also had higher rates of having been arrested and were more likely to have body piercings. The tattooed women in the Drews et al. sample were more likely to report using drugs other than alcohol, to have shoplifted, and to have piercings in body areas other than their ears.

What can we conclude from these results? Perhaps only that the students in this sample had a combination of strengths and weaknesses associated with tattooed status. The tattooed youth viewed themselves as being creative, free-spirited, attractive, and sexually engaged. These would appear to be strengths. However, they were also more likely to engage in illegal activity and risk-taking behaviors than their nontattooed peers. These would appear to be deficits.

DETERMINING WHEN BODY MODIFICATION
IS SELF-DESTRUCTIVE

Whereas discussing people who are pierced and tattooed is an interesting diversion, there are also practical clinical issues that need to be addressed in a book on self-injury. One way to assess whether or not body modification is in the service of self-destructive motivations is to refer to the classification scheme regarding direct and indirect self-harm. A checklist for assessing direct and indirect self-harm is provided at the end of Chapter 2. The clinician can employ this checklist, informally at least, when speaking with a client who has extensive tattoos, piercings, or other forms of body modification. A useful rule of thumb is: If an individual presents with multiple forms of direct and indirect self-harm, then the clinician should be alert for self-destructive motivations associated with the body modification. Otherwise, the client may just be part of the cultural phenomenon of body art and enjoy it as a form of self-expression. In the latter instance, it would be a mistake to pathologize the behavior. Two examples from clinical encounters bring home the distinction between dysfunctional versus normative body modification.

Eugena was a 15-year-old teen brought into treatment by her parents due to self-injury. For about 6 months she had been cutting her forearms and legs with a razor blade. Eugena reported hurting herself when she fought with peers at school or when she broke up with a boyfriend. She conceded that her relationships tended to be stormy and short-lived. Asked about other forms of self-harm, Eugena acknowledged smoking pot almost daily and taking physical risks with some frequency. She denied suicide ideation or attempts.

The therapist noticed that Eugena had many pierced earrings in the outer cartilage of both ears. Asked about these, Eugena said that she had acquired some of these professionally but had done others herself. She admitted that sometimes she pierced an ear as a variation to cutting. The precipitants were strong, unpleasant feelings and the results were emotional relief. The therapist concluded that Eugena occasionally used ear piercing as a self-injurious behavior. He decided to monitor both cutting and body piercing in his treatment with Eugena.

In the case of Eugena, the body modification was deemed to be a variant of the cutting behavior. In the case that follows, the conclusion was different.

For more conventional people, the first encounter with Buzz tended to produce shock. Buzz was a 30-year-old with tribal tattoos swirling about his face. He also sported a 3-inch bone-like protuberance through the cartilage at the base of his nostrils and symmetrical piercings on his eyebrows, cheeks, and forehead. Although Buzz felt no need for psychological treatment, he would talk at length with anyone who was interested in his unusual appearance. Buzz's profession was that of a tattoo artist and body piercer. He recognized that his extensive facial tattoos and piercings precluded him from interacting with a more conservative mainstream society. This was fine with Buzz. He spent the majority of his time working in his shop, having a beer in biker bars, or socializing with similarly body-modified peers. Buzz was quite comfortable within his niche in society. He had friends, a stable job, and little or no behavior that could be considered self-destructive.

THE EXTREME END OF THE CONTINUUM

What is one to make of individuals with *really* extensive tattoos and body piercings? How should professionals view individuals who have scores of piercings on their face, body, or genitals? What about those with multiple subcutaneous decorations, brandings, scarifications, and full body tattoos? Some individuals suspend heavy objects from their nipples or genitals in order to induce intense body sensations. Others have multiple penile or labial piercings decorated with jewelry that they employ for extra stimulation during sexual contact.

My own opinion is that these individuals are quirky adventurers on the frontiers of body art and modification, and there is much we can learn from them. Persons who push their bodies to their limits may have insights into the age-old mind–body dilemma that others cannot fathom. The mainstream is often informed and influenced by the exteriors. Those who test the limits of body modification rarely end up in psychological treatment. They do not view the consultation room as a relevant resource and therefore are neither a concern nor a challenge for psychotherapists.

PART II

Assessment and Treatment

CHAPTER 5

A Biopsychosocial Model
for Self-Injury

In this book self-injury is conceptualized as a biopsychosocial phenomenon. Based on this framework, the recommended approach to assessment
and treatment is a bio-cognitive-behavioral one. The simple, streamlined
model presented in this chapter is designed to be user friendly and leads
directly to the recommended assessment and treatment techniques discussed in subsequent chapters. For a much more complex, comprehensive
theoretical explanation of self-injury, consult Linehan's biosocial model
(1993a), which has been updated and applied exclusively to self-injury in
Brown (2002).

Self-injury as a biopsychosocial phenomenon includes five interrelated
dimensions.

1. Environmental
2. Biological
3. Cognitive
4. Affective
5. Behavioral

The etiology of the behavior can be understood by attending to the
interrelationships among these five dimensions. For the large majority of
individuals, all five dimensions play a role in the emergence and recurrence
of self-injury. The mix of dimensions is unique for each individual. For
some clients environmental and biological dimensions may be most important. For others, cognitive, affective, and behavioral dimensions may pre-
dominate. The task of assessment is to identify which are most important

and to prioritize these in the course of treatment—although all relevant dimensions need to be addressed eventually.

The five dimensions in the biopsychosocial field are discussed in the sections that follow.

ENVIRONMENTAL DIMENSION

The environmental dimension contributing to the occurrence of self-injury includes three basic categories: family historical elements, client historical elements, and current environmental elements. These elements, as contextual or environmental, are in some sense "outside" the individual, but nonetheless have a salient impact on the individual and his or her pattern of self-injury.

Family Historical Elements

"Family historical elements" refer to key aspects of the history of the nuclear, extended, or surrogate family that have been "observed" but not directly experienced. (Although relationships beyond the family can have a major influence on children, they tend to be less important than daily living environments.) For example, to observe violence or substance abuse in the family is different from being assaulted or ingesting substances oneself. The former may have a powerful *indirect* impact; the latter, a profound *direct* impact. Many aspects of family history have been linked in empirical research to the emergence of self-injury later in life. These include such variables as mental illness, substance abuse, violence, suicide, and self-injury in the family (e.g., Walsh & Rosen, 1988; Shapiro & Dominiak, 1992; Favazza, 1996, 1998).

On a daily basis family environments teach children behaviors via modeling, reinforcement, punishment, and extinction. For example, when family members tend to express emotions explosively, the child may learn to be explosive (or markedly inhibited). When family members deal with distress by using substances heavily, the child may acquire a pattern for this behavior and implement it at a later time. Clinicians are all too familiar with the latency-age child who swears he or she will never use alcohol or drugs, due to observing the effects of a parent's addiction. Then, years later, as if on automatic pilot, the now adolescent child begins abusing substances unmindful of previous convictions.

A particularly ominous pattern in family environments is self-destructive behavior. When parents or other family members model self-destructive behavior, such as suicide attempts or self-injury, these acts tend to have significant repercussions for children. Observing this behavior can have many connotations for a child. Witnessing self-destructive behavior in family members can convey such messages as:

"Life is overwhelmingly painful."
"Life is not worth living."
"Distress can be relieved by behaving self-destructively."
"Others cannot help my pain."
"My pain negates responsibilities I have to others."

These are only a few of the possible interpretations that children may attach to seeing family members behave self-destructively. While such behavior in the family must be understood and responded to with compassion, the long-term effects on children cannot be ignored. Children living with family members who behave self-destructively learn to consider self-harm as an option when life becomes challenging. Completed suicides are the most damaging of self-harm acts. The long-term profoundly negative effects on family and significant others are well documented (American Association of Suicidology, 2002). These effects include depression, despair, isolation, substance abuse, and the repetition of self-destructive behaviors across generations.

Client Historical Elements

"Client historical elements" include those elements in the individual's personal history that have been *directly* experienced, as opposed to observed. Those found to be associated empirically with self-injury include the death of a parent or other caregivers, loss through separation, divorce or placement outside the home, and experiences of neglect and/or emotional, physical, and sexual abuse (Walsh & Rosen, 1988; Shapiro & Dominiak, 1992; Miller, 1994; van der Kolk et al., 1996; Alderman, 1997; Favazza, 1998; Briere & Gil, 1998; Turell & Armsworth, 2000; Rodriquez-Srednicki, 2001; Gratz, Conrad, & Roemer, 2002; Paul et al., 2002).

The recent work by Gratz et al. (2002) has provided some new insights into family experiences associated with self-injury. In a racially diverse nonclinical sample of 133 college students, a remarkable 38% of the sample reported a history of direct self-harm (self-injury). Also striking was that the lifetime self-reported prevalence of self-injury was slightly greater for males than for females—a very rare finding, indeed: 36% of the women and 41% of the males reported having self-injured.

Gratz and colleagues (2002) hypothesized that self-injury would be associated with a number of aversive family experiences, including neglect, physical and sexual abuse, separation, loss, and related attachment problems. They also predicted that these negative family experiences would be linked to dissociation experiences, which in turn would be predictive of self-injury. The Gratz study found significant gender differences regarding family experiences. The predictors of self-injury for the *women* in the sample were, in order of importance, dissociation, insecure paternal attachment, childhood sexual abuse, maternal emotional neglect, and paternal emotional neglect (for which there was a significant inverse relationship). In contrast, for the *men* in the sample, the predictors of self-injury, in order of importance, were childhood separation (especially from father), dissociation, and physical abuse. Thus the findings suggested that a number of aversive experiences from childhood should be considered when assessing self-injury, including neglect, physical and sexual abuse, separation, and loss. Also, the possibility of gender differences should be given serious consideration.

Invalidating Environments within the Family

Linehan (1993a) has discussed somewhat subtler family antecedents to histories of self-injury (and other problems). She has described the "invalidating environment" in the family experiences of individuals diagnosed with borderline personality disorder. She contends that in many of these families, the affective experiences of children are often ignored, denied, ridiculed, or condemned (i.e., "invalidated"). Such experiences often result in children questioning the accuracy, and even the very existence, of their own internal feeling states. Moreover, such environments may differentially reinforce only the most extreme of affective responses. For example, if a child indicates in a subtle manner that he or she is distressed, the invalidating environment may ignore the communication. Only when the child presents with an extreme emotional behavior (e.g., a tantrum) does he or she receive a response. The entire pattern is conducive to reinforcing maladaptive behavior while extinguishing adaptive behavior. When such a pattern is repeated countless times for many years, the end result can be an emotionally dysregulated person. Such people may come to rely on self-invalidating behaviors such as self-injury to manage emotional distress (Linehan, 1993a).

Family and Environmental Strengths and Assets

Often missing in the discussion of the families of self-injurious individuals is an examination of their strengths. Even the most dysfunctional family has strengths that should be identified and reinforced. In many cases, the families of the "new generation of self-injurers" have considerable assets. The fact that a person self-injures does not mean that he or she comes from a family with marked dysfunction. Unlike the families often described in the empirical research, families of self-injuring persons can often be validating, non-neglectful, and nonabusive. Stated more positively, the families of self-injurers are often loving, committed, compassionate, and skillful at problem solving. The clinician should not assume dysfunction; rather, the clinician should conduct a careful strength-based analysis of each family. The areas to be assessed should include strengths within

- The home and extended family
- The neighborhood and related networks
- School and employment sectors
- Financial resources and management
- Cultural identity and resources
- Recreational activities and hobbies
- Religious and spiritual beliefs and institutional supports

The strengths within a family serve to mitigate the risk of self-injury. The more strengths that can be brought to bear within the family, the greater the positive impact on reducing self-destructive behavior. Families may often be a source of distress for a self-injuring member, but they can also provide the solutions to problems if they are respected and engaged as therapeutic allies.

Current Environmental Elements

"Current environmental elements" refers to circumstances in the present that tend to trigger self-injury. There are many environmental conditions that can precipitate self-injurious behavior. Common examples include experiencing loss or conflict in relationships, being abused by a present caregiver or partner, or being exposed to peers who self-injure. Performance problems in the functional areas of school, work, and athletics or other extracurricular activities can also be key elements. Persons who have experienced aversive conditions in the *family* and *personal historical elements* are especially sensitive to similar problems in the present. For example, an individual who has experienced loss of a parent during childhood may be especially reactive to losses in peer relationships during adolescence. In a similar vein, those who have been physically abused or sexually assaulted as children may be exquisitely sensitive to threats of abuse or assault in the present. They may also be reactive to even normal forms of sexual approach from others. Not surprisingly, poly-self-destructive individuals often come from histories of poly-abuse. The more complicated and aversive the individual's historical context, the more vulnerable he or she is likely to be in the present to negative experiences.

BIOLOGICAL DIMENSION

The understanding of self-injurious behavior from a biological perspective has changed with the increasing advances in brain imaging studies. For many years clinicians accepted a distinction between so-called "organic" and "functional" disorders. It is clear today that such a distinction arose from the limits of assessment technology in a given era. For instance, in the days of Kraepelin, some psychiatric disorders, such as general paresis (tertiary syphilis), were associated with changes in brain structure that were visible with the microscopy of the time. Those examining brain tissues from patients who died of schizophrenia or manic–depressive disease could find no differences from the appearance of the brains of healthy comparison subjects. So the "organic" versus "functional" distinction arose and lasted for most of the 20th century.

In the last 20 years, with a rapidly increasing pace of discovery in the brain sciences, these distinctions are obsolete. Demonstration of altered brain structure or function in living subjects as well as in postmortem brains through brain imaging or metabolic studies suddenly removed a disorder previously judged "functional," such as obsessive–compulsive disorder or autism, from that category. Obsessive–compulsive disorder has, in fact, provided one of the most provocative findings, in that interventions in preliminary studies were found to "move" brain imaging abnormalities in the direction of patterns seen in control subjects. Most strikingly, these changes with treatment were seen with both pharmacological and cognitive-behavioral interventions.

In retrospect, the old functional–organic distinction was faulty in principle, not just in the light of today's neuroimaging. All behavior arises in the brain. The old distinctions differentiated not disorders that were fundamentally different but only those in which we could measure a difference in the brain from those in which we could not.

The complex relationships between biology and self-injury are an important and emerging focus of empirical research. A number of psychiatric diagnoses associated with self-injury have been shown to have biochemical components, including borderline personality disorder, depression, bipolar illness, and schizophrenia. Many extreme forms of self-injury have often been found to be associated with psychoses such as schizophrenia

(Simeon & Hollander, 2001). Other physiological problems commonly associated with self-injury include physical illness (e.g., diabetes, asthma, ortho-
pedic disease), sleep disorder, eating disorder, and a tendency to somaticize
distress.

Biological Vulnerability to Emotional Dysregulation

Linehan (1993a) has written about the biological vulnerabilities of individuals with borderline personality disorder. She has suggested that the emotional dysregulation that characterizes this disorder in all likelihood has
biological underpinnings. As she stated, "Biological causes could conceiv-
ably range from genetic influences to disadvantageous intrauterine events
to early childhood environmental effects on development of the brain and
nervous system" (p. 47).

Limbic System Dysfunction

Research from Gardner and Cowdry (1985) suggested that deficiencies in
the limbic system of the brain may be associated with repetitive self-injury.
The limbic system is known to play a key role in the regulation of emotion.
Gardner and Cowdry have suggested that the link between the limbic system dysfunction and emotional dysregulation may account for why some
self-injurers respond well to anticonvulsant medications (e.g., carbamaz-
epine/Tegretol) that are known to impact the limbic system. However, as
noted by Favazza (1996), only a relatively small proportion of self-injurers
appear to respond to anticonvulsant pharmacotherapy.

Serotonin Level Dysfunction

The most extensive discussion to date of the biological underpinnings of
self-injury is presented in Simeon and Hollander's edited volume (2001).
Within that work, Grossman and Siever (2001) review the research regarding the biological factors associated with "impulsive" self-injury. Because
impulsive self-injury is closest to the focus of this book, their discussion is
briefly summarized here. One area of research that appears promising in
understanding the biology of self-injury concerns serotonin levels in the
brain. A number of empirical studies have linked diminished serotonin levels with impulsive aggression and self-injury (e.g., Simeon, Stanley, & Frances, 1992; Markowitz, 1995). Both Simeon and colleagues and Markowitz
measured serotonin levels in self-destructive people, and both found lower
than normal serotonin levels. They independently concluded that such levels may facilitate self-injury. The use of selective serotonin reuptake inhibi-

tors (SSRIs; e.g., Prozac, Zoloft, Paxil, Celexa) is designed to assist the body in using existing serotonin levels (however diminished) most efficiently (Medinfo.co.uk website, 2003). Some indirect support regarding the possible role of serotonin in self-injury has been obtained via the reduction of depression, impulsivity, and self-injury in some individuals using SSRIs (Grossman & Siever, 2001).

Endogenous Opioid System Dysfunction

Another biological explanation for self-injury concerns the endogenous opioid system (EOS). Many clients who self-injure report an absence of pain at the time of the act (Favazza, 1996, 1998; Alderman, 1997; Conterio & Lader, 1998). As noted by Grossman and Siever (2001), "Abundant evidence indicates EOS involvement in pain perception, particularly in stress-induced analgesia" (p. 125). A number of researchers have hypothesized that enhanced brain opioid activity may support self-injury. Stated in lay-persons' terms, when an individual harms his or her body, the brain may release naturally occurring opiate-like chemicals (e.g., endorphins) that are experienced as pleasurable and/or as a relief from emotional distress.

As noted by Grossman and Siever (2001), there are two main hypotheses regarding the relationship between the EOS and self-injury: *the addiction hypothesis* and *the pain hypothesis*.

> The addiction hypothesis suggests that there exists essentially a normal EOS that has been chronically overstimulated by frequent SIB [self-injurious behavior] for the purpose of relieving dysphoria. The individual develops a tolerance for the outpouring of endogenous opioids, cyclically suffers a withdrawal reaction, and is driven to further EOS stimulation by means of impulsive SIB. (p. 125)

> The pain hypothesis suggests a constitutional abnormality in the EOS that is unmasked by the environment such that pain sensitivity is diminished. This may involve a lack of negative feedback in the EOS and/or overproduction of endogenous opioids. This heightened opiatergic tone could eventually lead to dysphoric experiences of numbness and dissociation. SIB may present a stimulus that breaks through a self-alienating dissociative state, brought on by a environmental and/or intrapsychic stressors, and thereby allows the self-injurer to feel again. (p. 125)

Some support for the addiction hypothesis is provided indirectly by reported success in treating self-injury using naltrexone, a medication originally developed to block opiate "highs" in substance abusers. The use of naltrexone for self-injurers is intended to block the positive sensations associated with endogenous opioid release. The hypothesis is that blocking the EOS response may eliminate the biochemical "payoff" of self-injury for the more "addicted" individuals. We might also speculate that when naltrexone fails to work, the pain hypothesis might be the more accurate explanation for those individuals.

Diminished Pain Sensitivity

There is also empirical evidence that some self-injurers have diminished responsiveness to physical pain. Bohus and colleagues (2000) have reported that about 60% of self-injurers report no pain at the time of the act. Russ and colleagues (Russ et al., 1992; Russ, Roth, Kakuma, Harrison, & Hull, 1994) have conducted experiments comparing physical pain tolerance in self-injuring persons (who report an absence of pain during the act) with self-injurers who report experiencing pain and other non-self-injuring controls. In experiments that deliberately induced closely measured physical pain, Russ and colleagues reported a significantly diminished experience of physical discomfort for the "no pain" self-injurers.

Bohus and colleagues (2000) have also found diminished pain sensation in self-injurers with borderline personality disorder. They compared a sample of 12 female self-injurers with borderline personality disorder (BPD) who reported analgesia during self-injury with 19 "healthy controls." They administered both the cold pressor test and the tourniquet pain test in order to measure perception of physical pain in the study subjects. Subjects were tested both when they were feeling calm and when they were markedly distressed. In order to control for possible effects of psychotropic medication on pain sensitivity, none of the subjects as receiving pharmacotherapy. Bohus and colleagues reported:

> Even during self-reported calmness, patients with BPD showed a significantly reduced perception of pain compared to healthy control subjects in both tests. During distress, pain perception in BPD patients was further significantly reduced as compared with self-reported calmness. The present findings show that self-mutilating patients with BPD who experience analgesia during self-injury show an increased threshold for pain even in the absence of distress. (p. 251)

The Russ and Bohus studies are especially intriguing in that they move beyond psychological hypothesizing about dissociation or pain tolerance to physiological experiments. Clearly, there is an emerging body of evidence regarding the biological underpinnings of self-injury. This conclusion points to pharmacotherapy as an important tool in the treatment of self-injury.

(This topic is addressed in Chapter 14.) However, as noted by Grossman and Siever (2001), pharmacotherapy is unlikely to be a sufficient treatment, in and of itself. Complementary psychological interventions are usually required as well. They stated:

> Histories of sexual abuse and other traumatic/chaotic experiences often populate these patients' formative years. The lack of appropriate interpersonal experiences and the attendant conflicts in the areas of trust, self-esteem, mood regulation, and self-soothing cannot be resolved with medication. Rather, appropriate pharmacologic treatment can lessen the intensity of certain experiences and create a more favorable setting for psychotherapy and long-term characterologic/behavioral changes. (p. 128)

These words are an appropriate segue to discussing the cognitive, affective, and behavioral dimensions of self-injury.

COGNITIVE DIMENSION

The cognitive dimension associated with self-injury falls into two basic categories: *cognitive interpretations of environmental events* and *self-generated cognitions*. Environmental events are problematic only if the self-injuring person interprets them to be aversive, painful, or disorganizing. Of course, some environmental circumstances are so overwhelming as to have very compelling cognitive implications. It is a very rare individual who can be on the receiving end of physical or sexual abuse and not end up with problematic, self-defeating thoughts. I did encounter one such individual who had been sexually assaulted as a prisoner of war during the Desert Storm war in 1991. She dismissed the groping behavior she had received as insignificant because "the death and destruction around me were so much worse." She stated that the assault had no untoward repercussions for her thereafter. However, most individuals who are sexually abused develop complicated thoughts and judgments regarding their experiences. Very common are irrational self-blaming thoughts such as, "I should have done something to stop the abuse," or "I must have wanted it to happen for it to go on so long." Assisting clients to give up such irrational self-blaming cognitions is often at the heart of treatment for self-injuring trauma survivors.

Other thoughts that are dysfunctional may be derived from less powerful environmental conditions and more within the immediate power of the individual to challenge and modify. Examples include such thoughts as "I must get an A on every paper and test," or "I have to get along with all my friends all the time or I'll be totally alone." These are cognitions that can cause individuals untoward pain and discomfort because of their unattainable perfectionism. Such thoughts are often far more amenable to gentle challenging than more complex trauma-based thoughts and beliefs.

Self-generated cognitions are triggered by internal cues as opposed to external events and circumstances. On awakening, a client might start the day with the thought, "Another grim, empty day. How will I get through it?" These are cognitions for which there may have been no conceivable environmental triggers. The day has just begun; there has been no time for aversive environmental events. Some self-injurers carry with them an extensive roster of thoughts and judgments that predict nothing but discomfort and pain. Assessment of these recurrent negative, pessimistic cognitions is fundamental to moving forward psychotherapeutically; they need to be identified and modified if the client is to experience more success and less anguish.

In addition, self-injuring persons generate a wide range of cognitions that trigger their acts of self-harm. Identifying these thoughts is another key step in assessment. Typical thoughts that precede self-injury include "I have to do something," or "I deserve this," or "I hate my body so much," or "This will show people that I'm really hurting," or "This is the *only* way to deal with this problem." Supplanting such thoughts with ideas regarding alternative courses of action is fundamental to moving away from lives of self-harm.

The cognitive dimension related to self-injury is discussed in much greater detail in Chapter 10.

AFFECTIVE DIMENSION

Closely linked to the cognitive dimension is the affective dimension. Emotions emerge from the irrational, self-blaming, distorted cognitions that precede them. Emotions are often centrally important in assessing and treating self-injury. Most individuals self-injure in order to reduce or eliminate affective distress. As noted in Chapter 1, self-injuring persons identify a wide range of emotions as preceding their acts of self-harm, including anger, anxiety, tension, sadness, depression, shame, worry, and contempt (Favazza, 1987; Walsh & Rosen, 1988; Alderman, 1997; Conterio & Lader, 1998; Brown, 1998; Simeon & Hollander, 2001). I have yet to encounter a self-injurer who identified a positive emotion as triggering self-harm. No one is likely to say that they cut or burned themselves because they were feeling too relaxed or joyous. Self-injury is about negative emotion.

Assessment needs to identify, very specifically, the most important and recurrent affective triggers for each individual. In turn, treatment needs to teach skills to endure, manage, and reduce powerful affects without resorting to self-harm.

BEHAVIORAL DIMENSION

The behavioral dimension consists of overt actions that immediately precede, accompany, and follow acts of self-injury. These are the behaviors that are strongly and recurrently associated with the acts of self-harm. Typical behavioral antecedents include conflicts with family or peers, isolation, failure at an activity, sexual behavior, substance abuse, or eating-disordered behavior. The behavioral dimension also includes actions that prepare for self-injury, such as choosing the physical location, securing it to prevent interruption, and selecting a tool. Other behavioral components include actions that immediately follow self-injury, such as deciding whether or not to provide self-care, disposing of or hiding tools, and communicating with others. The aftermath of self-injury is very important to assess. Some individuals report falling asleep immediately after self-injuring; others return to normal activities; some remain agitated and seek other forms of release. The behavioral "results" of self-injury provide a great deal of information about why the behavior is repeated.

INTEGRATION OF THE FIVE DIMENSIONS

As I noted at the beginning of the chapter, the five dimensions of this biopsychosocial model do not function in isolation. They are entirely interrelated and even interdependent. For example, biological vulnerabilities affect the responsiveness of the individual to environmental conditions. A biologically compromised individual will be more negatively impacted by aversive experiences in the environment than one who is constitutionally strong. Conversely, there is evidence that recurrent traumatic experiences have sustained physiological effects, including changes in brain chemistry (van der Kolk et al. 1996). In addition, environmental conditions and physiology have a major impact on cognitions in terms of positivity, negativity, and self-efficacy. Cognitions, in turn, trigger and "refire" emotions; and emotions reciprocally impact future cognitions. Cognitions and emotions precipitate behaviors which, depending in their results, affect subsequent thoughts and feelings. A tabular summary of the five dimensions is depicted in Table 5.1.

TABLE 5.1. Biopsychosocial Model for Self-Injury

Environmental dimension

- Family historical elements (e.g., mental illness, violence, substance abuse, self-injury, suicide in family)
- Client historical elements (e.g., neglect, attachment problems, loss of parent, physical and sexual abuse)
- Invalidating environment within the family
- Family and environmental strengths and assets
- Current aversive environmental elements (e.g., loss, relationship conflict, abuse, peers who self-injure)

Biological dimension

- Biological vulnerability to emotional dysregulation
- Limbic system dysfunction?
- Serotonin level dysfunction?
- Endogenous opioid system dysfunction?
- Diminished pain sensitivity?

Cognitive dimension

- Interpretations of environmental elements, especially negative, pessimistic thoughts, judgments, beliefs (e.g., "All my relationships end badly," "No one understands me," "I'm all alone")
- Self-generated cognitions regarding self and self-injury (e.g., "I have to do this," "Only self-injury helps," "I deserve this," "I hate my body," "Now others will understand how much pain I'm in")
- Thoughts, images, flashbacks related to trauma

Affective dimension

- Susceptibility to frequent, intense, sustained emotions
- Negative emotions trigger self-injury, especially anger, anxiety, tension, shame, depression, sadness, contempt, worry
- Emotions and/or dissociation related to thoughts, images, flashbacks from trauma

Behavioral dimension

- Major behavioral antecedents, such as conflicts with others, substance use, isolation
- Preparation for self-injury, such as choosing location, obtaining tool, ensuring privacy
- Aftermath behaviors, such as returning to activities, falling asleep, communicating with others regarding self-injury

CONCLUSION

This chapter has set the stage for the next section on assessment and treatment. In order to conduct a thorough assessment of self-injury, clinicians need to understand the environmental, biological, cognitive, affective, and behavioral concomitants to the acts of self-harm. This chapter has reviewed the five key dimensions that influence, trigger, and serve to maintain the behavior. These five dimensions must be addressed when providing treatment. The "mix" of the five dimensions is idiosyncratic for each individual; therefore treatment strategies need to be individualized to meet the needs of each self-injuring client.

CHAPTER 6

Initial Therapeutic Responses

The early clinical responses to self-injury set the stage for the remainder of assessment and treatment. Skillful management at the outset can gain the confidence of the client, comfort family members in a time of intense stress, and correctly delineate the unique features of self-injury. Conversely, mishandling the initial responses to self-injury can have long-term negative repercussions. Misdiagnosis can lead to labeling the behavior as suicidal, resulting in unnecessary psychiatric hospitalizations and related stigmatization. This chapter discusses using language strategically and adopting an appropriate interpersonal demeanor in responding to self-injury.

AVOIDING THE USE OF SUICIDE TERMINOLOGY

Chapter 1 emphasized the major points of distinction between self-injury and suicide. Consistent with this emphasis, in speaking with clients about their self-injury, it is important, first and foremost, to avoid the language of suicide. Unfortunately, many professionals use terms such as a "suicide gesture" or "suicide attempts" to refer to self-injury. The use of "suicide gesture" is not only misleading but is generally "countertransferential" (Maltsberger, 1986) or "therapy interfering" (Linehan, 1993a). A gesture is a slight movement, a minor act of motion, an insignificant behavior in the grand scheme of things. Professionals use the term "suicide gesture" to convey that a behavior is "not a real suicide attempt" and therefore not deserving of serious alarm. Often, an additional implication of the term "gesture" is that the act is "manipulative." The position of this book is that self-injury is neither insignificant nor manipulative. The behavior is important, deserving of full attention and a concerted therapeutic strategy. Self-injury should not be dismissed or minimized; it is not a mere gesture; it is a significant act.

Although the equally common term "suicide attempt" does not suffer from countertransferential implications, it is inappropriate because it leads the professional and the client down the suicide path. If, as discussed in Chapter 1, the behavior of self-injury generally has little to do with suicide, why use suicide terminology? Calling a self-injurious act such as arm or body cutting a "suicide attempt" creates a needless misdirection, fosters confusion, and runs the risk of excessive stigmatization. Therefore, it is desirable to keep the language of suicide out of the professional response to self-injury.

Another problematic term commonly used to refer to self-injury is "parasuicide." Coined by Norman Kreitman (1977), it has been employed by many other researchers, including Shneidman (1985) and Linehan (1993a). There are two main problems with the term "parasuicide." The first is its definition, which is "similar to or alongside suicide" (Kreitman, 1977). My contention is that self-injury is neither similar to nor alongside suicide. Self-injury is distinct from suicide, and emphasizing similarities between the two behaviors is misleading and inaccurate.

Furthermore, when researchers or clinicians use the term "parasuicide," they include within its boundaries an astonishingly large range of self-destructive behaviors. Linehan (1993a), for example, includes behaviors ranging from a superficial scratch on the arm with a paper clip (that fails to break the skin) to a high-lethality suicide attempt that fails to end in death only by accident (e.g., a nonfatal self-inflicted gunshot wound to the head). Including such a broad range of self-destructive behaviors under the rubric of a single term is not useful because it is too heterogeneous. The average clinician finds it bafflingly complex to use the same term in referring equally to such behaviors as modest, low-lethality hair pulling and high-lethality attempts at hanging. Inevitably we are left wondering, Does it refer to a low- or high-lethality act in this case? A far more useful way to organize information about self-destructive acts is Pattison and Kahan's (1983) multidimensional schema regarding direct and indirect self-harm presented in Chapter 2, which offers gradations as to intent, lethality, and frequency. The schema does not comingle acts of high lethality with those that have little or no lethality.

EMPLOYING THE CLIENT'S LANGUAGE STRATEGICALLY

If the language of suicide gesture, suicide attempt, and parasuicide should be avoided in discussing self-injury, what language *should* be used? It is often very helpful to employ the language of the self-injurers themselves, with certain exceptions. Most self-injuring persons use behaviorally descriptive language when they speak or write of their self-harm. They will refer to it as "cutting," "scratching," "carving," "burning," "picking," "hitting," and so on. When the therapist responds to the client by using such language, it has distinct advantages. First, it is a joining strategy to use the client's own terminology. It is also respectful of, and empowering to, the client to accept his or her language. The implicit message from the therapist is "I am giving respectful attention to your view of this and using your own language in discussing it."

An additional advantage of mirroring a client's language is that it is a preliminary step in entering the psychological space of that individual. This entrance is crucial in coming to understand and assist the person with his or her self-injury. Language that reflects the speech of another is one of the most basic and affirming of empathic behaviors.

However, there are exceptions to this rule. There are times when using the language of self-injuring persons is ill advised. These exceptions involve two types of language: the minimizing and the ultrasubjective. Language of minimization occurs when the individual is performing considerable harm to his or her body and the language does not reflect the damage inflicted. For example, I worked with a woman in her 30s whose scars were extensive and permanent on both arms. The scars were jagged, random, thick, white keloidic records of 15 years of self-mutilation (the damage went beyond self-injury). Many of her scars came from wounds that should have been sutured at the time of the acts. However, she had cared for the wounds herself, worsening the extent and permanence of her scarring. When this woman first began therapy, she referred to her self-mutilation as "scratching" or "picking." I found this language to be quite minimizing, given the extent of her scars. Moreover, these scars were stigmatizing when noticed by others. People would recoil and avoid her once they had seen the tangled mass of scars on her arms.

Once I had built a positive alliance with the client, I chose to challenge, gently, her use of language. I was careful to avoid shaming or chastising her, but I felt I needed to insert a sense of reality into our dialogue. On one occasion when the time seemed right, I said that in my opinion her "self-harm went way beyond 'scratching' or 'picking.'" Although initially surprised by my comment, she was able to accept my questioning of her use of language. Later, I asked her what words might be more accurate in referring to her self-harm. She suggested that we use "cutting" or "slashing," and I agreed. Her coming to view the extent of the damage more accurately was part of the therapeutic process. She became more motivated to reduce the behavior as she acknowledged the social cost. She began to conceal her scars from others when she was concerned about social repercussions. With those she knew well and felt more comfortable, she took no such precautions.

Another problem with language occurs when clients refer to the behavior in an ultrasubjective way. Most commonly, the use of idiosyncratic language emerges from people who suffer from some form of psychosis. For example, I worked for a number of years with a man who mutilated himself by punching his face, head, and eyes. (This individual's dilemma is presented at length in Chapter 18.) Years of this self-inflicted abuse resulted in this individual's becoming legally blind. His explanations for these acts of self-harm were entirely consistent year after year. His language referring to his self-mutilation was related to a very fixed delusion. He stated that evil spirits took over his body and punished him for his sins; he had no control over the acts of self-punching. In the course of treatment, I often explored his delusional thoughts; however, I never endorsed them and made them my own. I would use his language about spirits from time to time but always added qualifiers, such as, "I know *your view* is that spirits caused this self-assault. Or "What, *in your view*, were you being punished for today?" I attempted to walk a narrow narrow path with this client whereby I was respectful of his experience of the world without endorsing or affirming it. Chapter 18 presents other aspects of responding to delusional thought and language in strategic, therapeutic ways.

THE IMPORTANCE OF INTERPERSONAL DEMEANOR

A second aspect of initially responding to self-injury concerns the importance of interpersonal demeanor. People tend to respond to self-injury with affectively charged behaviors. These include such reactions as

- Intense concern and effusive support
- Anguish and fear
- Recoil, shock, and avoidance
- Condemnation, ridicule, and threats

Most people react to self-injury with positive emotions such as concern and support. These are responses that convey to the self-injurer a desire to help and protect. Unfortunately, over time, positive responses from others can become a form of secondary reinforcement for the behavior. The first level of reinforcement for self-injury is the relief obtained from emotional distress. Markedly and rapidly reducing intense emotional discomfort is intensely reinforcing. However, inadvertent social reinforcement can also play an important secondary role. For this reason, even positive reactions of concern and support can be problematic. This is especially the case when the reactions are effusive. The more intense the emotional response, the greater the risk of inadvertent reinforcement.

Of course, many people react to self-injury with behavior that goes beyond concern and support. Hysterical behavior that involves anguish and fear is not uncommon. For example:

A mother with an only child, a 12-year-old daughter, called a therapist sobbing on the phone. She said that she had just discovered that her daughter had been cutting herself from time to time over a 6-month period. Between gasps for breath, the mother said that she lived for her daughter and didn't know if she could survive if her daughter killed herself. The clinician tried to comfort the mother, expressing how important her daughter must be to her. Then he asked what the daughter was doing at that moment. The mother said she was outside playing happily. Ascertaining that the daughter was at no immediate risk, the clinician attempted to reassure the mother. Through a series of questions, the clinician discovered that the extent of the girl's self-injury was occasional scratches on her wrists and ankles that required no first aid. The clinician then explained to the mother that although self-injury is alarming and needs treatment, it usually has little to do with suicide. The mother calmed down markedly in response to this statement. The mother and the clinician made an appointment for the next day. Before hanging up, the therapist gave the mother a phone number for a local psychiatric emergency unit, should any major problem arise in the interim.

In this case, the therapist's job was to calm the mother and provide some brief education about self-injury. Hysterical reactions are rarely helpful in responding to the behavior. They interfere with problem solving and may inadvertently reinforce the behavior in those who find intense reactions in others to be rewarding. Particularly for those who have been ignored or punished frequently, hysterical protective reactions can be quite gratifying.

Another common reaction to self-injury is some combination of recoil, shock, and avoidance. In these circumstances, the people encountering self-injury are overwhelmed by the behavior and feel compelled to leave the emotional field. In these situations, the responders behave in a way that is more protective of themselves than the self-injurers. They may want to help but find the notion of self-injury to be too upsetting and disorganizing to endure. As a result, they abandon the self-injurer and flee to safer ground. Sometimes even seasoned therapists respond in this manner to self-injury.

A 21-year-old male described his previous therapist's handling of his self-injury. "She never liked to talk about it. If I brought it up—or worse—if I walked into her office with short sleeves on, her face kind of scrunched up and she looked stressed out. She would start moving around in her chair and breathing like she was real uptight. Then she would make me promise never to do it again and say something like, 'Let's move on to more positive things. . . .'"

Conveying shock, followed by recoil and retreat, is destructive to self-injurers. Too many have encountered multiple losses and rejections in their lives and do not need additional abandonment experiences. Professionals need to assess why they might be so triggered by self-injury and strive to overcome it. For many, a tendency to be shocked by self-injury fades over time with exposure to, and a greater understanding of, the behavior. If avoidant reactions cannot be neutralized, it is best for clinicians to transfer self-injuring clients elsewhere.

Some individuals go beyond recoil and avoidance to downright hostility. In this case the excessive affect is the opposite of too much support and empathy. It is punitive and rejecting. For example:

A father's reaction to first learning about his daughter's cutting and burning herself was to call her "a stupid idiot." He added, "If you're going to do that kind of sick behavior, you can move out of here and into a mental hospital right now! You know and I know you're just doing it for attention! Get out of my sight!"

It is hard to imagine a less helpful response than this father's—unless violence came into play. It is not surprising that encountering self-injury—particularly when it is unexpected—causes intense emotional reactions in others. The behavior involves tissue damage and blood, which most human beings understandably prefer to avoid. Moreover, the behavior is self-inflicted, which runs counter to normal human expectations regarding self-protection. In addition, the behavior may stir up in others fears of body fragility or fragmentation, and threaten a sense of bodily wholeness or integrity. They may also fear (usually irrationally) that the self-injuring person will attack them.

USING A LOW-KEY, DISPASSIONATE DEMEANOR

The first of several alternative strategic courses of action in responding to self-injury is to use a low-key dispassionate demeanor. The affect-laden responses cited above are doubly harmful to self-injuring people. First, the responses, be they supportive or condemning, may shame or embarrass the self-injurer. Emotional reactions in others may make the self-injuring person less likely to communicate about the behavior in the future. Also, in many cases, the intense reactions may inadvertently reinforce the behavior (i.e., make it more likely to recur in the future). On the one hand, the nurturing, overly solicitous response may be immensely gratifying for people who have been neglected, ignored, or abused. On the other hand, condemnation and recoil may be paradoxically rewarding, especially for adolescents who take some gratification in provoking strong reactions in adults.

For all these reasons it is clinically advisable to use a calm, dispassionate demeanor in responding to the behavior. Achieving some form of equanimity may take practice, but it has the double advantages of (1) not adding additional affect to an already emotionally charged situation, and (2) not inadvertently reinforcing a behavior that the clinician wants very much to see decline and cease.

RESPECTFUL CURIOSITY

Caroline Kettlewell (1999) has suggested another helpful way to respond to self-injury: with "respectful curiosity." She said that she preferred that response when presenting a therapist with information about her cutting (personal communication, 2002). Curiosity conveys an attitude of wanting to know more about the problem rather than wanting the problem to go away quickly. To be helpful, curiosity has to be tempered and respectful. Interest that comes across as prurient or thrill seeking is aversive (or too reinforcing) for most self-injurers. The exception can be in peer groups where contagion is developing, as is discussed in Chapter 16.

NONJUDGMENTAL COMPASSION

Another therapeutic response to self-injury is nonjudgmental compassion. Time and again self-injurers have encountered harsh pejorative judgments related to their self-injury. They are deemed to be mentally ill, impulsive, explosive, dangerous, etc. When a therapist responds with nonjudgmental compassion, it can be immensely relieving for the self-injurer. Such a stance positions the therapist to hear the rest of the client's story with some assurance of full disclosure.

A very legitimate question is: What is the difference between compassion, which is recommended, and concern and support, which are not?

Granted, both types of positive responses are not easily differentiated. The main difference is one that is subtle in tone. Concern and support suggest a certain amount of affective intensity, a yearning to be of assistance, and a desire to quickly protect and intervene. Compassion is more about acceptance, about being with the client in a neutral, nonjudgmental way with no immediate expectations for change.

An example of this nonjudgmental, compassionate demeanor—which is both hard to describe and to achieve—is provided in the following dialogue from an initial therapy session:

> THERAPIST: It's good to hear those details about your life. Could we move now to discussing why you came?
>
> CLIENT: (*looking embarrassed*) Well, I cut myself all the time . . .
>
> THERAPIST: (*low-key demeanor, compassionate tone*) How often do you do it?
>
> CLIENT: Almost every day.
>
> THERAPIST: That is quite frequent. [not minimizing] Where do you tend to cut yourself? [respectful curiosity]
>
> CLIENT: (*even more embarrassed*) Everywhere, I guess.
>
> THERAPIST: I see. Do you have favorite body areas to cut? [respectful curiosity]
>
> CLIENT: Yeah, my arms and legs.
>
> THERAPIST: I see. What do you think cutting does for you?
>
> CLIENT: It gets my feelings out and calms me down.
>
> THERAPIST: Okay. Is it one of the most effective ways you have to deal with your feelings?
>
> CLIENT: (*enthusiastically*) Definitely!
>
> THERAPIST: Well, it's no wonder you do it so often then, is it? [nonjudgmental]
>
> CLIENT: Thanks for understanding. Most people think I'm a jerk or a nut.

This therapy is off to a promising start. The therapist has conveyed to the client that self-injury can be discussed matter-of-factly and compassionately. There is no evidence of excessive empathy, hysteria, shock, recoil, or condemnation. The therapist has even acknowledged, nonjudgmentally, that self-injury has adaptive features in that it is effective in managing painful emotions. The client appears to feel understood in a preliminary way.

They are now in a position to move on to discussing self-injury using the client's own language.

CONCLUSION

In summary, in responding to self-injury, it is generally most helpful if clinicians and others

- Avoid the use of suicide terminology.
- Use the client's own descriptive language.
- Gently challenge language that is minimizing or too idiosyncratic.
- Are aware of the risks of inadvertently providing secondary reinforcement.
- Employ a low-key, dispassionate demeanor.
- Convey respectful curiosity.
- Are nonjudgmental and compassionate.

CHAPTER 7

Cognitive-Behavioral Assessment

This chapter employs the biopsychosocial model (discussed in Chapter 5) to demonstrate how to conduct an assessment of self-injury. The model addresses five interrelated dimensions that assist us in understanding and treating self-injury: environmental, biological, cognitive, affective, and behavioral. Assessment begins with the last of these dimensions—behavioral—because it is important to evaluate the specifics of the self-injury at the outset. Then the clinician can begin to identify the conditions that precipitate and maintain the behavior.

The assessment procedures presented here are based on the principles of conducting a thorough behavioral analysis, which involve a three-step process of collecting measurable data and descriptive information regarding (1) the *antecedents* to the behavior, (2) the *behavior* itself, and (3) the *consequences* thereafter (Kazdin, 1994).

ASSESSING THE SELF-INJURY BEHAVIOR

Using a Self-Injury Log

One way to collect accurate information regarding self-injury is to ask clients to complete a Self-Injury Log, as shown in Figure 7.1. Many clients in outpatient treatment are willing and able to complete such a log between weekly psychotherapy sessions. Clients living in supported living and residential programs can also use logs quite productively. Such clients may require and benefit from being prompted or assisted by their support staff.

Name: _____

Week of: _____

Category	Monday	Tuesday	Wednesday	Thursday	Friday	Saturday	Sunday
Environmental antecedents							
Biological antecedents							
Cognitive, Affective, and Behavioral antecedents							
Number of wounds							
Start time of SIB episode							
End time of SIB episode							
Extent of physical damage (length, width; were sutures obtained?); (if yes, how many?)							
Body area(s)							
Pattern to wounds (yes/no; if yes, type)							
Use of tool (yes/no; if yes, type)							
Room or place of SIB							
Alone or with others during SIB?							
Aftermath of SIB (thoughts, feelings, behaviors)							
Aftermath of SIB (biological elements)							
Aftermath of SIB (events in environment)							
Reactions of others to your SIB							
Comments							

FIGURE 7.1. Self-Injury Log.

81

The information generated from the use of the log is far more reliable than recall alone. My experience is that adults who are motivated to stop self-injuring are quite reliable about remembering to complete the log and bring it to sessions. In contrast, adolescent clients can be highly variable; some lose the log, forget to complete it, or fail to bring it to sessions. For clients who tend to forget to complete their logs, a prompt from the therapist via a phone call or e-mail two to three times per week can be helpful. Permission to make this brief contact should be obtained in advance from the client. When clients *still* forget their homework, the best course of action is to ask them to complete the grid in the session from memory as best they can. The clinician may need to assist clients in this process with suggestions and clarifying questions.

It should be emphasized to clients that it is far more helpful if they complete the log themselves on a daily basis between sessions. When clients have been able to do so, they should receive considerable acknowledgment and praise for making this important contribution to the treatment process. The reasons for failing to complete the log should be pursued in detail. Sometimes clients are worried that other members of the household will discover the log. In other cases, clients need time to recover from the intensity of a psychotherapy session by not thinking about challenging problems for a few days. In trying to obtain the most accurate information possible, clients should be addressed compassionately but persistently in this area.

I almost always review the Self-Injury Log with clients early in a session. I begin with the number of wounds, the length of episodes, and the extent of physical damage. First and foremost I want to know the amount and extent of physical harm done to the body. Later on I move to antecedents and consequences of the behavior.

It is important to routinely ask if there are behaviors that the client has *omitted* from the log. Some clients will write down the more typical forms of self-injury, such as arm and body cutting, but will leave out atypical forms, such as wounds to the breasts or genitals. I have found that asking about additional behaviors may elicit important information about self-injury that clients are too embarrassed to acknowledge in writing.

Another important detail is to ask clients to put zeros in the row for number of wounds when there has been no self-injury. Writing "0" serves to make explicit the fact that the client has not self-injured on that day. It can be quite reinforcing for clients to be able to look at a row of zeros over the course of a week as visible evidence of having successfully resisted self-injury.

DEFINITIONS FOR THE SELF-INJURY LOG

The following are definitions and related explanations for the various items contained on the Self-Injury Log. Even if the therapist chooses not to use a

Self-Injury Log, the categories should be reviewed informally as part of a thorough assessment.

Baseline Frequency Regarding Wounds and Episodes

Collecting baseline data regarding self-injury involves counting both the number of wounds and the duration of episodes. Accurate information can only come from the client. No therapist, counselor, or significant other can be privy to all of the details pertaining to self-injury.

Wounds

A *"wound" is defined as each discrete instance of tissue damage*. A wound can be a 2-inch scratch, a 10-inch cut, a single cigarette burn, or a self-inflicted tattoo.

Episodes

An *"episode" is defined as a time period during which an individual is involved in relatively uninterrupted self-injury*. A single episode of self-injury can result in multiple wounds.

The client is asked to count the number of wounds that are inflicted during an episode and to estimate the start and end time of the episode. The following example includes both types of baseline data:

After a bad day at work, Jim has a habit of coming home and retreating to his bedroom. He often removes an X-acto knife from his art supplies and makes a series of cuts on his left arm. Jim states that he cuts until he feels relief. Sometimes he cuts himself two or three times and feels better. Other times it takes 8 or 10 cuts. The time period that Jim cuts varies from about 10 minutes to a half an hour. Therefore, in terms of baseline data for Jim, a single episode lasts from 10 to 30 minutes and results in 2 to 10 wounds.

Collecting baseline data of this type can be complicated. Some configurations of wounds are hard to count; some episodes are ambiguous as to when they start and end. The following case vignette includes both types of ambiguity:

Nikki's pattern of self-injuring involved making cuts on her forearms that resembled graph-paper-like grids. Episodes of cutting sometimes took 3–4 hours. During her lengthier episodes, she often "took a break" from cutting to eat or do an errand. Several hours later she resumed executing the grid-

like pattern on her arm. In such instances, it was difficult to determine whether the behavior represented single or multiple episodes. In Nikki's view, an episode began when she stared incising her arm and ended when she completed the entire design of the grid. The therapist accepted this definition of an episode.

The number of wounds also was difficult to determine. Quite often several days after she had cut the grid-like designs into her arm, she would excoriate the wounds. This involved scraping a blade over the length of her arm and reopening the wounds considerably. It was essentially impossible to quantify the number of wounds in such an episode. After such instances, Nikki tended to write "many" in the Self-Injury Log.

Although precise counts are preferable, they are not necessary. The goal is to obtain accurate information about the general frequency of self-injury and the length of episodes. The client should be encouraged to be as clear as possible, but there is no need for extreme precision. The "comments" row in the Self-Injury Log is provided to deal with ambiguous circumstances. In this space, the client can provide brief details that explain ambiguities in defining an episode or number of wounds. The blank reverse side of the Self-Injury Log can also be used to record additional information.

The start time of a self-injury episode is an important detail in the life of a self-injuring person, because it can provide crucial information about antecedents to the behavior. It can also provide important opportunities to interrupt the habit of self-injury and to practice replacement behaviors.

I am not aware of any empirical studies regarding the time of day that people self-injure. In my clinical experience there appears to be considerable variation. Some people begin inflicting self-harm as soon as they wake up in the morning. Others hurt themselves at any time of day when stressful events occur or unpleasant feelings emerge. Some prefer self-injuring immediately after they get home from school or work—when they have their home to themselves. The majority of people with whom I have worked report harming themselves in the evenings, often right before going to sleep.

Why is bedtime the preferred time of day for so many people who self-injure? Clients provide many different explanations. One is that they tend to reflect on the events of the day at the time of its conclusion. Unfortunately, many self-injuring people tend to put a negative spin on daily events—and they do so day after day. These individuals tend to view a day as series of failures, rejections, or embarrassments; self-injury provides some solace for them before bedtime.

For others, bedtime has the obvious association with sexuality. As people prepare to retire, they are likely to think of other experiences they have had in bedrooms. If individuals are trauma survivors who have been abused in bedroom contexts, they may be especially likely to have a series of mental images or flashbacks. Many people report having been abused at night when others in the their household were asleep. For these people, entering the bedroom and preparing for sleep is a time of day fraught with danger and painful memories.

For other individuals, hour of sleep symbolizes a time of vulnerability and loss of control. Sleep is a time when one is not alert, when one's defenses are down and sense organs are quiescent. For those who are able to feel safe and secure in the world, sleep is a time of renewal and rest. In contrast, for those who feel chronically unsafe and vulnerable, nighttime is a period to be endured until the light of day returns.

Hannah often discussed her night terrors in therapy. She felt a need to speak again and again about the memory of the sound of her father's footsteps coming down the hall around midnight, when he got home from his night job. Sometimes he came into her room and molested her; other times he went to her mother's room and left Hannah undisturbed. For Hannah as a child, midnight was the most terrifying time of the day. Twenty years later, it still is.

Extent of Physical Damage

"Extent of physical damage" is defined as the amount of tissue damage or disfigurement associated with a self-injurious act or episode. Amount of physical damage is one of the most important elements in a behavioral analysis of self-injury. When clients are completing a self-injury log, the key detail is whether the self-injury required medical intervention such as suturing. Clients are not expected to do a medical assessment of their self-injury, but they can write down the dimensions of the wounds and whether sutures were obtained. The extent of physical damage conveys crucial information about

1. The level of risk presented by the individual, and whether or not the individual may need emergency medical treatment, psychiatric assessment, and protective intervention.
2. Whether the individual is relatively stable or escalating in level of distress.
3. Important diagnostic information.

As noted in Chapter 5, the large majority—90% or more—of self-injuring acts result in modest physical damage. The large majority of persons who harm themselves recurrently in low-lethality ways choose to cut themselves, excoriate their wounds, or hit themselves. They also exercise a level of control over what they do to their bodies. Granted, they are in considerable distress and act in alarming ways by hurting their bodies. Nonetheless, they have a modicum of control over their acts in that their assaults do not require suturing, other medical intervention, and do not result in extensive permanent scarring.

An additional feature of self-injurious behavior is that self-injurers are somewhat selective about the areas of the body that they assault. Most commonly they cut their arms and legs and may then pick at their wounds as they are healing (excoriation). These are body parts that can be hidden with long sleeves or pants, indicating an awareness of the social repercussions of the behavior.

However, some individuals—the minority—also perform acts of self-harm on their bodies that require suturing and/or are permanently disfiguring. These forms of self-harm differ from the self-injury scenario and suggest a level of dyscontrol that is alarming. When people cut themselves more deeply or burn themselves extensively or cause other forms of significant scarring, they *are* mutilating their bodies. The scars are there for a lifetime unless they are removed through cosmetic surgery (and even then, restoration tends to be only partially effective). Self-inflicted burns also tend to cause permanent scarring. For example, most cigarette burns on the skin leave reddish-blue, circular scars that are unsightly and disfiguring.

When physical damage is more serious, protective intervention may be necessary, such as obtaining medical treatment and utilizing a psychiatric inpatient unit, hospital diversion program, or respite service. The general rule-of-thumb as to what defines "serious" is the need for suturing or other professional medical intervention. Another rule-of-thumb is the inflicting of many cuts or burns suggesting considerable emotional agitation and distress. For example, a client once cut both of her arms over 40 times within a 2-hour period. She did not do a level of damage that required suturing, but the sheer volume of cuts suggested that a psychiatric assessment at an emergency mental health unit was in order.

Extent of physical damage can also provide important information about escalation of psychological distress. For example, if an individual usually scratches her arm with a paper clip, barely breaking the skin, and she shifts to using a razor blade and inflicting deeper cuts, this is an important development. The level of physical damage may still be modest but the increased damage suggests a greater level of distress. This modest increase in physical damage should be explored in detail as part of the behavioral analysis.

When individuals self-inflict massive trauma or disfigurement, they are usually floridly psychotic or in an acute manic state. In these cases the individuals have passed over from self-injury into self-mutilation. Examples of these behaviors are among the most unpleasant in the annals of humankind; they include self-enucleation, autocastration, autocannibalism, and self-amputation. Preventing extreme acts of this type is discussed in Chapter 18.

Body Area

"Body area" is defined as the location on the body where the self-injury is inflicted. Body area or topography is an especially important piece of information. The two most common areas assaulted are arms and legs. Often the arms are selected because of easy accessibility. A person holding a blade or hot object in one hand can very conveniently harm the other wrist or forearm. It takes no great contortion or physical discomfort to reach this body area. Secondly, self-injurers often state that they harm the arms or legs because the wounds can be hidden under clothing.

The wrist and forearm may also be popular because "cutting your wrists" has long had connotations of suicide. Although the position of this book and many others (e.g., Ross & McKay, 1979; Favazza, 1987; Walsh & Rosen, 1988; Alderman, 1997; Conterio & Lader, 1998) is that wrist cutting is rarely likely to result in death, the behavior can convey a message of desperation. Self-injurers often wish to communicate to others that they are in considerable psychic pain. Although their message may include implications of suicide, the actual risk to life is modest. Therefore, "cutting the wrists" can have considerable communicative utility, with the additional advantage of posing little or no risk to life.

Although some generalizations can be made about many self-injuring people, it is nonetheless crucial to assess each individual afresh. Each person should be asked why he or she selects a particular body area for self-harm. A few brief examples of the types of highly individualized responses are provided below:

Twenty-five-year-old Sarah almost always cut her forearms. Her explanation was that she loves to look at the blue veins on her arms. She said that only on her arms is the blood under the skin visible in that transparent way. She gets a rush when, under the pressure of the blade, "all that blue turns to red."

Twenty-two-year-old Gina said that she prefers to cut her abdomen because she can still wear short sleeves and shorts in the summer. She added that she would "never get caught dead in a bathing suit," so her abdomen is the place for her.

Seventeen-year-old Joel had been cutting for about 6 months. To date he had cut his right and left calves exclusively. Asked why he chose these two body areas so consistently, Joel, a born comic, said in an exaggerated Shakespearean voice, "Doctor, I regret to say, yet again, 'I do not know!' " Cajoled to say more, Joel eventually explained that he likes to lift weights at the gym and he doesn't want his "lifting buddies asking a lot of stupid questions"—so he leaves his arms alone. Joel added that he always wears sweat pants to cover his legs.

For most clients, the body areas selected involve a combination of symbolic meaning and practical utility. The therapist should seek to learn these idiosyncratic aspects for each individual. In so doing, the therapist begins to learn important information about the client's relationship with his or her own body. For many individuals, body image may become a central focus in treatment, as explored in the chapters on body alienation and trauma resolution (Chapters 11 and 12).

It should be noted that clients who select a body area, in part, for purposes of concealment are showing a level of control that others do not. Although cutting or burning oneself may seem like a completely out-of-control act, this may not be true for those who take great care to injure a body area covered by clothing. Despite their anguish and pain, such self-injurers are nevertheless exercising a substantial level of control in keeping subsequent social repercussions in mind. Such "future planning" is a good prognostic sign. For others, the self-injury can be much more impulsive with little regard for social consequences. For example:

Anne stated, "When I have one of my bad cutting times, I just let it rip. When I'm really out of control, I cut any part of my body. Sometimes I've cut my face and scalp. Sometimes I've cut my left breast and pubic area. Afterwards, I'm freaked out at all the damage and the blood around, but at the time I'm doing it, there's no stopping the helter skelter."

An important detail in the assessment of self-injury occurs when a client shifts to self-injuring a new body area. Such a change usually indicates a psychological shift in the self-injurer. Sometimes the alteration can suggest an exacerbation of distress, requiring psychiatric emergency assessment. For example, when the self-injurer shifts to harming face, eyes, breasts, or genitals, it often should be considered an emergency requiring immediate psychiatric assessment (explained immediately below). In other cases, the shift is essentially parallel in nature, for example, when a self-injurer moves from arms to legs, or from left bicep to right. As stated before, the key information can be found in the details, which should be sought with persistence.

Especially Alarming Body Areas

In my experience, injury to any one of four areas of the body is cause for special concern. These are face, eyes, breasts (in females) and genitals (in either gender). Harming the face is a very ominous sign suggesting a profound lack of regard for personal attractiveness and social repercussions. Cutting or otherwise harming the face may convey the message "I hate how I look and I hate myself." It also conveys "I don't care if I'm excluded from many social contexts." Harming the face suggests an alarming level of both psychological distress and social disconnectedness.

Harming the eyes is even worse. Eyesight is fundamental to daily life. To run the risk of reducing or eliminating sight is an extreme act. Eye tissue is fragile and its healing abilities are modest. Permanent damage is easy to inflict.

Harming the breasts and genitals is cause for concern for different reasons. These parts of the body usually remain hidden from public view, so social repercussions for the injuries may be less of an issue. Nonetheless, the symbolic meaning of breast or genital self-harm, and the level of distress it implies, is cause for special alarm. Breasts and genitals are sensitive regions with nerve endings that are very responsive to stimulation and pain. To deliberately harm these areas, the person has to have somehow "turned off" the normal physiological pain responses (Bohus et al., 2000; Russ et al., 1992, 1994). Intense distress or dissociation may neutralize pain responses, enabling people to harm these body locations. There is also the symbolic significance of harming these areas. Extreme distress about sexuality is usually indicated. Psychotic decompensation or primitive trauma reenactment may be involved in such self-injury. The link between psychosis and major self-injury is discussed in Chapter 18; the topic of trauma and self-injury is reviewed in Chapters 11 and 12.

In general, when persons injure the face, eyes, breasts, or genitals, an emergency psychiatric evaluation should be considered. The level of distress accompanying such behavior is often considerable, meriting protective intervention and close supervision.

Visual Inspection

A final comment about assessing body area concerns whether or not the therapist chooses to look at wounds. Seeing wounds for oneself often provides far more information than hearing verbal descriptions. Therefore, I routinely ask to see wounds, while emphasizing that it entirely up to the client to grant or deny the request. If clients are approached politely and respectfully, they rarely say "no." I justify the request by explaining that seeing the wounds may be helpful in understanding and helping the individual. Obvious exceptions to my asking to look at the wounds occur in the circumstances when the body areas are beyond the bounds of modesty— that is, breasts, thighs, genitals, abdomen.

However, I do *not* go as far as Levenkron (1998) who often provides first-aid-like attention to his clients' wounds. He has written that he applies ointment and bandages to the wounds of cutters and that he believes his clients benefit psychologically from this intervention. He has speculated that his physical attentions to the wounds may be crucial in successful treatment (personal communication, 2000).

Each therapist must define his or her own limits. I am not comfortable in administering to clients physically. I am a therapist who rarely physically touches clients out a sense of caution and respect. The main exception to this rule occurs when I sometimes hug a client goodbye at the termination of an extended, multiyear treatment. Some may find this formality too aloof. Others may deem it common sense in a litigious age. I believe that many clients are relieved to be in a treatment where there is no physical contact, especially those who have histories of physical and/or sexual abuse.

Pattern of Wounds

"Pattern of wounds" is defined as the visual arrangement of wounds inflicted during a single episode. Self-injuring people often inflict more than one wound on their bodies during an episode. In such cases, it is useful to ascertain whether the wounds are organized into some sort of pattern. Multiple-wound episodes can be said to fall into four general categories: (1) random or disorganized, (2) organized, (3) symbolic, and (4) verbal/numerical. In my experience the majority of wounds inflicted by self-injuring people are either random or organized. The use of symbols, words, or numbers is much rarer. Many people inflict wounds that have no discernible pattern. For example, an individual may inflict five wounds during a single episode, confined to a single body area, the forearm. Although the wounds are clustered in a common area, they are neither parallel nor at right angles nor otherwise patterned. They display no discernible design. Therefore, this configuration can be considered random.

A second especially common type of self-injury is one that reflects a modest type of organization. For example, a person my inflict four cuts on the forearm that have been precisely executed in parallel fashion. They are the same length and width. Such precision in execution is usually no accident. To create such a design, the individual has to have been focused and taking considerable care to inflict the self-harm "in just the right amount, in just the right way." Thus it is often the case that the self-injurer who inflicts an organized pattern may be in greater control of his or her actions than the individual who inflicts random, disorganized wounds. The later type of self-injury suggests some type of ritual or at least a precise, focused process. The former type indicates a more random "let's see where this takes us" experience. Either way, if the presence or absence of a pattern to the self-injury wound is scrutinized, valuable information can be obtained.

Ironically, wounds that involve symbols or words tend to be associated with less control and greater level of disturbance. That is to say, although symbols and words require greater attention to detail than simple, non-representational patterns, they tend to occur in people who are significantly distressed. There are probably many exceptions to this observation, but I will share what I have encountered about these types of wounds.

People who inflict symbols on their bodies tend to use such markings as crosses, stars, lightning bolts, flowers, and tears. They may execute the designs with sharp blades, producing patterned scars, or use needles and ink to create crude self-inflicted tattoos. I have never encountered a self-injurer who was a master craftsman in the creation of a design on his or her skin. The large majority of self-injurers whom I have met who make symbols on their bodies have been adolescents. It may well be rare for adults to make such designs on their bodies, except for persons in institutions such as psychiatric hospitals or correctional facilities.

When therapists encounter self-injurious symbols on clients' bodies, they should inquire in detail as to their meanings. I like to ask the client how he or she selected that specific symbol among all the possible options, how it came out, how he or she likes it now that it's healing, and especially, what that symbol means to him or her. Self-injuring people can provide some poignant and startling explanations regarding these symbolic designs.

James was a 14-year-old boy who carved a star onto his lower neck and another on his forearm. Asked why he chose a star design for his body, he initially replied with the not entirely unexpected, "I don't know." Encouraged to say more, he explained that he and his girlfriend had each carved stars on their bodies and that they had done so together. He said it pointed to their love for each other in an otherwise "shitty, fucked-up world."

Keekee had many symbols, words, and numbers on her body, mostly in the form of self-inflicted tattoos. The designs included multiple inverted crosses, tears (identifiable only with her assistance), the words "hate" and "LOVE," and the numbers 666. Keekee stated she was a satanist and was proud of it and wanted the world to know. Then again, she said, she didn't really care what anyone else thought. "It's my body and I'll do what I want with it. Bodies eventually rot, anyway!"

Keekee is an especially interesting example because she presents with both symbols and words. Words are a special and relatively rare category of self-inflicted injury. It is quite telling when someone feels a need to give a word such emphasis as to carve, tattoo, or burn it into the skin. We all encounter thousands of words every day via conversation, advertisements, radio, television, Internet, letters, phone calls, mail, etc. To take from these thousands of words a single one and inflict it on one's body is a dramatic and significant act. In some cases the self-injuring person inscribes the name of a beloved in order to convey passion or commitment. In others the inscription is designed to impress someone they are pursuing or attempting to regain. Sometimes the name or word is carved to express grief or rage or both.

Using a cigarette, Beth burned the word "MOM" into the back of one hand and "HATE" into the back of the other. Asked about her intentions, Beth said, in the sardonic tone she used when she wasn't upset, "Actually, it's multipurpose! It means, 'I hate Mom,' but it also means, 'Mom hates me!' or 'Mom equals hate,' or 'Hate equals Mom!' And that's just a few of the possibilities!"

Beth had great rage and deep sadness in relation to her mother because of years of sexual abuse and her mother's recurrent failure to protect her. Beth's feelings for her mother were so overwhelmingly complex and painful that she felt the words "mom" and "hate" deserved to be permanently burned into her skin. No other form of verbal expression was powerful, vivid, and dramatic enough to convey the depth and rawness of her feelings. Beth once said that she would have liked to burn "love" into her body as well, then added with bitterness, "I don't really have the word in my vocabulary."

Some of those who inscribe words into their bodies are experiencing a psychotic process. These are individuals who may be descending into psychological disorganization and decompensation. For these persons the inscription of words may be a desperate attempt to hold onto some centrally important concept or sense of identity. For example:

Cecily had been convinced since her early teens that she would die before her 20th birthday. At times she felt she would die due to a physical illness such as cancer—even though she showed no evidence of the disease. At other times she said she was likely to kill herself because of all the pain in her life. As she approached age 20, she became increasingly agitated and frightened. Once again she began to hear voices calling her "bitch" and "slut." The voices also instructed her with the single-word command, "Die!" One morning she took a shard of glass and carved her birth date into her upper arm, including month, day, and year. Cecily stated that this act symbolically helped her to accept that she might survive her 20th birthday and live beyond it—which she, in fact, did.

Sidney had an especially bad case of schizophrenia with serious, persistent symptoms that seldom remitted. Almost every day involved hours of intrusive auditory hallucinations. He also suffered from persecutory delusions involving devils taking over his body and "causing" self-destructive acts. When Sidney's psychosis exacerbated, he became mute. During these times he occasionally cut or scratched a word into his body, such as "No" or "Yes" or "Gone." In these cases, the best his caregivers could deduce was that he was desperately holding onto language in his state of deterioration. By inscribing a word into his body, he seemed to be striving to retain his capacity as a speaking human subject.

Use of a Tool

"Use of a tool" is defined as whether or not the person has used an implement other than his or her own body to inflict self-harm. As with other details of self-injury, the use of a tool or implement conveys a great deal of information regarding the state of mind and level of disturbance of the person. It is very informative to ask whether or not a tool is used, and if so, what type. Details about the recurrent use of the same implement, the cleaning of the implement, where it was obtained, and where it is stored when not in use can be quite illuminating.

In general, self-injuring persons who do *not* use a tool are suffering from a more primitive level of disturbance. Persons who hit themselves with their fists, scratch themselves with their fingernails, or bite themselves with their teeth are often in more impulsive, explosive states than those who use an implement. People experiencing psychotic decompensation or those with significant mental retardation often hurt themselves repetitively using only their fists, fingers, or teeth. The absence of a tool can point to problems of biological origin that must be diagnosed and addressed.

In contrast, persons who employ razor blades, small knives, or burning cigarettes are generally in more precise control of the damage they inflict. The same is true for those who use paper clips, pocket knives, and the hot metallic ends of butane lighters. Still, there are so many exceptions to this rule-of-thumb that it can be considered no more than tentative. The examples provided below are "exceptions to the rule" about the use of tools, in three different ways: (1) non-use of a tool due to environmental factors, (2) non-use of a tool, with only precise, modest damage inflicted, and (3) use of a tool in an impulsive, out-of-control way.

Gustav had a long history of cutting himself. It was his only mode of self-harm when he was living in the community. However, when he was hospitalized for mania or suicidal impulses, he sometimes resorted to self-hitting. Gustav stated that in the hospital there was tight security and blades were unavailable to him. He did not prefer to hit himself, but when the tension built up, "something had to give."

Tina used only her fingers to extract hair from her head. For several months her hair pulling resulted in multiple bald spots that were disfiguring. Tina never used a tool to extract hair or to harm herself in any other way.

Angela, an eighth-grade student in regular education, became so enraged in class one day that she took sharp-pointed scissors from her desk and began assaulting her legs with high-arcing blows. The tips of the scissors penetrated her clothing and made wounds in her thighs that required suturing. Angela ended up hospitalized for her self-harm.

The *type* of tool also conveys important information about the mindset of the self-injurer or the environment in which he or she lives. For example, use of a very sharp X-acto knife suggests a different state of mind than employing a burning cigarette. Use of a paper clip to inflict superficial scratches is very different from employing the tip of a meat cleaver to inflict the very same wounds. A paper clip has little potential to inflict massive self-harm at a later date, whereas the cleaver has considerable potential. Questions about the selection of a particular tool can provide all kinds of amplifications that aid the treatment and move it to a different level of specificity.

Room or Place of the Self-Injury

"Room or place of the self-injury" is defined as the physical space in which the self-injury occurs. Most people perform acts of self-injury indoors. The most common location reported is within a person's private space, usually a bedroom. Those who share a bedroom with a sibling, roommate, spouse, or partner may select a bathroom as an alternative private space to self-injure. Others choose a basement or garage as a preferred location. The key issue for most persons is finding a space where they are unlikely to be interrupted during the self-injury episode.

Whereas most individuals prefer privacy, others do not care and take little precaution to prevent discovery during the episode of self-injury. Obtaining information regarding place is important because it provides some information about the social connectedness of the self-injurer. In some cases a self-injuring person may do little to prevent discovery because he or she has ceased caring what others think; other people may prefer to be discovered; the behavior has a communicative function, and the self-injurer wants the interpersonal message to be delivered.

It is useful to ask self-injuring persons *where* they self-injure and *why* they selected that location. Often the explanation is a matter of pragmatics, but the place may have other significance, as evidenced in the following:

Stacy said, "I usually cut myself at school, which is why I don't cut myself much during the summer. I hate school. All the pressure about grades, all the cliques, all the worrying about what to wear, the loud jokes, the stupid, loud guys trying to outdo each other with their sarcastic putdowns. Most days it feels like the most negative pressure pot in the world. I go into the girls' room, lock the door in my favorite stall (can you believe I have a favorite?!), and cut away. I get really upset if somebody's in my stall. How dare they! I wait until they come out and give them a really dirty look."

Joseph preferred to harm himself outside, usually deep in the woods. He stated, "I usually burn or scratch myself behind my family's barn. I go far away where it's peaceful and quiet. When I hurt myself I get quiet inside, just like it is on the outside. Then I tend to feel good for a while. It's my one peaceful place."

Social Context

"Social context" is defined as whether the person self-injures alone or with other persons. This detail often says a great deal about the conditions that maintain the individual's self-injurious behavior. The social context of self-injury can be viewed as occurring within six categories:

1. Persons who self-injure alone and keep it secret from all others.
2. Persons who self-injure alone and disclose it to a few others.
3. Persons who self-injure alone and disclose it to most others.
4. Persons who self-injure with others and keep it secret from all others.

5. Persons who self-injure with others and disclose it to a few others.
6. Persons who self-injure with others and disclose it to most others.

The majority of people appear to fall in category 2. These are individuals for whom the self-injury has primarily a tension-reduction function; they are concerned about the social repercussions of disclosing the behavior and are very selective to whom they disclose. They also have some normative social ties and are not part of a social network that endorses self-harm. They may be adolescents or adults. They tend to have some close friends or intimates who know about their self-injury and attempt to help them overcome it.

As the above list suggests, there are many other variations. Some people are secretive from all others all the time. Hyman discusses examples of such individuals in her book *Women Living with Self-Injury* (1999). She provides examples of self-injurers who have concealed their acts from all others for years, including spouses or partners with whom they reside on a daily basis.

For others, the behavior pattern of self-injury is the opposite. Their self-injury only occurs with others, and they choose to fully disclose this group behavior to many other persons who do not self-injure. Persons in categories 4, 5, and 6 tend to participate in active contagion episodes (discussed at length in Chapter 16).

There is no need to discuss each of the six categories because the content is self-evident. Suffice it to say that the therapist should assess for social context as an important variable in the self-injury behavior of any individual.

ANTECEDENTS TO THE SELF-INJURY

Having completed the assessment of the details of self-injury, the clinician now turns to the antecedents of the behavior. The biopsychosocial model includes five dimensions: environmental, biological, cognitive, affective, and behavioral.

Environmental Antecedents

"Environmental antecedents" are defined as events or activities in the environment of the self-injurer that trigger an episode. Some individuals are consistently triggered by external events; others self-injure primarily in response to internal psychological conditions. It is crucially important to determine what, if any, events set the self-injuring sequence in motion. Once identified, these events can be employed as opportunities to practice healthier behaviors in place of the self-injury. External events that clients commonly identify as precipitating self-injury include:

- Loss or threat of loss of a relationship
- Interpersonal conflict
- Performance pressure
- Frustration about unmet needs
- Social isolation
- Seemingly neutral events that trigger associations with trauma

Loss

It has been noted for decades in the literature on self-mutilation (now more commonly referred to as self-injury) that loss is a frequent precipitant to self-harm. Loss can take many forms, ranging from the complete and permanent, such as death of loved one, to the nuanced and subtle, such as an almost imperceptible slight in a relationship. Authors have noted that the histories of self-injurers include high rates of death of a parent and/or marital separation or divorce of parents (e.g., Walsh & Rosen, 1988). Self-injurers have also experienced high rates of foster home placements, psychiatric hospitalizations, and residential placements, all of which involve multiple moves and relationship disruptions (Walsh & Rosen, 1988). Researchers on self-injury have cited histories of physical and sexual abuse as associated factors (Walsh & Rosen, 1988; Shapiro & Dominiak, 1992; Favazza, 1998). In these cases, the loss takes the form of psychological abandonment and recurrent victimization.

Linehan (1993a) has noted that persons with a diagnosis of borderline personality disorder may be easily triggered into episodes of emotional dysregulation and may be slow to return to baseline. For these persons, relatively modest forms of loss, such as a disdainful look or a person's failure to return a phone call promptly, can be experienced as a deliberate affront or terrifying rejection.

More recently, self-injury has emerged as a major problem in psychologically healthier populations of middle school, high school, and college students (see Chapter 3). Often these individuals do *not* have the histories of significant loss and trauma previously reported to be associated with self-injury. They may have not experienced the death of, or separation from, a significant other and may have no history of physical or sexual abuse trauma. Nonetheless, these healthier, less traumatized self-injurers may be exquisitely sensitive to interpersonal slights and use self-injury repeatedly to deal with their psychological pain. In some cases it may be difficult to understand why a seemingly innocuous event is experienced as grievously hurtful, but the old truism applies: "Pain is pain." If the client experiences the playful taunting of peers as an overwhelming humiliation, then it must be responded to with a sense of empathy that is congruent with the client's level of discomfort. The key deficiency in the psychological functioning of these individuals is the lack of self-soothing skills to deal with perceived loss, hence they use self-injury.

Interpersonal Conflict

Many self-injurers report harming themselves immediately after a disagreement with a partner, peer, or parent. In response to this conflict, there is often an intense rage and a desire to attack. The sequence for these persons can resemble the following:

Interpersonal conflict → Cognitive interpretation of slight or unfairness → Affective response of rage (or other intense emotion) → Decision to act on rage → Decision to self-injure → Self-injurious behavior

When a client and therapist are able to identify a pattern such as the one above, the therapeutic course can be fairly direct. The client can be helped to reduce the incidence of self-injury by (1) learning more effective interpersonal negotiation skills (thereby reducing the potential for interpersonal conflict), and (2) learning more effective affect management skills related to anger (thereby reducing the affective dysregulation). Of course, clearly identifying the goals for treatment does not mean that they are easy to accomplish.

Performance Pressure

Other clients cite pressures related to performance as key precipitants to self-injury. Among the most common forms of external pressure related to self-injury are academic demands in middle school, high school, college, or graduate school. Other examples include deadlines or productivity demands at work, athletic competition, preparation for a prom or other big social event, etc. Individuals who self-injure in response to performance pressure often have perfectionistic expectations for themselves. Uncovering irrational expectations related to performance can lead to productive work in treatment designed to reduce such self-imposed pressure.

Frustration about Unmet Needs

This antecedent does not entail loss, per se. Rather, it involves expectations that are not fulfilled. One of the most common complaints of adolescents is that they are misunderstood. They convey what they want and subsequently discover that they have not received what they want. This may result in frustration and rage that are subsequently relieved via self-injury. An effective behavior analysis attempts to identify recurrent sources of frustration that precede self-injury. Once again, skills can be targeted to assist clients in becoming more effective in getting what they want and in dealing with frustration when they do not. Cognitive restructuring becomes necessary when the desired goals are unrealistic, grandiose, or based on entitlement misconceptions.

Social Isolation

Aloneness is a trigger to self-injury for some clients. These are people who work hard to avoid time alone and become desperately agitated when confronted with isolation. Although this is not the most common pattern, it can be found fairly often in trauma survivors. Such individuals may fear being attacked when alone and take solace in having others around to protect them or at least distract them.

Seemingly Neutral Events

Some individuals are triggered into self-injury by events that seem utterly innocuous to others. A good behavioral analysis of self-injury can identify precipitants that no therapist would expect to find. In such cases, neutral events may have been paired with traumatic circumstances in the past, resulting in conditioned responses to benign antecedents. For example:

Reanne approached all elevators with great caution. She would scan the entire area to avoid being alone on an elevator with a man. If a man approached the elevator while she was waiting, she would look preoccupied and wait for the next one. However, if a man entered an elevator after she had already traveled a floor or two toward her destination, she would experience great anxiety. Not infrequently, she would cut her body afterward. Reanne stated, "Too many memories of being alone with my father invade my consciousness and need to be cut out."

Beth hated it when men made an upward motion with their heads, indicating direction. When she encountered such behavior out in the world, she usually hurt herself within 24 hours. Upward head motions in men reminded her quite powerfully of her abusive father's head gestures from her childhood. These movements indicated her father's ultimatum that they were to go upstairs to have sex. Years later, if Beth saw such a motion in a restaurant or store, she usually would have to leave. She preferred one-story buildings where men were less likely to make such head motions. She was not reactive to similar gestures made by women.

Biological Antecedents

"Biological antecedents" refer both to chronic physical problems or vulnerabilities and more immediate physical conditions. As discussed in Chapter 5, a thorough assessment considers biological vulnerabilities that may predispose an individual to self-injury. These can include forms of mental illness thought to have a strong biological component, such as depression, borderline personality disorder, bipolar disorder, and schizophrenia. Behavioral assessment involves identifying the warning signs associated with such mental illness toward the goal of preventing and managing relapse. Many clients cycle in and out of episodes of intense anxiety, sadness, rage, mania, or psychotic decompensation. Once clients are able to acknowledge that they have such vulnerabilities, they can strive to avoid relapse by avoiding or managing key triggers. Some of these triggers are biological. Short-term triggers include fatigue, insomnia, over- or undereating, excessive exercise, and abuse of alcohol or drugs. Other common, more immediate, biological triggers include failure to comply with prescribed psychotropic medication regimens or abuse of these psychotropic drugs.

Also discussed in Chapter 5 are specific biological vulnerabilities that research has linked to self-injury. These include limbic system dysfunction, diminished serotonin levels, endogenous opioid system factors, and reduced sensitivity to physical pain. Recurrent self-injurers should be assessed for

- Emotional dysregulation (which may respond to anticonvulsant medications such as Tegretol or mood stabilizers such as Depakote)
- Depression, anxiety, and impulsive aggression (which may respond to an SSRI or a selective norepinephrine reuptake inhibitor)
- "Addiction" to the release of endogenous opioids associated with self-injury (which may respond to naltrexone)
- Diminished sensitivity to physical pain (for which there is no known pharmacological treatment)

Each of these areas of dysfunction can be an important biological contributor to the recurrence of self-injury. Awareness of these elements allows their being targeted for treatment, along with environmental and psychological contributors.

Cognitive Antecedents

"Cognitive antecedents" are defined as thoughts and beliefs that trigger episodes of self-injury. Using Beck's (1995) cognitive model, the types of cognitions that precede self-injury include the following:

- Interpretations of external events
- Automatic thoughts
- Intermediate beliefs
- Core beliefs
- Cognitions and other mental activity related to trauma

In performing a behavioral analysis of self-injury, assessing cognitions is centrally important. What people think and believe about their experiences in the world and their internal experiences has much to do with the recurrent pattern of self-injury. Interpretations of events, automatic thoughts, intermediate and core beliefs, and trauma-related cognitions often occur right before acts of self-injury.

Interpretations of Events

The environmental antecedents to self-injury have been discussed in the preceding section. It should be noted that whatever the external events, it is the *interpretation* of the self-injurer that determines their power and influence. Assessing the person's interpretation of an event that precedes self-injury adds subjective world to observable world. Some people encounter devastating losses and interpret them benignly; others run into modest challenges and view them as catastrophic. The cognitive mindset of the self-injurer determines a great deal about the nature of the coping responses (i.e., positive vs. negative). Unfortunately, many self-injurers suffer from the negative cognitive triad characteristic of depression, which involves persistent pessimism about self, world, and future (Beck et al., 1979; Rush & Nowells, 1994; Beck, 1995). The following is an example of an inaccurate, pessimistic interpretation that preceded an act of self-harm.

Liz was at school when she noticed her friends clustering at the side of the dining hall. She perceived them to be looking at her and laughing. Liz assumed they were ridiculing what she was wearing as well as her weight. Embarrassed and enraged, Liz left school early, went home, and excoriated several wounds she had inflicted earlier in the week. Only the next day did Liz discover that her friends' conversation had had nothing to do with her.

Assessing interpretations of events and identifying gross distortions are important parts of cognitive assessment.

Automatic Thoughts

Automatic thoughts are the most immediate form of thought; they are situation specific (Beck, 1995). An example of an automatic thought that preceded a client's self-injury is "What my boyfriend said was so unfair, I must cut myself right now!"

Many thoughts become so routinized as to become automatic. A simple analogy is the process of learning to drive a car. At first, driving requires a great deal of self-instruction. Beginning drivers talk to themselves, using self-instructions such as "Okay, now put on the brake," or "next, put on the left blinker." Eventually explicit self-instructions fade because the thoughts have become automatic. The thoughts are still operational in some semiconscious manner, but they do not require full attention.

For some individuals, self-injury is so frequent that the thoughts that precede the acts have become automatic. Thoughts such as "This is too much to bear," "I need to find my blade," "Only cutting will do the job" become so commonplace as to be essentially out of consciousness.

The task for the clinician assessing self-injury is to bring such automatic cognitions back into conscious awareness. Persistent, respectful questioning can identify thoughts that support and immediately precede the self-injuring episode. Recovering these out-of-awareness cognitions is a necessary component of behavior analysis. For example:

> CLINICIAN: So, tell me what you were thinking just before you burned your leg.
>
> CLIENT: I wasn't thinking anything. It just happened.
>
> CLINICIAN: Well, maybe there were some steps that happened so fast, you weren't aware of them.
>
> CLIENT: I don't think so.
>
> CLINICIAN: You mentioned that you hung up the phone feeling frustrated after talking to your boyfriend.
>
> CLIENT: (*sarcastically*) Don't I always?
>
> CLINICIAN: Did anything pass through your mind before you hurt yourself?
>
> CLIENT: No, I just did it.

CLINICIAN: Let's break it down into small steps. As you were walking from the phone to your room, did you have anything on your mind at all about your boyfriend?

CLIENT: Now that you mention it, I was thinking, "He's going to break up with me again."

CLINICIAN: And what did you think about that?

CLIENT: I guess I thought it sucked and he sucked and life sucks, and that I might as well hurt myself because what's the use?

Intermediate Beliefs

Intermediate beliefs include attitudes, rules, and assumptions that are fundamental to an individual's thought process (Beck, 1995). Intermediate beliefs serve as linkages between automatic thoughts and core beliefs. Examples of intermediate beliefs that precede self-injury include (1) the attitude, "I deserve this pain," (2) the rule, "Cutting myself relieves distress better than anything else," and (3) the assumption, "It will always be this way."

Core Beliefs

Core beliefs are persistent convictions about self, world, and future. As Beck (1995, p. 16) has indicated, core beliefs tend to be global, firmly held, and not easily revised. They are often derived from patterns of affirmation and support (or lack thereof) that individuals experienced in childhood. An example of a core belief shared by a chronically self-injuring client is "I'm an unlovable loser."

Many self-injuring persons are prone to excessively negative self-evaluations. Linehan (1993a) considers this problem to be so central to treating borderline personality disorder that she includes being "nonjudgmental" as one of six components of mindfulness training. For many self-injurers, their thoughts involve recurrent, exaggerated self-criticism. These self-statements may be chronic, pessimistic, and brutally self-denigrating.

One useful way to elicit such negative judgments is to ask clients to share "favorite ways of putting themselves down." Many clients respond immediately with an extensive list of critical self-statements. The rapidity with which they rattle off these negative thoughts and judgments points to the frequency of their occurrence and the conviction with which they are held. The following is an excerpt from a transcript of a skills training group that illustrates the sharing of "favorite" negative core beliefs.

GROUP LEADER: Since we're talking about being judgmental today, I'm wondering if any of you have favorite ways of putting yourselves down? (*Four of seven members nod enthusiastically or say things like "Oh, yeah!"*) Okay, well, these may be important. Who would be willing to share one of these putdowns?

MEMBER 1: (*with conviction and disgust*) I call myself a baby.

GROUP LEADER: A baby? What do you mean by that?

MEMBER 1: Because I'm immature, can't do anything. I'm anxious all the time. I just can't handle anything.

GROUP LEADER: All those putdowns sound like quite a burden to be carrying around. Remember those, okay? Who else would be willing to share theirs?

MEMBER 2: I'm always saying to myself how fat, ugly, and stupid looking I am!

MEMBER 3: (*to Member 2*) You think *you're* fat? Look at me. I'm a pig, plus I also call myself a loser.

MEMBER 4: My favorite way of putting myself down is to say "You're a burden to society. You don't deserve to live!"

GROUP LEADER: Well, I guess we have some excellent examples of being judgmental here. Let's get to work on the skill of letting go of these judgments.

Cognitions and Other Forms of Mental Activity Related to Trauma

Trauma-related cognitions refer to thoughts, images, flashbacks, memories and dreams derived from trauma that precede acts of self-harm. These various forms of mental activity are especially challenging because clients often experience them as being entirely out of their control. Persons with trauma histories report experiencing flashbacks at any time during waking hours and may also report intrusive trauma-linked nightmares during sleep. It is no wonder that trauma survivors feel anguished that their histories may revisit them at any moment. Also complicating the picture is that these mental activities can take so many forms, including visual images, tactile sensations, odors, sounds, flashback dialogues, and so on.

Assessing these forms of cognitive antecedents to self-injury has to be done skillfully because the client has to be ready to do detailed disclosure work related to trauma. Knowing when to proceed with trauma resolution work is discussed in Chapter 12. If the client is not ready, probing for details may be too much for him or her to handle and may, in fact, cause the self-injury to worsen. If the clinician notices any escalating pattern of self-harm in the client, he or she should evaluate whether the behavioral analysis is inadvertently playing a role in the exacerbation. Retreating from such probing may be necessary until the client has acquired the skills necessary to discuss trauma in detail. In such cases, the clinician may have to confine analysis of cognitive antecedents to interpretations of events, automatic self-statements, and intermediate and core beliefs related to self-injury.

This topic of cognitive antecedents to self-injury is discussed in considerably more detail in Chapter 10, which is devoted to cognitive treatment.

Affective Antecedents

"Affective antecedents" refer to the emotions experienced prior to self-injury. In some cases, these emotions can build for an extended period of time, even several days; in others the emotions flash in an instant. For most persons the primary function of self-injury is to reduce the intensity of these painful emotions. Brown (1998) has provided a thorough review of reports that link negative emotions with self-injury. Almost any conceivable negative emotion has been identified as precipitating self-injury, but the primary ones noted by Brown are:

- Anxiety, tension, or panic
- Anger
- Sadness or depression
- Shame
- Guilt
- Frustration
- Contempt

Although not cited in the literature, I have also heard self-injuring persons refer to fear, worry, embarrassment, disgust, and excitement as preceding their self-harm.

A smaller proportion of people self-injure in order to rid themselves of feeling too *little* emotion. These are the individuals who report feeling "dead," "empty," "like a robot," or "like a zombie." The self-injuring is comforting for these people because it restores a sense of being alive. For example:

A client stated, "Yesterday when I cut I was feeling nothing. I was feeling absolutely dead inside. I went to the mirror to see if I still looked the same. I thought I might have turned into a machine or something. But there I was, same old shitty me. When I cut myself, I felt so much better. The blood really helped. I looked down at my arm and saw the blood and realized I was still alive, even though I felt nothing."

Identifying the emotions that precede self-injury is important because the primary motivation for the behavior is reducing unpleasant feelings. Sometimes clients have difficulty identifying specific emotions. The best they can do is to indicate that they are experiencing an intense generalized discomfort. For these persons, a list of emotions such as provided in Linehan's dialectical behavior therapy (DBT) workbook (1993b, pp. 139–152) can be helpful. For younger clients or those with intellectual challenges, a chart with faces and accompanying emotion names can facilitate identifying key emotional antecedents.

Another important consideration is to evaluate whether particular forms of self-injury are tied to specific emotions. For example, some clients tend to cut themselves when they are anxious but burn themselves when they are enraged. For others the emotional antecedent to cutting versus burning are the exact opposite. An important question can be, "Are there specific emotions tied to specific forms of self-injury for you?" A relevant follow-up question is, "Is this link consistent or does it vary over time?"

Behavioral Antecedents

"Behavioral antecedents" are defined as observable actions by the self-injurer that trigger episodes of self-injury. These behaviors are key in the sequence that culminates in self-injury. For example, some people self-injure only when they are high on marijuana or intoxicated on alcohol. Some tend to cut or burn themselves only after they have made the decision to stop taking their medication, and the psychotropic effects have worn off. Some self-injure after they have consumed a great deal of food and are thinking judgmentally and feeling disgusted with themselves. Still others self-injure immediately after they have behaved in a way that embarrasses them. One client I knew tended to self-injure after masturbating. He found himself unable to resist the impulse to masturbate, but immediately afterward became extremely judgmental and felt shame and disgust about the behavior. The self-injury served to punish him and his body for the "evils" of his masturbation behavior.

Whereas all of these behavioral antecedents have thoughts and feelings that accompany them, the behaviors themselves can be the key element that triggers the self-injury. In many cases, if the therapist does not know the specific behavioral antecedents, the cognitive and affective antecedents will not come to light. Thus it is important for the therapist to learn what the client was *doing* right before self-injury

THERAPIST: What were you doing right before you opened those wounds?

CLIENT: Lots of stuff. I was racing around.

THERAPIST: Okay, but was there anything you did that seemed to get you going in the direction of hurting yourself?

CLIENT: Hmm (*thinking*). Well, I was getting pretty uptight, so I smoked some grass.

THERAPIST: Do you think that smoking grass plays a role in your hurting yourself?

CLIENT: I don't think so. They both do the same thing for me. They chill me out.

THERAPIST: Well, how often do you think you smoke grass right before you cut yourself or pick at your wounds?

CLIENT: I guess most of the time, actually.

THERAPIST: What do you make of that connection?

CLIENT: I think being stoned makes me brave enough to do it.

THERAPIST: Well, do you want to keep doing it?

CLIENT: That's the big question, isn't it?

CONSEQUENCES OR AFTERMATH
OF THE SELF-INJURY

The consequences or aftermath of self-injury can be discussed in terms of the following components:

- Specifics of the psychological relief
- Presence/absence of self-care after the self-injury
- Presence/absence of excoriation after the self-injury
- Presence/absence of communication regarding the self-injury
- Demeanor of the client describing the self-injury
- Social reinforcement

Specifics of the Psychological Relief

"Specifics of the psychological relief" refer to the alleviation of affective discomfort provided by the self-injury. Although it has been stated repeatedly in this book that the prime reason for self-injury is reduction of affective distress, this element of behavioral analysis should go beyond that insight. The question for this part of assessment is what specific type of psychological relief does the self-injury provide? It is helpful if the client can describe exactly how she or he feels after self-injury. The type of relief provided is key because the positive replacement behaviors to be sought in treatment should "echo" or "mimic" this type of relief. For example, if the client says self-injury produces feelings of deep relaxation, then self-soothing activities that produce similar feelings should be taught. If the client says self-injury produces peaceful sleep, then sleep-induction techniques may be helpful. If the client says the self-injury reduces anger to manageable proportions, then a focus on anger management is key. Behavioral analysis must move from the general concept of obtaining relief to the specific details of the *type* of relief.

A helpful question related to analyzing the aftermath of self-injury is: "After you have self-injured, where in your body do you feel relief?" This question can yield some unexpected answers, as shown in this dialogue with a 22-year-old female client.

THERAPIST: What sort of relief does cutting yourself provide?

CLIENT: It stops the pain.

THERAPIST: Do you mean psychological pain?

CLIENT: Sort of. Different kinds of pain, I guess.

THERAPIST: What are the different kinds?

CLIENT: Well, some of it's physical.

THERAPIST: Where do you feel this physical pain in your body?

CLIENT: (*noticeably uncomfortable*) Right up the middle of it.

THERAPIST: Starting where?

CLIENT: (*pointing*) Down there.

THERAPIST: Are you pointing to your genitals?

CLIENT: (*embarrassed*) Yes.

THERAPIST: Are you saying you have pain in your genitals and that cutting your arms relieves that?

CLIENT: (*showing some relief*) Yes.

This dialogue led to a disclosure of sexual abuse that involved her father digitally penetrating her vagina. This abuse, which occurred about 10 years previous and lasted for 2 years, not only caused her great shame and rage, but also considerable physical pain. Years later, when she experienced pain in her genitals as a trauma-related symptom, she cut herself.

Cutting immediately relieved both the physical pain and the emotions of shame and rage related to the abuse.

Presence/Absence of Self-Care after Self-Injury

"Presence/absence of self-care after self-injury" refers to whether or not the client cares for wounds after acts of self-harm. Many clients take at least basic precautions to ensure that their wounds do not become infected. They keep the wounds clean and may apply an antiseptic salve and bandage, if necessary. Therapists should be reassured when clients take care to prevent their wounds from becoming infected.

However, other clients provide little self-care to wounds or may even deliberately attempt to induce infection. For these individuals the lack of care to wounds after self-injury may represent an extension of the self-harm episode. For example:

Sula was a 16-year-old who had a 3-year history of cutting her arms and legs. On one occasion when she was especially agitated, she pierced both of her nipples. She did this without sterilizing the needle she employed to make the holes. In addition, she made no attempt to treat her nipples with antiseptic salve after the piercings. Eventually, her piercings came to the attention of the nurse in the residential program where she resided. The nurse discovered that Sula had developed an infection in one of her nipples due to the absence of self-care.

There are multiple aspects to the self-injury episode in a case such as Sula's: (1) failure to use sterile procedures, (2) harming a body area deemed atypical and alarming, and (3) failure to use self-care after the self-injury. These details, in combination, point to an intense level of distress that requires assessment for psychiatric hospitalization/diversion.

Presence/Absence of Excoriation after the Self-Injury

"Presence/absence of excoriation after the self-injury" refers to whether or not the client deliberately reopens wounds after self-injury. Failure to care for wounds is a passive form of self-injury; excoriation is an active form. There may be symbolic meanings for clients who reopen the same wound time after time. What is striking is that self-injuring people always have the option of moving on to a different, unharmed body area (even if it is only centimeters away), yet some reopen the same wounds repeatedly. The therapist needs to explore the meaning of these repetitions. Is the message one of unfinished business, of unresolved probings, or the need to go deeper? The answer is different for each individual and always important to assess.

Presence/Absence of Communication Regarding the Self-Injury

"Presence/absence of communication regarding the self-injury" refers to whether or not the individual chooses to inform others of the self-injury after the act. This detail is an important one in determining whether the behavior is essentially intrapersonally motivated or, at least in part, intended to have an interpersonal communicative function. As stated above, in the section on social context, the majority of self-injurers harm themselves when alone but disclose the self-harm to a small number of people thereafter. In adolescents, these confidants are usually peers. Eventually, the parents or caregivers of these adolescents tend to find out about the self-injury, but the disclosure is usually delayed and/or quasi-accidental. In adults, the confidants are friends, partners, or psychological caregivers.

For all but the most secretive of self-injurers, the behavior has a communicative function. First and foremost the behavior may be driven by internal psychological distress, but it may also be intended secondarily to speak to others. The job of the therapist is to discover (1) the intended recipient of the self-injurious message, and (2) the content of the message. An example of two such communicative functions of self-injury is provided in the following vignette.

Amelia's message in the form of self-injury was delivered with aggressiveness. Her pattern was to cut jagged wounds into both arms using razor blades. Afterward, Amelia made no attempt to conceal the wounds. Rather, she wore short-sleeve shirts at home and school. The message to her parents was that she was in intense emotional pain. When her parents ignored the wounds, dismissing her as "just doing it for attention," Amelia cut deeper and more often. Amelia's message to her parents was one of rageful unhappiness and an appeal for help.

Amelia's self-injury had a different communicative function at school, where she had been belittled and ridiculed for years. Asked why she made no attempt to conceal her wounds at school, she stated she didn't care if they called her "freak" or "psycho." Amelia was beyond social connectedness in her school setting. The exhibition of her wounds conveyed a defiant and revengeful message.

Often the intended recipient of the self-injurious message is someone in the day-to-day life of the client. However, a therapist can also become the intended recipient. In such cases, the therapist may be unintentionally reinforcing the behavior. When this occurs, the therapist needs to perform behavioral analysis on his or her own actions.

Inge disclosed in therapy that she sometimes cut herself right before coming for a session. She stated that the therapist appeared to like talking about self-injury, and she wanted to make sure she "wasn't boring." In response to this disclosure, the therapist indicated that he liked talking about many issues with Inge, not just self-injury. He also deliberately muted his response to Inge's discussion of self-injury for several sessions thereafter.

Demeanor of the Client Describing the Self-Injury

"Demeanor of the client describing the self-injury" refers to the behavior of the self-injurer when describing or exhibiting the wounds. This demeanor conveys a great deal of information about the client's motivation to stop, or at least reduce, the frequency of the behavior. Some clients express remorse that they have lapsed into self-injury again; others are bland about having committed the act, considering it a routine and entirely unavoidable action; still others are openly defiant of external disapproval, clearly indicating a commitment to continuing. The best advice for the clinician is to put aside assumptions and listen to the self-injuring person with great care. Asking the client how he or she feels about a particular wound or episode can be quite illuminating. The following as an example of an unexpected disclosure from a self-injuring person.

Betsy is a 13-year-old who has been self-injuring for 6 months. In the course of the second interview, the therapist asked to see the wounds on her arm. She complied quite agreeably. After she rolled up the long sleeve on her left arm, two types of scars became visible: a series of five or six finely executed parallel scars on the forearm and four or five random, jagged, discolored wounds near inside of the elbow. The therapist commented that there seemed to be two types of wounds on her arm. She responded, "When I'm really nervous I cut myself, but when I'm really angry, I gouge myself with my finger nails."

As Betsy was saying these words, the therapist noticed her looking at her wounds with a beatific smile on her face. Curious about this seemingly incongruous response, the therapist asked her what she thinks of when she looks at her scars. She said, "To me they're beautiful. They remind of everything I've learned from all the pain in my life."

Social Reinforcement

"Social reinforcement" refers to behavior on the part of others that increases the likelihood of self-injury recurring. Any sort of attentional response to self-injury may reinforce the behavior. Social reinforcement can be intentional or unintentional. If a peer says to a self-injurer, "Oh, those cuts look so cool!" the social reinforcement is direct and intentional. However, unintentional reinforcement can be just as powerful, such as when people are very supportive or condemning of self-injurious acts. This is why the recommendation made in Chapter 6 is to use a low-key, dispassionate demeanor in responding to self-injury. The strategy is to be compassionate but to try to avoid inadvertent social reinforcement.

It is important to emphasize that obtaining social reinforcement is rarely the primary motivation for self-injury. However, the social responses of others can be important *secondary* motivators. Almost all self-injurious behavior requires some measure of psychological distress. People do not self-injure "just to get attention." Although this argument is frequently proposed, it is specious. People may self-injure because it meets their internal psychological needs *and* it is socially reinforced, but they are unlikely to self-injure for the interpersonal "rewards" alone. There are too many other methods available to "get attention from others" to justify self-injury as a means to that end.

A thorough analysis of self-injury focuses on the reactions of everyone in the person's environment, including peers, partners, spouses, fellow students, coworkers, siblings, parents, teachers, supervisors, other therapists, and so on. Those who inadvertently reinforce the behavior may need to become part of the treatment; they need to be educated in the basic management of self-injury, as presented in Chapter 6. They need to become allies in the treatment if the effort to reduce and terminate self-injury is to be successful.

PRIORITIZING ELEMENTS WITHIN THE ASSESSMENT

The first step in performing an assessment of self-injury is to ask the client to complete the Self-Injury Log between sessions for multiple weeks. This step in the assessment process considers the entire field of environmental, biological, and psychological events associated with self-injury. It takes a broad approach and does not initially assign priority to any particular events.

A second step involves asking the client to complete a Brief Self-Injury Log, as shown in Figure 7.2. This log is a concise version of the full log that adds the additional component of prioritization. I ask clients to shift to using the Brief Self-Injury Log only after a thorough assessment has been conducted and a reliable baseline has been obtained. Although individual practice varies widely, it is not unusual to switch to using the Brief Self-Injury Log after 8–10 sessions.

The language used in the Brief Self-Injury Log is identical to that used in the full log in that it refers to antecedents, events associated with self-injury, and aftermath For younger or more intellectually challenged clients, the language can be changed to something simpler, such as *triggers, behaviors*, and *results*.

The brief log allows the client and clinician to prioritize using a scale of 1–5. This prioritization can be done by the client alone, the clinician alone, or in collaboration. At the outset, a collaborative approach is generally the recommended course. Later the client can assume sole responsibility for its completion. Use of the Brief Self-Injury Log ensures that treatment focuses initially on the primary elements that precipitate self-injury. Later on the treatment moves to less important items that are nonetheless contributors.

The log presented in Figure 7.3 has been completed for a hypothetical case. In this case, under "Antecedents" the client has identified the top two

Name: _____

Dimension	Antecedents	SIB events	Aftermath
Environmental			
Biological			
Cognitive			
Affective			
Behavioral			

Rank order in each column the item that had the strongest role in producing or reinforcing the self-injury. 1 = most important; 2 = very important; 3 = moderately important; 4 = somewhat important; 5 = least important.

FIGURE 7.2. Brief Self-Injury Log.

priorities as fighting with a peer in school and feeling sad, empty, and panicked. Treatment therefore might well target reducing peer conflicts, improving social skills, as well as teaching emotion regulation and self-soothing skills.

In a similar vein, under "SIB Events" the client has prioritized the excitement of anticipating self-injury and the insistent thought of "I must do this." Treatment would prioritize learning to endure or reduce these anticipatory feelings and cognitively restructuring the maladaptive thought.

Under "Aftermath" the client has prioritized the feelings of calmness and relief and the thought "I deserved that." Treatment would prioritize teaching the client alternative self-soothing skills and restructuring thoughts regarding self-punishment and self-blame.

This simple assessment tool can be used on an ongoing basis. It is dropped only when the client has ceased self-injuring for extended periods. When a relapse occurs, the clinician must decide whether to reinstitute a full or brief log as the preferred assessment tool.

Name: 16-year-old female

Dimension	Antecedents	SIB events	Aftermath
Environmental	Fight with a peer at school 1	Looked for blade hidden in bedroom 4	No consequences at first; alone in bedroom 5
Biological	Already overtired; not high 5	Still overtired; headache starting 5	Headache gone; slept better later 4
Cognitive	"I'm all alone; I have no friends." 3	"I have to do this!" 2	"I deserved that! Phew!" 2
Affective	Felt sad, empty, panicked 2	Excited, feelings of anticipation 1	Felt much calmer; obtained relief 1
Behavioral	Retreated to bedroom; intentionally isolated self 4	Cut forearm four times, causing tissue damage without need for first aid 3	Washed cuts; applied Band-Aid; later was able to do homework 3

Rank order in each column the item that had the strongest role in producing or reinforcing the self-injury. 1 = most important; 2 = very important; 3 = moderately important; 4 = somewhat important; 5 = least important.

FIGURE 7.3. Example of a completed Brief Self-Injury Log.

CONCLUSION

In summary, in the assessment of self-injury, it is generally most helpful if clinicians and others:

- Use a Self-Injury Log to collect information systematically, if possible.
- Be especially attentive to extent of physical damage and body area affected.
- Identify idiosyncratic details about the self-injury, such as number of wounds, patterns or symbols, use of a tool, physical location.
- Identify recurrent environmental, cognitive, affective, and behavioral antecedents to the self-injury.
- Identify consequences of the self-injury, such as emotional relief.
- Be alert for social reinforcers in the environment.
- With the client's assistance, identify the most important variables in triggering and maintaining the self-injury and target these in treatment.

CHAPTER 8

Contingency Management

After a baseline assessment has been obtained, the first level of intervention in treating self-injury is contingency management: either the informal or systematic dispensing of reinforcement in relation to self-injury. Managing informal reinforcement of self-injury has already been discussed in Chapter 6, where I recommended employing a low-key, dispassionate demeanor along with a respectful curiosity in responding to self-injury. As a treatment intervention, formal contingency management is useful in reducing the frequency of self-injury, but it is unlikely to eliminate the behavior. One advantage of contingency management is that it can be used with clients who are unmotivated to stop self-injuring. In these instances the focus is on analyzing and modifying the environmental conditions that support to the behavior.

Oddly, sometimes the mere activity of collecting baseline data in preparation for contingency management can result in a reduction or extinction of the behavior. This has been referred to as the "reactivity effect" (O'Leary & Wilson, 1987, p. 27). Several years ago I worked with a client who had multiple problems with self-harm behaviors. She was a chronic cutter who frequently lacerated her arms, legs, and abdomen. In addition, she was involved in daily hair pulling (trichotillomania), which produced multiple disfiguring bald spots on her head and related wounds from persistent skin picking on her scalp. This client also presented with a variety of indirect forms of self-harm such as medication discontinuance, risk-taking behavior, and peer relationships in which she was exploited and disrespected. Having conducted an assessment of her forms of direct and indirect self-harm, I asked her which of these problems she wanted to address first, and she said the hair pulling. She explained that it caused her the most embarrassment socially and therefore she wanted to stop it.

Based on this preference, we began collecting baseline data regarding her hair pulling. I employed Keuthen's protocol (Keuthen, Stein, & Christenson, 2001) for charting daily hair removal. This involved asking the client to count as precisely as possible and record on a simple chart the number of hairs she removed from her head each day. Despite being quite disorganized in many aspects of her daily life, the client was remarkably consistent in responding to this request. Over a 3-week period, she never failed to record the number of hairs she had removed. The counts ranged from 0 to 360 hairs per day, with a mean of about 185.

At the conclusion of this period the client announced to a surprised therapist that she was no longer removing her hair. She explained that the data collection had been so annoying and time consuming that it was "no longer worth the trouble." This cessation of hair pulling continued for months afterward and, to my knowledge, has not recurred. Also worth noting is that there was no evidence that her other self-destructive behaviors increased during the hair-pulling data collection period of time.

Why was the act of data collection effective in eliminating the behavior? There are several possible answers:

1. The data collection was aversive, and she stopped hair pulling based on negative reinforcement principles.
2. The data collection was a recurrent, time-consuming activity that was both different and dramatic enough to interrupt a chronic pattern.
3. The client was already motivated to stop the behavior, and the data collection may have distracted her from hair pulling or allowed her to self-soothe in other ways; the counting itself might have been somewhat self-soothing.
4. There may have been other factors beyond my knowledge that influenced her, such as additional pressure from peers regarding her appearance.

I experienced a similar reactivity effect in doing baseline data collection with a 17-year-old male encopretic. Although this behavior was a form of *indirect* self-harm for this young man, rather than self-injury, the case is still relevant as an example of the therapeutic effect of assessment per se. In this case the data collection was informal (as opposed to quantitative) and involved only one session—which made the result especially surprising. This young man, despite having an IQ of 140, had an extensive problem with soiling himself and either walking about with feces in his pants for extended periods of time or storing his soiled underwear in family bureaus, closets, or school lockers, etc. Not surprisingly, this behavior caused him to be shunned in any setting where it occurred. It also caused some mild tissue damage to his buttocks.

I conducted my preliminary assessment interview of the youth with his parents present. The assessment consisted of asking the client a series of very detailed questions about the soiling behavior. The progression of questions included the following:

> "How often do you store soiled underwear in your parents' house?"
> "How often do you store soiled underwear on school property?"
> "How do you decide when to walk about with feces in your pants as opposed to using the toilet?"
> "Please describe the physical sensation of having feces in your pants. Is it uncomfortable? Pleasant? Neutral?"
> "Are you aware of the feces all the time or every so often?"
> "Are you aware of any odor?"
> "Does the looseness or firmness of the stool affect whether you decide to keep the feces on your person?"
> "Are there types of feces you prefer?"

I continued in this vein for 40 minutes or more, careful to employ a low-key, dispassionate demeanor. I believe I came across as nonjudgmental and respectful as well as intensely curious. That the client was becoming ever more uncomfortable was quite evident during this series of questions. I noticed him increasingly squirming in his seat and beginning to sweat on his forehead. I wanted to spare him discomfort but also felt that completing the assessment was important. He had suffered from his encopresis problem for years and had spent months in psychiatric hospitals because of it. What was remarkable about the interview was that after its conclusion, he never soiled himself again. Although many other explanations for this cessation are possible, I believe the assessment process played a key role. Somehow, the detailed questioning interrupted a chronic, self-destructive pattern. Clinicians therefore should be alert to the possibility of a reactivity effect derived from baseline data collection—and although dramatic cessation of self-harm behaviors during the assessment process is rare, subtler changes in behavior are quite common.

CONTINGENCY MANAGEMENT CONTRACTS

The far more typical experience is for baseline data collection to yield valuable information but no immediate therapeutic effect. Baseline data can be used to construct simple contingency management contracts designed to reduce the frequency of the self-injury. I find that generally at least 4–5 weeks are necessary to collect adequate baseline data. However, for clients who self-injure infrequently, such as every 3 months, a much more extended time period may be needed. For clients who self-injure very infrequently (e.g., every six months), behavioral contracting is unlikely to be helpful. In such cases, reducing the frequency of the behavior is more likely to require cognitive restructuring and replacement skills training than contingency management. The baseline frequency is just too modest to target reduction as a primary treatment goal.

For clients with a high rate of self-injury a baseline of a few weeks can be quite adequate. As presented in Chapter 7, the therapist and client should begin by using a Self-Injury Log. After detailed baseline data have been obtained, they can shift to using the Brief Self-Injury Log. The client and the therapist are then in a good position to construct a simple "Self-Protection Contract." I prefer the term "Self-Protection" to "Self-Injury Contract" because it is worded positively. Moreover, the same contract can be used later to target other self-destructive and self-defeating behaviors.

The basic principle in using a Self-Protection Contract is for the client to commit to *reducing* the frequency of the behavior. The goal need not be extinction of the behavior at the outset. Note that I am not talking about "Contracting for Safety," which is a very different strategy that is discussed below. A Self-Protection Contract should have a least the following elements:

1. Quantitative baseline data
2. A clearly stated, measurable goal
3. Identification of needed replacement skills
4. Identification of a reward if the goal is reached
5. A "hold harmless" statement if the goal is not reached
6. Commitment statement involving signature, witness, date, and time period

An example of a simple Self-Protection Contract for a 33-year-old recurrently self-injuring person is provided in Figure 8.1.

Note that the contract is very individualized, using recent baseline data and a measurable goal. The contract identifies self-soothing and distraction skills that the client has previously noted as useful in fending off self-injury. In addition, the contract is a written document that makes the commitment of the client and therapist both formal and concrete. It is also a short-term agreement (1 week) that rewards the client if she is successful and holds the client harmless if she is not. Why is it important to hold the client harmless? If the client is punished for disclosing self-injury, he or she

Baseline data: My rate of self-injury over the past 4 weeks has been an average of 3 episodes per week with 3 to 8 cuts per episode.

Goal: I agree to attempt to reduce the frequency of my cutting over the coming week to 1 time per week with 2 to 3 cuts per episode.

Skills: In order to do so, I commit to using the following self-soothing or distraction skills when I feel angry or anxious:

1. Listening to music

2. Patting my cat

3. Calling my friend Sam

4. Listening to my relaxation tape

Reward: If I am able to fulfill this contract, I will treat myself to a new haircut. If I am not able to fulfill the contract, there is no penalty.

Commitment:

Signature: _____

Witness (therapist, counselor, etc.): _____

Date: _____

For the time period of _____ to _____

FIGURE 8.1. Example of a completed Self-Protection Contract for a 33-year-old.

may choose to hide self-harm thereafter. This risk is discussed more extensively in the section below on safety contracts.

Another example of a Self-Protection Contract was used with an adolescent client residing in a group home (see Figure 8.2). This 16-year-old male had been in residential treatment for 3 months. He was placed in the program due to violence toward others, destruction of property, and recurrent self-injury (burning, cutting, self-inflicted tattoos). Other contracts and treatment strategies were used to target his aggression, and residential staff developed the following contract with him to address his recurrent self-injury. This client was quite adept at obtaining tools and self-injuring despite close staff supervision.

In this case the goal is more ambitious (only one episode of self-injury) because the client has been in treatment for 3 months and has learned and practiced many replacement skills. All the other elements of the Self-Protection Contract are the same as those in Figure 8.1, including the hold

Baseline data: My rate of self-injury over the past 3 months has been 3 episodes per week with 2 to 4 burns or 4 to 6 cuts per episode (no tattoos).

Goal: I agree to attempt to reduce the frequency of my self-injury over the coming week to 1 episode.

Skills: In order to do so, I commit to using the following self-soothing or distraction skills when I feel angry or depressed

1. Lifting weights

2. Talking with my residential counselor, Jim

3. Practicing deep breathing

4. Listening to nonviolent music

Reward: If I am able to fulfill this contract, I will be eligible for a pass from the program without staff supervision. (I must also be on the proper level in the program.) If I am not able to fulfill the contract, I will not be dropped a level unless my level of self-harm requires medical intervention.

Commitment: [same as in Figure 8.1]

FIGURE 8.2. Example of a completed Self-Protection Contract for a 16-year-old.

harmless provision—which is unusual in most residential treatment settings.

CONTRACTING FOR SAFETY WITH SELF-INJURY

A common question is whether to use contracting for safety in responding to self-injury. This strategy usually takes the form of obtaining commitment from a client to refrain from self-injuring for a period of time, such as a day or week. Using Safety Contracts for self-injury is a common strategy in many settings such as outpatient clinics, psychiatric emergency rooms, and group homes. The purpose of Safety Contracts is generally to (1) attempt to prevent the behavior from recurring, and (2) protect the professional from liability should subsequent self-harm occur. As noted by Shea (1999), Safety Contracts may *not* do a very good job of either. There is little empirical evidence that Safety Contracts serve a deterrent function. Moreover, the protection against liability by having employed a safety contract is, at best, modest (Shea, 1999).

I generally recommend *against* using Safety Contracts as a strategy to deal with self-injury, because they often have more risks than benefits. The main risk is that contracting for safety often drives the behavior underground by fostering dishonesty. For the most part clients are unable to stop self-injuring until they have acquired effective replacement skills. Asking them to forgo the behavior before they have incorporated these skills is requesting the near impossible. The expectation (or demand) is that they endure their usual intense level of emotional distress (or emptiness) without using their preferred management technique. This is generally asking way too much.

Therapists have a tendency to place extensive pressure on clients to stop self-injuring. They may communicate this pressure by offering effusive praise when the client does not self-injure or by expressing disappointment, dismay, frustration, or condemnation when the client has self-injured. Clients react to such pressure by feeling misunderstood, resentful, and like a failure; they learn very quickly how to solicit praise and avoid condemnation. They may attempt to please the therapist (or other professional) by saying that they have not self-injured when, in fact, they have. When this kind of deception occurs, the therapeutic alliance is seriously compromised. Clients have learned to avoid negative responses from the therapist but at the cost of providing accurate information. The therapy may not recover from this setback. A therapy based on misinformation cannot proceed productively.

Another result of therapists inappropriately using Safety Contracts is that clients drop out of therapy, feeling that they have failed the therapist (and themselves) by not meeting the therapist's expectations. The last thing most self-injuring clients need is another experience with failure. When clients prematurely drop out of therapy, they may be even less likely to seek out treatment in the future. Thus multiple adverse effects can be the result of "forbidding" self-injury too early in treatment.

My general rule-of-thumb is: *Do not ask self-injurers to give up the behavior before they are ready, unless the behavior involves extensive tissue damage or alarming body areas.* In these cases, Safety Contracts are beside the point. Protective intervention involving inpatient psychiatric care or residential respite services is necessary.

This is not to say that the use of Safety Contracts is *never* indicated. Sometimes clients *ask* to use Safety Contracts, saying that they are helpful in fending off self-injury. When clients makes this request, I am usually willing to develop a Safety Contract with them, making sure to incorporate the features they prefer.

Shea (1999) has provided an invaluable review of safety contracting with suicidal individuals. A number of his suggestions are useful in designing Safety Contracts regarding self-injury as well. He indicates that if a clinician is going to use safety contracting, it should be viewed primarily as an assessment tool as opposed to a preventive intervention. He also suggests that a clinician wishing to develop a valid Safety Contract should look for good eye contact, genuine affect, and a natural and unhesitant tone of voice from the client.

According to Shea, an effective Safety Contract often concludes with a firm handshake and the signing of a formal, written document. Any signs of hesitancy, ambivalence, or deceit should result in the clinician starting over or abandoning the pursuit of a Safety Contract in favor of other strategies.

One client who used a Safety Contract productively with me was a 29-year-old woman with a long history of self-injury. She requested that I develop a Safety Contract with her, saying that it had previously helped in other therapy. She wrote the Safety Contract shown in Figure 8.3, which I agreed to witness and sign.

Although this contract did not include all the elements I like to see in a Self-Protection Contract, I still accepted it because the client wanted to design her own vehicle. The client subsequently stated that the contract was quite helpful in decreasing her self-injury. She reported that when she had impulses to cut, she gently reminded herself that she had promised herself and me that she would not do so. This prompt was effective in helping her postpone or altogether avoid self-harm. Over time, Safety Contracts, in combination with replacement skills, enabled her to give up self-injury permanently.

With most populations, the most effective contingency management procedure is informal social reinforcement. Many self-injuring clients come from backgrounds of abuse and neglect. They are not used to warm, empathic attention and positive feedback. My strategy is to extend the majority of social reinforcement not on the *absence* of self-injury but on the *presence* of clients' use of healthy cognitive restructuring techniques and replacement skills. These key areas of treatment are the foci of the next two chapters.

I, _____, have been cutting myself about 2 or 3 times per month recently and want to stop. I realize that cutting indicates disrespect for myself and my body. I want to learn to respect and love myself for who I am. I promise not to cut myself over the next week. I will report on my progress at my next therapy appointment on Wednesday.

Signed:_____ Date: _____

Witness: _____ Time period: _____ to _____

FIGURE 8.3. Safety Contract.

CONCLUSION

In summary, in the contingency management of self-injury, it is generally most helpful if clinicians and others:

- Collect baseline data regarding the frequency of self-injury for several weeks.
- Use Self-Protection Contracts that have clearly stated measurable goals, identify replacement skills to be employed, and specify any rewards to be obtained.
- Include a "hold harmless" statement if the goal is not reached in order to foster full disclosure.
- Employ a formal commitment statement involving signature, witness, date, and time period.

CHAPTER 9

Replacement Skills Training

A central focus in the treatment of self-injury is teaching replacement skills. The therapist's role is to assist the client in identifying skills that will be a good match for that individual and to convey a sense of urgency about learning and using the skills. The client's role is to carefully select skills with the therapist and to practice them over and over again. Early in treatment, after the assessment has been completed, the therapist and client discuss skill options repeatedly and practice them together during sessions. Once some useful, relevant skills have been identified, the emphasis shifts to the client using the skills in his or her real-world living environments. Skills need to be practiced at home, school, work, and social settings. Over time the client finds that some skills are not particularly helpful, whereas others are especially effective. The client frequently revises his or her roster of skills as some skills fade in importance and others take prominence. The goal is for the client to develop a core set of skills that can be counted on when really needed.

It would be nice to be able to say that considerable empirical support has emerged regarding the effectiveness of a skills training approach to treating self-injury. The reality is that the literature is still in its infancy regarding the effectiveness of skills training. Linehan et al. (1991) have demonstrated the effectiveness of dialectical behavior therapy (DBT) in treating self-injury, among other problems. Their study of adult women with a diagnosis of borderline personality disorder found that subjects receiving DBT had significantly fewer "parasuicidal acts" during the treatment period than "treatment as usual" controls. (In this study, "parasuicide" referred to both suicide attempts and low-lethality self-injury.) Linehan reported that the parasuicidal behavior of subjects receiving DBT declined from 100 to about 37% during the 1-year treatment protocol. In contrast, the "treatment as usual controls" declined from 100 to 63%, still presenting with parasuicide. Thus a statistically significant, positive treatment effect was demonstrated for the DBT subjects, although more than a third were still presenting with parasuicidal behavior at the conclusion of treatment.

Comtois (2002) presented a recent review of interventions designed to reduce parasuicidal behavior. Her conclusion was that only four psychosocial studies have shown a positive impact on parasuicide. One was the previously cited DBT study; another was a cognitive-behavioral study conducted in England; and the other two were home-visit models provided in England and Belgium (where the presenting problems were more suicidal than self-injurious). The DBT and cognitive-behavioral therapy studies shared a focus on problem solving and compliance with treatment protocol. Given this dirth of outcome studies, the field clearly needs much more in the way of empirical research regarding the treatment of self-injury using skills training approaches.

In the meantime this chapter presents a skills training approach that has been found anecdotally to be helpful in treating self-injury. A skills training approach seems likely to be helpful in that other skills training interventions have been found to be effective in treating problems such as youth suicidal behavior (Miller, Rathus, Linehan, Wetzler, & Leigh, 1997) and substance abuse (Marlatt & Vandenbos, 1997; Marlatt, 2002).

BEGINNING REPLACEMENT SKILLS TRAINING

Early in treatment the client especially needs to practice skills when he or she is relatively calm and focused. This rehearsal will enable the client to use the skills at other times when emotional distress is high. The therapist needs to remind the client, "You can't learn to ride a bicycle away from a tornado."

SELECTING THE RIGHT SKILLS

If clients select the right skills and practice them diligently, they are very likely to get better; conversely, if they practice halfheartedly or not at all, their problems with self-injury are likely to continue. This is not to say that individuals cannot recover through other means that do not involve treatment (see Shaw, 2002), but learning replacement skills is the most direct route.

If clients are going to overcome self-injury, they need to acquire skills that manage their emotional distress (or emptiness) *at least as effectively* as self-harm behaviors. Initially, clients may be understandably skeptical that anything will work as well as cutting, burning, excoriation, or whatever their preferred methods may be. The therapist's role is to emphasize how many others have been helped by these skills. The therapist needs to repeat a basic mantra: "Replacement skills have worked for many others, and they will work for you if you find the right skills and practice, practice, practice" (see Linehan, 1993b, and Segal, Williams, & Teasdale, 2002, regarding the crucial importance of practice).

NINE TYPES OF REPLACEMENT SKILLS

There is a wealth of resources that review different types of skills that can be used to deal with emotional distress (e.g., Nhat Hanh, 1975, 1991; Davis, Eshelman, & McKay, 1982; Kabat-Zinn, 1990; Levey & Levey, 1991, 1999; Linehan, 1993b; Alderman, 1997; Conterio & Lader, 1998; Segal et al., 2002). Although there are myriad possibilities, I have found nine different types of skills to be especially useful in treating self-injury. I am not claiming that these are uniquely effective, only stating that they have repeatedly worked with clients. They are:

1. Negative replacement behaviors
2. Mindful breathing skills
3. Visualization techniques
4. Physical exercise
5. Writing
6. Artistic expression
7. Playing or listening to music
8. Communicating with others
9. Diversion techniques

These are discussed in the order presented.

Negative Replacement Behaviors

A controversial set of skills that some individuals use to fend off impulses to self-injure are behaviors that resemble self-injury. Conterio and Lader (personal communication, 2000) have argued against using what they call "negative replacement behaviors" because they believe such activities are too fraught with associations to self-injury. They contend that negative replacement behaviors are likely to trigger relapse because they maintain the client's focus on, or preoccupation with, self-harm. They recommend that therapists avoid or even forbid clients from using such techniques. Although their concerns are understandable, I have found that many clients use such replacement behaviors productively—at least, in the short term. I would certainly agree that no individual should depend on negative replacement behaviors exclusively to eliminate self-injury. However, some clients use negative replacement behaviors early in treatment because they represent such familiar territory and serve an important *transitional* function. Examples of negative replacement behaviors include:

- Marking one's body with a red-colored marker rather than cutting or burning (symbolic representation of wounding, without tissue damage).
- Applying Ben Gay or other topical stimulants to a body area previously self-injured (tactile sensation but without tissue damage).
- Snapping a rubber band on the area of an arm or leg that is usually cut or burned (tactile sensation and a stinging discomfort but without tissue damage).
- Briefly applying ice or portable cool packs to body areas usually assaulted (physical stimulation and discomfort but without tissue damage).
- Applying a temporary tattoo to a portion of the body and scratching it off with a finger nail (tactile stimulation of the area usually harmed, but without tissue damage).
- Gently stroking a body area previously assaulted with a soft cosmetics brush or other soft implement (soothing that which was previously harmed).
- Drawing a picture depicting the self-injury of a body area (visual cues representing self-injury without tissue damage).
- Writing about the act of self-injuring in great detail, from start to finish of an episode, without implementing the scenario (begins transition to verbal mastery while distancing the client from the immediacy of self-harm).
- Dictating a self-injury sequence into a recording device (verbal mastery and distancing).

Note that these strategies include tactile, visual, and auditory options. For some clients self-injury is primarily tactile; for others it is a more visual or even self-instructional experience. I believe for most it is a combination. In choosing such skills, clients need to select an option that intuitively feels right for them.

The assumption with all of these examples is that the act of self-injury is symbolically represented but that no tissue damage is inflicted. The cli-

ent experiences something that resembles the act of self-harm but is sufficiently in control to go through the sequence without harming the body.
The advantage of these techniques is that for some clients the activities
seem vivid and "real" enough to take the place of actual self-harm. The disadvantage is that the behaviors may cue actual self-injury because the
replacement behaviors are so similar to the real thing. Using negative
replacement skills may seem a bit like suggesting to an alcoholic that he or
she enter a bar and order a soda water as part of becoming sober. For some
clients the stimulus cues can be too triggering. Nonetheless, other clients
report that negative replacement behaviors have played a key role in helping them transition away from self-injury. For example:

*Nikki's pattern of self-injury was to incise precisely executed grid designs on
her forearms. She conceived of a replacement behavior that she used to fend
off impulses to self-harm. From her art supplies she took three sheets of con-
struction paper. She colored the first sheet deep red, the second, yellow and
orange, and the third, skin tone. She then stapled the three sheets together at
the corners. Using her X-acto knife, Nikki cut a grid pattern into the layers of
paper. The resulting design was identical to what she had previously incised
into her arms. She reported that this technique helped her avoid self-injuring
several times before she moved onto other replacement skills.*

Nikki's experience is not atypical. Clients often find that using behaviors that resemble self-injury may be useful transitionally, but they are not
likely to use these techniques for extended periods of time successfully.

Mindful Breathing Skills

Mindful breathing skills are often the most important in learning to give up
self-injury. The term "mindful" requires some explanation. Mindfulness
skills have increasingly been identified as playing an important role in the
empirically validated treatments of diverse disorders. Kabat-Zinn has reported using mindfulness skills in treating chronic illness, physical pain,
and psychological stress (Kabat-Zinn, 1990). Linehan considers mindfulness a "core component" of her DBT for individuals diagnosed with borderline personality disorder (Linehan et al., 1991; Linehan, 1993a, 1993b).
Segal and colleagues (2002) assign mindfulness training a central role in
their treatment of recurrent depression. Hayes (2004) has gone so far as to
identify mindfulness as central to the new "third wave" of behavior therapy.
There are also extensive writings about mindfulness that have a philosophical and religious orientation, such as those by the Buddhist monk Thich
Nhat Hanh (1975, 1991).

When I present the term "mindfulness" to clients, I generally keep the discussion simple because most clients are interested in practical results as opposed to philosophical discussions. The explanation that I provide is that "mindfulness" refers to being calm and relaxed while also being fully alert (Nhat Hanh, 1975; Linehan, 1993b). I also explain that mindfulness is about doing one activity *in the present*. Multitasking is the opposite of mindfulness, as are reminiscing or anticipating. As Nhat Hahn wrote:

> While we practice conscious breathing, our thinking will slow down, and we can give ourselves a real rest. Most of the time, we think too much, and mindful breathing helps us to be calm, relaxed and peaceful. It helps us stop thinking so much and stop being possessed by sorrows of the past and worries about the future. (1991, p. 8)

I explain that learning mindfulness is generally a good match for self-injurers because they experience the opposite of mindfulness so frequently. Rather than calm, they are frequently intensely distressed; rather than focused, they are often confused and distracted. All too frequently the lives of self-injurers are dominated by emotional lability and cognitive disjointedness. Clients learn to be mindful in order to calm themselves and solve problems more effectively.

Although any activity can be done mindfully (e.g., eating, walking, doing the dishes, mowing the lawn), mindful breathing skills are particularly recommended because:

- They are easy to learn.
- They enable individuals to physically calm themselves by reducing heart and respiration rates.
- They can be practiced and used at almost any time.
- There is no cost or need for equipment.
- There are no side effects.
- The skills require no assistance or participation from others.
- With a modest amount of practice, they produce very quick results.

Some clients, particularly adolescents, express distrust or discomfort when first presented with mindful breathing skills. They label the activity as "weird" or "strange" and indicate no intention of trying it. Other clients state at the outset that they have tried breathing skills before and the skills did not work. It is important to be patient with doubters and to assure them that if they *practice* breathing, they will be surprised by the results. I sometimes say to skeptics that "the first step in using breathing skills is being convinced they will *not* work." I tell them of many clients who have stated that mindful breathing skills did not work for them, only to acknowledge 6 months later how useful they had become.

It is often productive for therapists to refer to their own use of mindful breathing skills in order to encourage clients. When therapists indicate that mindful breathing is a "living skill" that anyone can use and not just some therapeutic technique, clients may become more receptive. I sometimes share this story with clients:

> "Several years ago, I was driving south along the California coast. It was a beautiful but frightening ride, with miles of road along cliffs that dropped off hundreds of feet to the ocean. There were no guardrails on many sections of road, and it was clear that even a slight mistake could result in a catastrophic accident and death. Although not normally a nervous driver, I became increasingly fearful. My forehead began sweating and my hands gripped the steering wheel more and more tightly. My driving slowed to about 15 m.p.h. as I negotiated hairpin turns on the edge of the ocean. Fortunately, there were no cars behind me.
>
> "One thing and one thing only got me through this driving experience. As I realized how stressed I was becoming, I began deliberately using my mindful breathing skills while I was driving. Within several minutes I calmed down and was able to drive with much less fear and improved concentration."

I conclude this story by asking clients if they ever feel afraid or have too much emotion.

I tell many other stories about former clients who have successfully used mindful breathing skills during sports competitions, when taking exams, talking with an intimidating boss, having an argument with a partner, and most importantly, as an alternative to self-injuring. This is one example of a story that clients appreciate.

A 15-year-old male came into therapy because he had been cutting himself about every 2 weeks for a year. This young man was an excellent high school baseball player. He was the star pitcher, even though he was one of the youngest players on the team. One area of his life he really wanted to work on was dealing with stress during competition. Very frequently, if he made a bad pitch that was hit hard, he would become furious with himself and launch into a series of self-denigrating judgments, such as "You're an idiot! You don't belong on the field. You're going to lose the game for the team," etc.

This client learned mindful breathing as part of treatment. He practiced diligently every evening before going to bed. He found the skill so useful he began deliberately slowing his breathing while on the mound. He also focused on his breathing while sitting on the bench between innings, as an alternative to making negative judgments about himself. Use of breathing skills enabled this client to experience much less stress on the baseball field. It also helped him give up self-injury within about 8 months.

Teaching Mindful Breathing

It is particularly important to teach and practice mindful breathing skills *in vivo* with clients. Descriptions are not as effective as demonstrations. Practicing *together* teaches the skills in a specific, vivid way and models for the client how to overcome any sense of awkwardness or skepticism. If the therapist is willing to look "weird" or "strange," why not the client?

Early in treatment, I begin the practice of mindful breathing with these basic instructions:

> "Let's begin by sitting in a chair or on a cushion in a balanced way. Find a comfortable alignment. The spine should be straight but not rigid. Try not to lean right or left. If you are in a chair, it is recommended that you place your feet flat on the floor. Place your hands and arms on your legs or the arms of the chair. It is best to sit rather than lie down, because people tend to fall asleep when reclining; mindfulness is about being both calm and alert.
>
> "Bring your attention gently to your breathing. Notice the physical sensations of your abdomen and chest expanding and contracting with each breath. . . . Notice the air entering and leaving your mouth, nose, and throat. . . . Become aware of the basic rhythm of the body and the breath.
>
> "When you experience distractions such as thoughts, feelings, worries, anticipations and the like, gently return your attention to your breathing. Distractions are inevitable but can be reduced with practice."

After providing these basic instructions, I like to teach four different types of mindful breathing within the first month or two of treatment. The pace of instruction depends on the client's readiness to learn and willingness to practice. Some clients learn all four breathing techniques within the first few weeks. Others need a much more time.

I should emphasize that there is no empirical support for the specific breathing exercises selected. They are comfortable for me to teach, and I find that many clients respond to them. Clinicians should feel free to select

other breathing exercises that they prefer. Following are the four types of
breathing.

IN . . . OUT BREATHING

The instructions are: "As you breathe in, say 'in' inside your mind; as you
breathe out, say 'out' inside your mind. Continue for several minutes."

Comment. This is the simplest breathing exercise. Many like it because
they quickly grasp that learning mindful breathing is not difficult and that
they "can do it." I have taught this technique to a wide range of people,
including mentally retarded and developmentally delayed adults, emotionally disturbed adolescents, seriously and persistently mentally ill adults,
and many therapists and residential counselors. For clients who are more
cognitively limited, "In . . . Out Breathing" is the preferred technique.
However, the simplicity of this breathing technique is also its weakness.
Clients often report that they prefer a more complex breathing skill
because they are better able to remain focused on breathing and not
become distracted.

1–10 EXHALE BREATHING

The instructions are: "As you breathe in, say nothing inside your mind; as
you breathe out, say '1.' Next, as you breathe in, say nothing again, and as
you breathe out, say '2.' Continue in this manner up to 10, counting only on
the exhalations. When you reach 10, return to 1. If you lose count or go
beyond 10, return to 1 and start over."

Comment: This is a good alternative introductory exercise to "In . . .
Out Breathing." It is more complex and requires more attention; however,
it is still quite simple and easily remembered. The counting aspect of this
breathing dispels any concerns clients may have that mindful breathing will
be weird, strange, or cult-like. There are no religious mantras or foreign
words to learn; it is just counting. It should be noted, though, that this form
of breathing has been practiced for 2,500 years by serious meditators
(Rosenberg, 1998).

DEEPER BREATHING

The instructions are: "Most of us breathe throughout the day in a fairly
shallow way, using only a modest percentage of lung capacity. This exercise
involves intentionally deepening the breath. Taking calm, deep breaths not
only increases relaxation; it also increases oxygen to the brain, making you
more alert. Begin by focusing on your breath. Deliberately slow down the

breath and make your 'in breath' fuller. Next, as you breathe out, do so more fully; deliberately expel more of the air from your lungs than you normally do. As you practice this exercise, find a comfortable new rhythm for breathing deeply."

Comment: This technique is an excellent way to induce a sense of greater relaxation and calm. Most people report feeling much more relaxed after 10 minutes of "Deeper Breathing." One risk is that some people report feeling lightheaded. Heavy smokers or those who are trying too hard and breathing too fast may experience some discomfort. Instruct people to return to normal "shallow" breathing if they start to feel any shortness of breath or other unpleasant sensations.

LETTING GO OF . . . BREATHING

This breathing technique is a modification of one presented by Nhat Hanh (1975). The instructions are: "As you breathe in, say inside your mind, 'Mindfully breathing.' As you breathe out, say inside your mind: 'Letting go of X. . . . ' Here X represents whatever feeling or thoughts you'd like to have less of, such as anxiety, tension, anger, judgments, perfectionism. The X selected should be something that is powerful in the moment or is known to be a key antecedent to self-injury. As you breathe out, imagine the feeling or thought leaving your body as you become more and more relaxed. You can select one thing to 'let go of' and say that recurrently, or you can let go of a series of different feelings or thoughts. Thus the first time you might say, 'Mindfully breathing, letting go of anxiety,' and the second time, 'Mindfully breathing, letting go of judgments,' etc. After doing this exercise for several minutes, people tend to naturally transition to simply saying, 'Mindfully breathing' on the in breath, and 'Letting go' on the out breath."

Comment: The idea is not to "drive out" or forbid any thoughts or feelings, but rather to notice them and then let them pass. This exercise can be done quite successfully in groups with both staff and clients taking turns saying out loud, "Mindfully breathing, letting go of X." This activity builds a sense of group cohesion and conveys the message that everyone has feelings and judgments they'd like to have less of; such an experience can be quite normalizing for clients who view their distress as unique or extreme. If a group has clients who are particularly anxious about speaking in front of others or disclosing personal feelings, the members can be told that they can say "pass" when it comes to their turn.

One disadvantage to this technique is that it is complex and requires good verbal skills. With some developmentally disabled clients, I've reduced the exercise to saying the word "breathing" on the in breath, and saying only X on the out breath (thus eliminating the words "mindfully" and "letting go of" for the sake of simplicity).

There are many other mindful breathing techniques that work well with clients. Appendix A is a Breathing Manual with diverse examples for teaching mindfulness skills. Please consult it for other techniques not presented here.

Some clients are particularly inspired by the link between mindful breathing and meditation. All of the world's great religions have meditative or contemplative traditions, including Buddhism, Christianity, Islam, and Judaism. For clients who respond to the spiritual aspects of mindful breathing and meditation, there are many helpful resources including Sekida (1985), Nhat Hanh (1975, 1991), Bayda (2002), Fontana (2001), and Rosenberg (1998). However, it should be emphasized one more time that mindful breathing can be taught in a completely secular manner that requires no reference to philosophical or religious traditions. The therapist's strategy is to understand the client's mindset and to proceed in a manner that is consistent with the client's attitudes and beliefs.

Tips Regarding Mindful Breathing Practice

In teaching mindful breathing skills it is also important to monitor the frequency and length of practice, the physical location, and the results obtained. In order for mindful breathing to become a useful skill, most people need to practice the behavior at least three times per week. A Mindful Breathing Tracking Card such as that presented in Figure 9.1 can be a useful way to monitor practice.

The length of practice is very important. Many clients may try the behavior for a minute or 2 and declare that it does not work. They are correct that 2 or 3 minutes of mindful breathing are unlikely to produce a deep sense of calm and enhanced alertness. Clients generally need to practice mindful breathing each time for 10 minutes or more in order for it to become a useful skill. Segal and colleagues' (2002) mindfulness-based cognitive therapy for depression requires that clients practice breathing for 40 minutes multiple times per week. Although I find this expectation too demanding for many clients (especially adolescents), I do think 15–20 minutes duration is an appropriate goal. In order for mindful breathing to work, clients need to move beyond the highly distractible first few minutes of mindful breathing into the calmness that emerges after 10 or more minutes. Clients need time to work up to more extended mindful breathing practice. Many can reach 15–20 minutes within a month or 2. After several months of practice the skill becomes increasingly effective and can be used in periods of high emotional arousal.

The physical location for the practice is also an important detail. Clients need to select a quiet place in their home or elsewhere where they are unlikely to be disturbed. Clients who live in a chaotic environment may need to seek out a library, prayer room, meditation center, or quiet outdoor location. They should use either a comfortable chair or meditation cushions. It is unwise to practice lying down for reasons previously stated. However, once mindful breathing has been well learned, it can be used quite productively as a sleep-induction technique for those with insomnia.

Another detail concerns whether the eyes should be open or closed. My opinion is that it does not matter. Some individuals prefer having their eyes open because they feel safe and are less likely to doze off. Others pre-

---

Name: _____

Week of: _____

	Mon.	Tues.	Wed.	Thurs.	Fri.	Sat.	Sun.
*Type of breathing							
Location							
Length of practice **Subjective units of distress (SUDs 0–10)							

*Type of breathing: In . . . out . . .
                     Counting 1–10 when breathing out
                     Deeper breathing
                     Letting go of
                     Other
**Note: 0 = the most relaxed you've ever been; 10 = the most distressed you've ever been; 5 is in the middle. Please rate yourself at both start and finish of the mindful breathing practice. Place the start SUD above the line, then finish SUD below.

FIGURE 9.1. Mindful Breathing Tracking Card.

---

fer having their eyes closed because they are better able to concentrate without visual stimuli. The client should decide which is the more comfortable practice.

It is also useful to monitor effectiveness with the client. I find a useful technique is to teach clients the concept of subjective units of distress, or SUDs (Wolpe, 1969). Clients can record on their Mindful Breathing Tracking Card how they are feeling immediately prior to and after breathing practice. Tracking breathing using SUDs involves teaching clients that 0 represents the most relaxed they have ever been in their lives and 10 the most distressed, with 5 approximately in the middle. Most clients report substantial reduction in SUDs after 10 or more minutes of mindful breathing.

For those who consistently report no change or even worse, an escalation of SUDs, it may be best to look toward other replacement behaviors. I encountered one client who consistently became more anxious while practicing mindful breathing. Initially, her only explanation was, "Breathing just doesn't work for me." Having heard this many times before, I plodded on, urging her to keep trying. Then she disclosed the following:

> "Breathing never works for me. It just makes things worse. Whenever I practice breathing, I *hear* my breath and it just reminds me of my abuser breathing hard in my ear while he raped me. I hear his breath all over again and everything comes back. Breathing will never work for me and now you know why."

Humbled by my misguided persistent attempts to teach her mindful breathing, I apologized for my insensitivity, and we moved onto other replacement skills (as well as trauma resolution work later in treatment).

Visualization Techniques

Visualization techniques involve identifying pleasant, relaxing scenes and retrieving them as a self-soothing strategy (Schwartz, 1995). Some clients experience the world in predominantly visual terms and respond especially well to techniques of this type. They will say quite clearly, "Visualization works better for me than any other skill." I find that there are two main types of visualization. One is "reality-based" and the other "fantasy-based." An example of a reality-based scene is the following:

At the Ocean
Close your eyes. . . . Imagine yourself leaving the area where you live . . . leave the daily hassles and the fast pace and demands behind. . . . Imagine

yourself taking an easy ride down back roads to the beach. . . . It is a pleasantly warm day and a relaxing day to drive. As you ride along, you can tell you are getting closer to the beach. The windows in the car are down and you can to smell the salt air and hear the sound of the ocean coming closer. . . .

Find a place on the road to the beach to stop. It is a pleasantly warm near the beach, with just enough of a breeze to make the warmth feel comfortable rather than hot. You get out of the car and begin walking down a path toward the beach, between sand dunes and high grasses that blow back and forth in the breeze. . . . Be aware of your surroundings. . . . Be aware of the pleasant feeling of warmth, a slight wind, and the fresh smell of the ocean. . . .

Now you are out of the dunes and onto the beach. . . . You discover that you have the beach to yourself. . . . Find yourself a pleasant spot where the sand is clean and soft and dry. Lay down your large towel and get settled. Feel the sun resting on you, pleasantly warming you. You feel more and more relaxed.

You can hear the ocean gently breaking on the shore. Occasionally you hear birds call in the distance. The breeze cools you. Before long you feel totally relaxed . . . calm . . . at peace with the world and yourself. This place is your own and you can return to it anytime you want to feel relaxed and at peace.

An example of a fantasy-based scene is the following:

Becoming Water

For this exercise you are asked to imagine that on a pleasantly cool day you are walking up a gently rising mountain. You are going on this hike alone. You have plenty of time to yourself and are feeling relaxed. There is a light breeze and the temperature in the air is just right.

After some time hiking up the path, you reach a large pool of water. On the far end of this pool is a stream that flows down the mountain. You decide to enter this pool of water and find that the water temperature is just right for you, neither too warm nor too cool. You lie down in the water, allowing the water to surround you. You just float and your breathing becomes more and more relaxed. Being in the water is calming and refreshing and soothing.

After some time you have an unusual, pleasant experience. You find that the water surrounding you is so relaxing and peaceful that you feel as if you are becoming more and more like the water and less and less yourself. Your sense of your own body temporarily dissolves as you become more and more water-like. This experience, although unusual, is a pleasant one. You feel more and more relaxed and at peace, as you can let everything go.

As you become more and more like water, you begin to drift through the pool as water. By now you are no longer yourself. For the time being—a brief time—you have become fully water. As water you drift through the pool and down into the stream. As water you flow gently and smoothly down the mountain in the stream bed. As water you flow by and around smooth stones and water plants. You flow around tree roots and pebbles. You flow over sand and around boulders. As water, you stop nowhere and rush nowhere.

Eventually you come to the end of the stream and enter another pool. This pool is like the other: calm and pure and pleasantly refreshing. While in this pool, you slowly begin to resume your normal shape as a person, a human being. You are less and less water and more and more yourself. Finally, you are fully yourself again and are water no more. You get up from the pool and walk back on the land. You feel refreshed, calm, and relaxed.

Some clients strongly prefer scenes that are feasible and derived from their personal experience; others enjoy something more imaginary and fantasy-based. A few individuals seem to like both.

I prefer to introduce visualization in treatment by using a real-world example such as "At the Ocean." If the client finds it relaxing and useful, I then suggest that the client develop his or her own "ideal" scene. This can be done initially during a session, with the client identifying a type of scene and the clinician helping to elicit details. In some instances, the client dictates a scene to the therapist, who types it up verbatim so that the client can take it home at the end of the session. An audio recording is also a good idea.

In treatment sessions or on their own, clients have generated wonderful examples of visualizations, including scenes in the mountains or meadows, sitting in a tulip field, swimming with dolphins, floating on a raft on pond, fly fishing, flying in a glider, etc.

Clients who like the more fantasy-based scenes have generated examples such as flying like a bird or soaring like a condor, floating in clouds, becoming the surf or wind, etc. Either way, clients are more apt to feel a sense of ownership if they develop their own examples.

Visualization can be combined with mindful breathing. Some clients get themselves settled and breathe mindfully for several minutes before retrieving a pleasant scene. Mindful breathing that focuses on counting or "letting go" can get stale with time and visualization can provide a fresh focus.

Rarely, clients develop scenes that are not soothing but counterproductive. For example, I discovered that one client was imagining scenes of violence—which he stated he found quite soothing. I questioned the appropriateness of these scenes and shaped him in the direction of more prosocial content (e.g., listening to guitar music in a cafe). Pastoral scenes would not work for this client; he had never been out of the city. The point is that it is important to monitor the scenes clients are using, lest they go astray into negative or destructive content.

Physical Exercise or Movement

Some clients prefer vigorous physical activity as one of their replacement skills. Adolescents, in particular, are understandably bored by too much sedentary activity. The affectively intense feeling states that dominate the lives of self-injuring people often include significant bursts of adrenaline. Clients may need the assistance of physical activity to bring the intensity of the adrenaline response back within normal limits. The full range of physical exercise options does not need a thorough review here. Suffice it to say that clients use such activities as walking, running, playing basketball, swimming, kayaking, martial arts, lifting weights, and so on, as replacement skills. Some clients use atypical forms of "exercise" as a replacement skill. For example, one client likes to vacuum her house when she feels agitated. She finds the physical movement calms her, the noise distracts her from emotional pain, and after the completion of the vacuuming, she feels a modest sense of accomplishment.

It is important that the preferred mode of exercise be accessible when the client becomes distressed. If the client selects swimming as a replacement skill but the pool is not open during evening hours, an alternative mode of exercise should be selected as a backup.

One recommendation is to avoid violent forms of physical exercise such as boxing or psychodrama activities that express aggressive impulses. The goal of treatment is to arrive at better forms of impulse control. Violent activities are too close to self-inflicted aggression and should be avoided.

Another pitfall that therapists should be aware of are clients who exercise in a self-destructive manner. Some individuals push themselves beyond normal levels of endurance and cause physical injury repeatedly. Not infrequently these are individuals for whom excessive physical exercise is related to an eating disorder. They may restrict their eating, induce vomiting, and exercise compulsively. Eating disorders have been found to be strongly associated with self-injury in a number of empirical studies (Walsh, 1987; Favazza et al., 1989; Warren et al., 1998; Favaro & Santonastaso, 1998, 2000; Rodriguez-Srednicki, 2001; Paul et al., 2002). Therefore, before encouraging exercise as a replacement behavior, the therapist should be careful to assess whether the behavior is within normal limits. Clients who repeatedly report exercise-related injuries may be using exercise in the service of self-destructiveness. The therapist and client can monitor the healthiness of the exercise selected by agreeing to an amount of time and frequency per week.

One form of physical movement that can be useful is walking meditation. This involves walking very slowly and deliberately while concentrating on the breath. Specific instructions for Walking Meditation are provided in the Breathing Manual in Appendix A.

Writing

Writing about the sequence of self-injury has previously been discussed under negative replacement behaviors. There are many other forms of writing that do not have self-injury content and assist individuals in fending off self-harm. Most typically this involves some type of journaling about day-to-day experience. Verbal expression is important because it provides a bedrock for mastery of overwhelming emotions. If the client can begin to distance him- or herself from the immediacy of an experience and write about it, it is a key step in moving toward expressing discomfort rather than acting on it.

Conterio and Lader (1998) have placed more emphasis on writing assignments in the treatment of self-injury than any other authors. In their inpatient treatment program for self-injurers, they require 15 written assignments in sequential order. Their assignments include such topics as an autobiography, a self-appraisal, discussion of the most influential female and male in one's life, the emotions surrounding self-injury, anger, nurturing oneself, saying goodbye to self-injury, and future plans. I have not used this sequence myself in treatment; however, Conterio and Lader report considerable success in their program in reducing and eliminating self-injury. Their writing activities serve as a cornerstone of their treatment approach. Clinicians would do well to read the Conterio and Lader volume and to consider using some or all of the writing assignments in their own treatment, if it is a good match for their clientele.

I have not used the assignments myself, in part, because many of my clients lack adequate verbal skills or organizational abilities. I think the structure and time-limited nature of Conterio and Lader's inpatient unit makes the completion of such assignments more practical than for many other client situations. However, if one's client is verbally adept enough, the Conterio and Lader approach deserves serious consideration.

I sometimes recommend to clients that they keep a "Success Journal" in the form of a written or electronic diary in which they agree to insert a note every day or two regarding a success or accomplishment. The intent of this journal is to direct the client away from thinking pessimistically about self, world, and future, and to celebrate positive steps. Clients initially report feeling that the exercise is awkward and embarrassing; they say they find it excruciatingly difficult to write positive statements about themselves. This difficulty points to their past negative mindset. Particular emphasis should be given in the Success Journal to days in which clients avoid self-injury and practice replacement skills. These days need to be acknowledged and celebrated.

Artistic Expression

Many clients use art as an effective replacement behavior. They do not need to be technically accomplished in order to use artistic expression productively. The client's willingness to use art when triggers occur is the only necessary feature. The therapist should ask if the client is artistically inclined and use the client's preferred medium during a session to assess its utility. The therapist may want to have a variety of art materials in the office in order to try the skill *in vivo*. This does not mean that the therapist becomes an art therapist, but rather that artistic expression is practiced as a possible replacement skill.

I worked with one client who was a talented sculptress. When she experienced key antecedents to self-injury, she chose consistently to work with clay. The physical, visceral sensation of manipulating the clay was very soothing for her. Sometimes she did uncanny self-portraits, at other times she created tortured, twisted, anguished abstract figures that were painful to behold. As she experienced cues that had in the past triggered self-injury, she routinely got out her art supplies and began sculpting. She found that if she worked for 30 minutes to an hour, the more intense urges to self-injure would pass. She could then return to other activities. When art failed to work for this client, she knew that she was especially distressed and needed to contact her therapist or friends for support, structure, and assistance.

Another client used art quite differently. Early in treatment she experienced high levels of stress on a daily basis. When she returned home from work, she developed a ritual of either practicing mindful breathing or drawing in a free-form manner. She found both behaviors to be quite soothing and meditative. Each day she selected one or the other depending on her mood or intuition. If she felt more agitated or "antsy," she tended to select the activity of drawing; if she felt more morose or contemplative, she did mindful breathing. This simple skill set was transforming for the client. Her self-injury dropped off to zero, and she experienced the added benefit of improving her artwork due to all the practice.

Playing or Listening to Music

Music is a key replacement skill for many individuals. In general, active participation is better than passive listening. Although one can listen to music quite mindfully, with full attention and concentration, playing an instrument is a more engaged, participatory skill. I have encountered only a few self-injurers who were accomplished musicians. One was a cello player who used playing as a form of expression and emotional regulation. On multiple occasions she was able to defer self-injuring by playing. However, music for her was also an arena of self-imposed perfectionistic demands, so playing "poorly" sometimes made her feel worse.

Most clients I have encountered use music as a replacement skill via listening. Listening to music can be problematic as a replacement skill because it tends to be done with partial attention. "Half-listening" to music is likely to have little effect on emotional distress. Clients can learn to listen to music mindfully by focusing deliberately and intensively on melody, specific instruments, dynamics, cadence, vocals, beat, harmony, etc. Adolescents often prefer listening to music to almost any other replacement skill. I urge them to develop more active, participatory skills such as mindful breathing, visualization, or creating art.

It is important to monitor music selection with adolescents. Some clients choose aggressive, violent music that makes them feel angrier or more agitated. Others listen to music that is maudlin and sad, thereby amplifying their feelings of depression and isolation.

Listening to music is often more of a diversion technique than a true self-soothing skill. It can be very productive but should be monitored closely so that it does not become a way of avoiding more active, engaged skills practice.

Communicating with Others

Communicating with others is obviously a useful alternative to self-injury, but it should be structured as to specifics. Details need to be identified as to who the others are, their availability, judgment and influence, supportiveness, and patience. If possible, these others should be trained in replacement skills, as discussed in the section above on engaging family members in treatment. The content of the talk is important as well. Too much aimless venting without a shift to skills practice is counterproductive. Some forms of communication can be clearly conducive to self-injury. For example:

One client, when she was depressed and inclined to cut herself, would call a "friend" who would belittle her. As soon as he heard her voice on the phone, he would begin mocking her as a "psycho" who was "so needy, stupid, and incompetent." This demeaning talk would go on for half an hour or more as the client became ever more depressed and hopeless. In her case, calling the male friend was not a replacement skill but part of her self-injuring sequence. During the assessment process, she identified these phone calls as a key antecedent that she needed to avoid. As an alternative, we developed a list of five nurturing people she should call in a prescribed order related to their likely availability and judgment.

The greatest assets are friends or family members who understand what triggers the self-injury of the client and will talk him or her through the urges to self-harm. These people can be at least as useful as clinicians because they are more available and likely to remain engaged for years. It is useful to bring these significant others into sessions when the client agrees and to use them as coaches and allies. They can be taught reinforcement principles regarding the behaviors they should especially reward and those to place on extinction. They can be very helpful in reducing any cues that they themselves provide to the self-injury sequence. Of course, friends and family members are not just ancillary therapists; their main role is to care and support with no specific strategic goals in mind.

One client who particularly used communication with others well was a 42-year-old female. With her best friend, who was of similar age, she could share almost anything. Her friend knew extensive details about the client's abuse history, related self-injury, divorce, and so on. When the client had strong urges to cut herself, she frequently called her friend and described the emotions she was experiencing. This friend had had her own challenges and was able to empathize and support. She also had a black sense of humor that was excellent in diffusing tension and panic. Over time, the client had shared the skills she had learned in therapy, and the friend would prompt her. Although I never met this friend, I considered her my co-therapist. She provided hours of support and good judgment that went way beyond my psychotherapeutic influence.

For clients who have very limited social skills and little or no social supports, hot lines can provide useful guidance. Many hotlines have the distinct advantage of being available 24 hours a day. Some hotlines are much better than others at tolerating what they call "frequent" or "regular callers." Hotline staff can consider recurrent callers a distraction from their main business, which is to save those in life-threatening crises. Other hotlines are quite willing to talk with the same caller several times per week and view it as consistent with their mission or "befriending role" (e.g., the Samaritans hotline). For more isolated clients, the therapist should locate a hotline that is receptive to regular callers and suggest it as a resource. For some clients the sound of a human voice is far more soothing than text in an e-mail.

Therapists should assess whether clients frequent chat rooms that focus on self-injury. More often than not, such chat rooms are venues for the sharing of lurid details about the methods of self-injury, the extent of wounds, the amount of blood, the length of scars, etc. A competitive one-upsmanship atmosphere can flourish in these sites that is clearly triggering.

Occasionally, I have heard clients talk about a small chat room where several individuals help each other with recovery. The therapist should assess whether the chat rooms are a help or part of the problem.

Diversion Techniques

Diversion techniques are means of deflecting attention from thoughts, plans, and urges to self-injure. This is a very idiosyncratic category of replacement skills. I have had clients who watch TV, pet their cat, groom their dog, play solitaire, clean the house, play video games, wash the car, make brownies, read a book, knit, quilt, and even one who reviewed new tax laws as a diversion.

Clients need to have multiple diversion techniques in their repertoire, because what works in one situation will be irrelevant in another. The main point that needs to be made about diversion techniques is that they are *not* a high-order replacement skill. They really serve to temporize and fend off rather than to solve. Diversion techniques generally do not have a major self-soothing function; they do not really compete with self-injury in terms of potential relief from affective distress or emptiness. Therefore, clients should be encouraged to have replacement skills other than this set. The limitations of diversion techniques are well indicated in the next example.

Scott, age 16, was not about to try mindful breathing or visualization. He called them "psychobabble" and laughed uproariously whenever they were suggested. Scott was only willing to use diversion techniques. He agreed to play video games, surf the net, and shoot a basketball when he started to feel like burning or cutting himself. He also decided to listen to music, primarily very vigorous punk rock. The problem with these activities for Scott was that he already did them quite frequently. They were so familiar he could do them and still think about self-injury.

Because his rate of self-injury was in no way declining, Scott decided to try a new diversion technique: walk to the mall, which was over 2 miles away from his home. This technique was modestly more successful, perhaps because it involved physical exercise and was novel enough to distract him. He found looking at people and passing cars sufficiently engaging to redirect his thoughts from themes of self-injury. However, Scott's treatment needed to move beyond diversion techniques in order for him to make real improvement.

Generally clients rely on diversion techniques before they have learned the new skills of negative replacement behaviors, mindful breathing, visualization, writing, artistic expression, and communicating with others. In order for clients to reduce and eliminate self-injury, they need to learn to calm themselves and to focus. Diversion techniques do not teach either element in a truly transformative way.

TRACKING THE USE OF SKILLS AS REPLACEMENT BEHAVIORS

Now that skills have been selected, practiced, and employed in the real world, it is important in treatment to monitor their use. In Chapter 7, a Brief Self-Injury Log was introduced to track the five types of antecedents and consequences for self-injury. This same format can now be used to monitor the use of skills as replacements for self-injury As with Figure 7.2 in Chapter 7, the Brief Skills Practice Log in Figure 9.2 tracks the environmental, biological, cognitive, affective, and behavioral antecedents for impulses to self-injure. However, now the emphasis shifts to which skills are utilized in the place of self-injury. Please refer to the end of Chapter 7 for the case example that is again employed here, with a new focus on replacement behaviors.

As the completed log in Figure 9.3 shows, the 16-year-old client used two main replacement skills in place of self-injuring. She did mindful breathing in the school library and communicated with her guidance counselor. These skills, along with some cognitive self-instruction ("I have to calm down"), helped her avoid cutting. These behaviors were reinforced in that she obtained a sense of relief and rewarded herself by saying, "Phew, I actually didn't cut myself!"

Name: _____

Dimension	Antecedents	Skills employed	Aftermath
Environmental			
Biological			
Cognitive			
Affective			
Behavioral			

FIGURE 9.2. Brief Skills Practice Log.

Name: <u>16-year-old female</u>

Dimension	Antecedents	Skills employed	Aftermath
Environmental	Argument with friend at school 1	Distanced from friend 4	No further contact with friend 5
Biological	Already overtired; not high; had a headache 5	Still overtired, but didn't smoke grass 5	Headache gone; slept better later 4
Cognitive	"I'm all alone; I have no friends" 3	"I have to calm down!" 2	"Phew! I actually didn't cut myself!" 2
Affective	Felt sad, empty, panicked 2	Very anxious; wanted to cut, wanted to avoid it 3	Felt much calmer; obtained relief 1
Behavioral	Decided not to do the usual cutting 4	Did mindful breathing in school library; talked with guidance counselor; returned to class one period later 1	Talked with friend about the conflict later; friend reassured me that we're still friends 3

FIGURE 9.3. Example of a completed Brief Skills Practice Log.

This simple assessment tool should be reviewed with clients early in each session. Clients should continue to complete this form on a weekly basis until skills are used so automatically that they no longer need to be monitored. Deciding to discontinue formal skills monitoring should be considered a "graduation" that can be celebrated in the therapy.

When a relapse of self-injury occurs, the clinician should ask the client to temporarily complete both a Brief Self-Injury Log and a Brief Skills Practice Log. When the acts of self-injury cease for several weeks, the completion of the Brief Self-Injury Log can be discontinued.

USING E-MAIL TO SUPPORT SKILLS

I find that e-mail serves as a useful support in assisting clients to learn and employ skills. When clients have access to an e-mail account, I obtain permission in the first session to contact them. I use e-mail to prompt practice and to exchange feedback between sessions. E-mail is far less intrusive than phone calls for both parties. It permits a reasonably prompt response without interrupting one's daily life for an extended phone conversation. In prompting clients to practice their skills, the therapist needs to strike the right balance. Clients do not want to feel nagged or coerced, but they do want to feel supported. The therapist can ask if the client would like a reminder regarding skills practice every few days. What happens most frequently over time is that the therapist and client exchange a couple of e-mails between sessions. The client briefly describes situations in his or her life and which skills have been tapped as coping measures. In turn, the therapist offers support and reinforcement and makes suggestions for improvements in using the skills. It is very important that the therapist emphasize skill acquisition and practice in e-mails rather than detailed discussion of life situations; these should be saved for therapy sessions. The therapist particularly wants to avoid reinforcing any venting or complaining that does not lead to skills practice. Of course, it is important that the clinician notify the client when he or she will be electronically unavailable. Also the client should be advised not to expect immediate responses from the therapist.

SIGNIFICANT OTHERS AS TREATMENT ALLIES

Treatment often involves significant others. It is very helpful when family members or friends actively practice skills with clients. The skills to be learned are generally "living skills" that almost anyone can use productively. For example, many family members report using mindful breathing skills themselves, although they originally learned them to support the client. Significant others can also play the important role of prompting the client to practice and reminding the client to use skills when he or she is distressed. Skills practice gives families a new arena for positive interaction and shifts their attention away from a problem focus. With adolescent clients, parents need to be judicious with their prompts; too many reminders can be counterproductive, producing an aversion to practice.

CONCLUSION

In summary, when teaching replacement skills to self-injurers, it is generally most helpful if clinicians and others:

- Select skills with the client that are relevant, appealing, developmentally appropriate, and effective.
- Draw from the nine categories of replacement skills.
- Downplay reliance on negative replacement skills, because these run the risk of triggering episodes.
- Identify and monitor a very specific practice schedule.
- Use the Brief Skills Practice Log when possible.
- Prompt and monitor practice via e-mail or assistance from significant others.
- Reinforce the client enthusiastically for ongoing skills practice.

CHAPTER 10

Cognitive Treatment

Cognitive treatment targets the thoughts, assumptions, rules, attitudes, and core beliefs that support self-injury. As discussed in Chapter 5, thoughts are one of the five key determinants of self-injury, along with environmental, biological, affective, and behavioral elements. Thoughts, in their myriad forms, play a fundamental role in the onset and continuation of self-injury. Cognitive processes always precede the emotions and behaviors associated with cutting, excoriation, self-burning, self-hitting, and so on. Cognitions need to be identified and targeted in order for treatment to be comprehensive and successful.

Cognitive therapies are among the most empirically supported available. They have the advantage of having undergone considerable replication. Cognitive treatment is structured, sequential, reasonably standardized, and sometimes manualized. It is also fairly simple, direct, and easy to learn.

Cognitive therapy has been documented to be effective in treating diverse problems, including depression and suicidality (Beck et al., 1979; Freeman & Reinecke, 1993), anxiety (Clark, 1986), eating disorders (Garner & Bemis, 1985; Garner, Vitousek, & Pike, 1997; Wilson, Fairburn, & Agras, 1997), trichotillomania (Rothbaum & Ninan, 1999; Keuthen et al., 2001), personality disorders (Beck & Freeman, 2003), posttraumatic stress disorder (Foa & Rothbaum, 1998; Rothbaum, Meadows, Resick, & Foy, 2000; Follette, Ruzek, & Abueg, 1998), and schizophrenia (Kingdon & Turkington, 1994).

J. S. Beck (1995) has provided a concise summary of the conceptualization on which cognitive therapy is based. A brief version of her diagrammatic presentation of the cognitive model is presented in Figure 10.1. In doing a cognitive assessment of self-injury, the therapist generally starts at

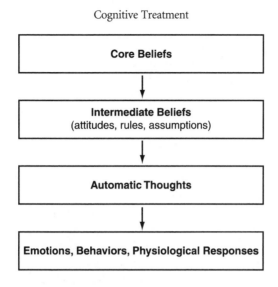

FIGURE 10.1. Cognitive model.

the bottom of the sequence and moves up. At the outset, the clinician ana-
lyzes the self-injury behavior itself, along with the emotions and physiological responses that precede and follow it. This aspect of assessment is discussed in Chapter 7. Next, the analysis considers the automatic thoughts,
followed by intermediate beliefs, and ending with core beliefs. These terms
require some explication.

AUTOMATIC THOUGHTS

Automatic thoughts are the actual words or images that go through a person's mind. They are the most immediate form of thought and are situation
specific (Beck, 1995). This form of thinking can be so fleeting and routinized that it becomes "automatic," hence the terminology. As noted in Chapter 7, an example of an automatic thought is the self-instruction that occurs
when one is driving a car, such as, "I need to put on my left blinker now."
This type of thought becomes so familiar and habitual that it often occurs
out of conscious awareness.

INTERMEDIATE BELIEFS

Intermediate beliefs are comprised of attitudes, rules, and assumptions
(Beck, 1995). These aspects of cognition serve as connections or linkages

between automatic thoughts and core beliefs. Using the same example, an attitude might be, "It is important to drive safely." A related rule might be, "Always put on the blinker before turning." And an assumption would be, "If I drive safely, I am unlikely to get into an accident."

CORE BELIEFS

Core beliefs are the most fundamental and pervasively influential form of thinking. They tend to be global, firmly held, not easily subject to revision, and "overgeneralized" (Beck, 1995, p. 16). Core beliefs are often fundamental convictions about the cognitive triad of self, world, and future (Beck et al., 1979; Rush & Nowells, 1994). Beck (1995) has suggested that counterproductive core beliefs tend to fall into the two basic categories of incompetence (e.g., "I'm stupid") and unlovability (e.g., "I have no friends"). An example of a core belief related to driving would be, "I am a competent person (and therefore likely to be a good driver)."

Not surprisingly, when the above conceptual model is employed in working with self-injurers, the cognitions identified are often pejorative in nature. When a thorough cognitive analysis is performed with self-injuring clients, complex layers of negative, pessimistic core beliefs, attitudes, rules, assumptions, and automatic thoughts often emerge. Provided below are examples of such thoughts and beliefs associated with self-injury using Beck's cognitive model.

In beginning to work on the cognitive antecedents and consequences that support self-injury, the therapist has to start with education by showing the client Figure 10.1 and explaining the content. For most clients, the material is easily understood, but for a few it can be too complex. The illustrative examples of cognitions should be tailored to the client's individual situation. Thus clients who do not drive may need an example such as brushing teeth, getting dressed, cooking, or feeding the cat. Once familiar nonthreatening examples of cognitions have been discussed (e.g., driving a car), examples related to self-injury can be identified, as shown in Figure 10.2.

In addition, the therapist needs to explain the following aspects of cognitive treatment to the client:

- Thoughts are important in maintaining self-injury; they precede feelings and behavior.
- Thoughts are multilayered, complex, and take time and work to understand.

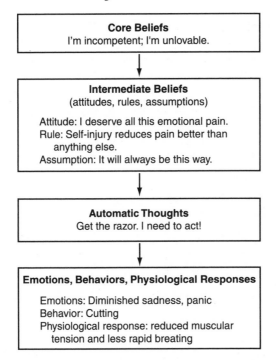

FIGURE 10.2. An example of the cognitive model for a self-injuring person.

- The therapist and client will employ "collaborative empiricism" as a method of proceeding in treatment (Belsher & Wilkes, 1994; Beck, 1995).
- Thoughts occur in the present (i.e., automatic thoughts) but are also derived from long-term personal history (i.e., core beliefs).
- Thoughts are not facts (Rush & Nowells, 1994; Beck, 1995), but they may be fueled by influential, powerful opinions.
- Dysfunctional thoughts that support self-injury can be, and need to be, changed over the course of treatment.
- The therapist will *not* challenge the client's thoughts cavalierly or label them as wrong or incorrect; the client will not hear, "It's all in your head" (Linehan, 1993a).
- Thoughts *will be* discussed in terms of whether they assist or hinder a client in reaching his or her goals.

Empathy, warmth, support, and validation are centrally important parts of cognitive therapy. If the client doesn't feel understood and supported, the therapy is unlikely to work and should be improved. The client is urged to communicate any deficiencies in this area to the therapist.

The assessment of thoughts that support self-injury occurs as part of the behavioral analysis. Eliciting automatic thoughts takes persistent, respectful questioning, given that clients often initially report that the self-injury "just happened." In addition to the example presented in the section on cognitive antecedents in Chapter 7, the following excerpt demonstrates the process of identifying automatic thoughts (and related core beliefs) tied to self-injury:

THERAPIST: So tell me about hitting yourself with the wire. What lead up to that?

CLIENT: Sam had just called and put me down, and I was feeling so low and useless.

THERAPIST: That must have been painful.

CLIENT: It was. I was just feeling so tired and hopeless and alone.

THERAPIST: How did hitting yourself affect those feelings?

CLIENT: It made me feel better and then worse.

THERAPIST: Explain, please.

CLIENT: At first I felt so much better. It got the anger and the sadness out. Now it was on the outside instead of inside. I looked at the welts on my back in the mirror and it was such a relief.

THERAPIST: I can see why you are drawn to hitting yourself, given that it provides so much relief.

CLIENTS: Yes.

THERAPIST: But you said it also made you feel worse. What do you mean?

CLIENT: Afterward I regretted doing it. I just felt, "You're such a loser. There you go hitting yourself again. That's not going to help anything."

THERAPIST: Good, I'm glad to see you starting to challenge the behavior of striking yourself. What were you thinking right *before* you hit yourself . . . right after you hung up the phone?

CLIENT: It wasn't good. I was thinking, "What a piece of shit! No one loves me, and no one ever will."

THERAPIST: Okay, those sound like the core beliefs we've talked about. What were you thinking *immediately* after you got off the phone.

CLIENT: I was thinking, "You're such a piece of shit! You should be whipped and struck until it hurts."

THERAPIST: Wow, what a sequence of thoughts. You must have been in a lot of emotional pain.

CLIENT: I was.

THERAPIST: Let's look very specifically at the automatic thought in this situation, which appears to be, "You should be whipped and struck until it hurts."

CLIENT: (*sarcastically*) Oh, that sounds like fun!

THERAPIST: (*mirroring*) Yes, doesn't it? I can see why you come here! It's so lighthearted!

In this sequence the therapist is careful to provide a lot of empathy and support. The dialogue has produced a lot of helpful information. Core beliefs are referenced when the client states, "No one loves me, and no one ever will." But beyond that are the cognitions that immediately preceded the self-flagellation, the automatic thought of "You should be whipped and struck until it hurts."

IDENTIFYING RECURRENT AUTOMATIC THOUGHTS RELATED TO SELF-INJURY

In identifying automatic thoughts, it is important to determine which are the recurrent "favorites." For the client above, the sequence of a core belief ("You're an unlovable piece of shit") was frequently followed by the *attitude* ("You deserve what you get"), a *rule* ("Self-injury is the only way to get relief"), and an *assumption* ("It will always be this way"). Concluding this sequence is the *automatic thought* ("You should be whipped and struck until it hurts").

Over the course of treatment, the recurrent automatic thoughts become cues for the client (1) to recognize that self-injury is about to occur, and (2) to practice replacement skills *immediately* as an alternative. Thus the automatic thought can be reframed as a "welcomed opportunity" to practice skills and escape the repetitive cycle of self-injury with all its sequelae. With the client above, we agreed that she would practice "Letting go of . . . breathing" (see Chapter 9) when she had thoughts of deserving to be whipped or struck. If using that skill proved too difficult or ineffective, she agreed to call a close friend or walk rapidly around the block until her urge to self-flagellate diminished. This was one among several strategies used in assisting her to give up self-harm.

Particularly important types of automatic thoughts are self-instructions that immediately precede self-injury. These are the thoughts related to the *mechanics* of inflicting self-harm. A sequence of thoughts including self-instructional details may resemble those presented in Figure 10.3. The self-instructional details often include automatic thoughts about whether or not to use a tool, where to inflict self-harm on the body, in what room, etc. A few specific details are often key to providing momentum to the self-injury sequence. For example, a person may always lock the door to her bedroom before self-injuring. This may be a powerful self-instructional cue or trigger to begin the self-harm sequence. Once the door is locked, the person feels "safe" to self-injure and is unlikely to stop. Working with the client to no longer lock the bedroom door may help reduce the rate of self-injury (assuming there are no other privacy considerations). Thus, eliciting automatic thoughts regarding self-instructional details can be important in interrupting established habits and designing treatment interventions.

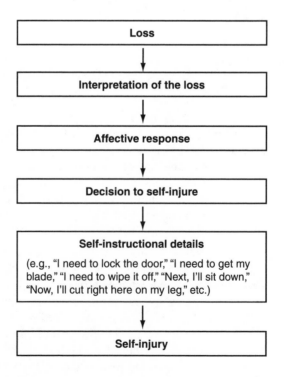

FIGURE 10.3. Cognitive processes in a self-injury sequence.

COLLABORATIVE EMPIRICISM

Automatic thoughts also need to be subjected to intensive empirical analysis in the course of treatment. Cognitive therapy emphasizes looking at the evidence with the client regarding thoughts that support self-injury. For example, the therapist can ask the client, quite supportively, for the evidence that she is "a piece of shit, unlovable, and deserving to be flogged." Being asked to provide evidence for their negative cognitions is enough for some clients to back off from unreasonable, distorted thoughts. They may say, "I know I don't really deserve it, but I sure feel that way sometimes."

However, if the client continues to endorse such beliefs and attitudes, the therapist can gently question the legitimacy of these statements by pointing out some of the client's positive features. Although many clients may initially respond to affirmative feedback with uneasy discomfort, most covertly relish it. They have so heard so little about their positive qualities over the years that experiencing praise is both gratifying and restorative. The following is an example of the therapist inserting supportive, positive statements in the course of evaluating the accuracy of automatic thoughts:

THERAPIST: You've said that immediately preceding whipping yourself, you thought, "You should be whipped and struck until it hurts." In using the strategy of collaborative empiricism, where is the evidence that this punishment "should" happen?

CLIENT: Well, there are many times when I feel like I've never done anything right in my life.

THERAPIST: Do you consider taking care of your mother doing something right?

CLIENT: Yes, I guess so. She needs a lot of help these days.

THERAPIST: Right, and you provide it. That is a major strength of yours. What about you as a friend? Do you bring any assets to being a friend?

CLIENT: I'm loyal and I don't give up on someone.

THERAPIST: Your friend Angie is a good example of that, wouldn't you say? You're always there for her.

CLIENT: (embarrassed) Hmm.

THERAPIST: I know you can't take too much positive feedback, but let me push your limits just a bit here. What about you as an employee? Are you dependable and dedicated?

CLIENT: (*laughing nervously*) All right, all right, enough already!

THERAPIST: A one-word answer would be fine on this one!

CLIENT: Yes, I'm a pretty good employee.

THERAPIST: If we were to do a positive versus negative chart here regarding "should be whipped until it hurts," where would we be right now?

CLIENT: Okay, I see your point. I guess I do have some strengths.

THERAPIST: You certainly do.

EVALUATING THOUGHTS AND BELIEFS

Another technique to deal with dysfunctional cognitions is evaluation. As suggested by Beck (1995), it is useful to ask an individual *how much* he or she believes a particular thought; this can be quantified on a scale from 0 to 100%. Thoughts held with considerable conviction (e.g., 70% or greater) need special attention if they have an important role in self-injury. The strategy is not to directly challenge the thoughts because this can be experienced as invalidating ("You're saying I'm wrong or stupid"). Rather, the therapist shapes the individual to take a more dispassionate, evaluative look at his or her own thoughts and to reach his or her own conclusions. The goal is to reduce the client's level of conviction regarding a dysfunctional thought or belief. Beck (1995) suggests that when clients say their belief in a particular thought declines to 30% or less, the "power" of that thought to deploy a dysfunctional behavior is generally of less concern.

QUESTIONING THOUGHTS AND BELIEFS

Beyond quantifying how much an individual *believes* a particular thought is the process of considering the evidence. Belief involves conviction and emotion. Evidence concerns *the facts*. Considering the evidence in this manner is often referred to as using the Socratic method (Belsher & Wilkes, 1994; Beck, 1995). This approach involves the therapist asking a series of incremental questions about the thoughts and beliefs that justify self-injury. In my experience one of the most common automatic thoughts that precedes self-injury is "Cutting [or other self-injury] is the only effective solution." Conterio and Lader (1998, pp. 228–236) have identified other thoughts that they believe are frequently associated with, and justify, self-injury.

"Self-injury doesn't hurt anyone."
"It's my body and I can do whatever I want."
"Giving up self-injury will only make me hurt more."
"The scars remind me of the battle."
"It's the best way to show others my pain."
"No one knows I self-injure anyway."
"It keeps people away."
"It's the only way to know if people really care about me."
"Negative attention is better than none."
"I need to be punished—I'm bad."
"If I don't self-injure, I'll kill myself."

Conterio and Lader's list shows the diversity of the thoughts and beliefs that support self-injurious behavior.

When the time is right, the therapist should question these thoughts and beliefs by asking gently worded questions that seek the evidence. The following list responds in order, to Conterio and Lader's examples:

"When you say that no one is hurt by your self-injury, what about your-self? Are there physical and emotional effects? Why don't you merit protection and safety?"
"What else reminds you of 'the battle' beyond your scars? I often think you have a vivid memory . . . do you agree?"
"What other skills do you sometimes use to let people know you're in pain?"
"Even if you no one else knows you self-injure, what do *you* deserve?"
"Is keeping people away *really* what you want in the long term? When you need space in the short term, what other techniques have you used that were effective?"
"You sometimes say that X cares about you. How does X show you that [he or she] cares even when you haven't self-injured?"
"Does self-injury ever cause those you care about to withdraw? What are some of the best ways to get attention from these people?"
"Haven't you been punished a lot in life already? What are some examples? Why would any more be justified?"
"Are they any other options or skills that can be used beyond suicide and self-injury? What are they? What are some of the skills we've been practicing?"

SHIFTING FROM DYSFUNCTIONAL THOUGHTS
AND BELIEFS TO ADAPTIVE COGNITIONS

Challenging dysfunctional thoughts and beliefs is designed to bring into question the processes that support self-injury. An additional key step is to identify, practice, and integrate more positive and adaptive thoughts and beliefs. A useful exercise to conduct with clients is to map out their automatic thoughts, intermediate beliefs, and core beliefs and to identify more effective cognitions. Like most new activities, at first the exercise may seem

---

Client's name ___A 22-year-old female___   Date ___November X___

Cognitions that support self-injury   ### Alternative adaptive thoughts

I. Key automatic thoughts

With these emotions I need to cut now.   I can use my new skills to manage emotions.

Self-injury provides such quick relief.   Self-injury has long-term negative effects.

Self-injury causes others to respond to me.   Self-injury causes many people to avoid me.

II. Intermediate beliefs

A. Attitudes

I deserve this rejection.   I deserve someone who treats me with respect.

I deserve to hurt myself.   I deserve to protect myself.

B. Rules

Self-injury is the best solution.   Self-injury is one of many solutions and not necessarily the best.

Self-injury works immediately.   I can live with some discomfort while I use my skills. I can surf the urge to self-injure.

C. Assumptions

It's hopeless. I can't change.   I've already made a number of important changes.

III. Core beliefs

I'm unlovable.   A number of people truly care for me.

I'm incompetent.   I'm a competent worker, cook, and gardener.

I'm a loser.   No more global putdowns! They are distorted and inaccurate!

FIGURE 10.4. Examples of a completed Before and After Cognition Chart: Changing the thoughts that support self-injury.

artificial and contrived. Only with practice and reinforcement from the therapist (and significant others) does the exercise become meaningful.

Figure 10.4 is an example of a completed Before and After Cognition Chart. This chart—in blank form (Figure 10.5)—can be used with any client to begin the shift to more adaptive thoughts and beliefs. The therapist should monitor the percentage of belief (0–100%) that the client has for the new thoughts, as described above.

This example of a Before and After Cognition Chart was not exhaustive for this particular client. She had had years of experience with self-

---

Client's name _____   Date _____

Cognitions that support self-injury   **Alternative adaptive thoughts**

I. Key automatic thoughts

II. Intermediate beliefs
A. Attitudes

B. Rules

C. Assumptions

III. Core beliefs

FIGURE 10.5. Before and After Cognition Chart: Changing the thoughts that support self-injury.

denigrating cognitions that were associated with hopelessness, depression, and self-injury. Nonetheless, the negative beliefs and automatic thoughts on the left-hand side of the table were her "favorites" that especially needed to be challenged. The client became convinced of the wisdom of this strategy and actively practiced both identifying the emergence of negative thoughts and substituting the more positive replacements. Not surprisingly, her commitment to this effort resulted in considerable progress in reducing the rate of her self-injury.

IDENTIFYING AND MODIFYING
OTHER COGNITIVE DISTORTIONS

The errors that clients make in their thinking often go way beyond those that are directly associated with self-injury. Clients may frequently experience recurrent negative, distorted cognitions that produce generalized emotional distress. In the process of treating self-injury, these cognitions need to be targeted because they play an important role in the diminished quality of life for clients. Chronic psychological pain derived from generalized distorted cognitions can foster such problems as substance abuse, risk-taking behaviors, withdrawal and isolation, interpersonal conflict, job loss, educational failure, etc.

Albert Ellis was a pioneer in identifying irrational thought patterns that trigger emotional pain (e.g., Ellis, 1962). Aaron T. Beck has further elaborated on these cognitions, as summarized by Judith S. Beck (1995). Some of the generalized cognitive distortions that commonly occur in self-injuring clients are provided below (adapted from J. Beck, 1995, p. 119). An example from clinical practice is provided for each type of cognitive distortion:

- All-or-nothing thinking—for example, "Either he loves everything about me or we can't continue dating."
- Catastrophizing—for example, "I feel under the weather. It must be cancer."
- Discounting the positive—for example, "If I did well at it, it must have been too easy. I bet my boss arranged this success to build my self-esteem. What a phony."
- Emotional reasoning—for example, "I believe this so deeply, it must be true."
- Labeling—for example, "I'm a borderline, how do you expect me to act normally?"

- Mental filter—for example, "One detail went wrong with the project; therefore the whole thing should be destroyed."
- Overgeneralization—for example, "This person repeatedly ignores me; therefore no one loves me."
- Personalization—for example, "When my teacher passed me in the hall today, she didn't even look at me. I must have offended her."
- Should or must statements—for example, "I should [or must] always do an excellent job on my schoolwork or I am incompetent, lazy, and hopeless."
- Tunnel vision—for example, "I am in so much pain right now that the other positives in my life are irrelevant, all but nonexistent."

Generalized cognitive distortions of this type need to be gently challenged. Using the process of collaborative empiricism, clinician and client need to examine the evidence that supports or disconfirms such thought processes. More often than not, there is little evidence in support of such generalized distortions, and they become self-invalidating. As noted above, the goal is to bring the client's belief in such distorted thoughts down to 30% or less so that their influence is diminished.

At times such distortions are so patently absurd that humor can be used to diffuse them. This must be done cautiously and skillfully, however, because it is all too easy for clients to mistake humor for ridicule. Nonetheless, when humor is employed effectively, it can provide both the client and therapist some much needed comic relief.

CLIENT: (*entering the session and sitting down opposite the therapist*): My stomach hurts.

THERAPIST: That's too bad. You seem to say that a lot when you first come in.

CLIENT: Yes, it happens almost every time. I bet it's cancer.

THERAPIST: Cancer! That's an alarming thought! Why cancer? Do you have any other symptoms, such as bleeding, vomiting, or inability to eat?

CLIENT: No.

THERAPIST: Do you experience this pain at other times when you're not in the office?

CLIENT: No, but I still think it's cancer.

THERAPIST: Hmm. Why not leprosy, an ulcer, or evil spirits?

CLIENT: (*laughing*) You're making fun of me!

THERAPIST: (*also laughing*) A little bit!

CLIENT: You're accusing me of, what do you call it, "catastrophizing?"

THERAPIST: Good memory! I'm not "accusing" you, but I am wondering . . .

CLIENT: Okay, maybe I'm exaggerating a little bit, but I do get anxious when I first come in.

THERAPIST: That's understandable. Does it tend to pass after a few minutes?

CLIENT: Yes, thank God.

THERAPIST: Good! You know I don't think cancer passes after a few minutes.

CLIENT: (*laughing again*) Okay, enough about cancer this week! But I may have it again next week.

MODIFYING CORE BELIEFS: BEYOND COGNITIVE STRATEGIES

In my opinion the most difficult part of cognitive therapy is challenging the core beliefs of self-injuring clients. By definition, core beliefs are the bedrock of cognitive processes. They are derived from early life history, tend to be firmly held, are not amenable to quick revision, and are fundamental to the additional layers of intermediate beliefs and automatic thoughts. Aaron Beck has proposed that dysfunctional core beliefs fall into the two general categories of incompetence and unlovability (as quoted in Beck, 1995). Examples of helplessness core beliefs are "I am helpless . . . powerless . . . weak . . . out of control . . . needy . . . incompetent . . . or defective." Examples of unlovable core beliefs include "I am unlovable . . . unlikable . . . undesirable . . . unattractive . . . not good enough . . . bad . . . different . . . crazy . . . easily left or abandoned" (modified version of Beck, 1995, p. 169).

My experience in trying to modify core beliefs is that cognitive strategies alone (e.g., collaborative empiricism; identifying, evaluating, and modifying beliefs; using before and after thinking exercises) are sometimes *not* sufficient. The core beliefs of some self-injurers—particularly those who are trauma survivors—are so profoundly self-denigrating and engrained that they are nearly impossible to modify with cognitive strategies alone. (This outcome may reflect my deficiencies as a cognitive therapist or point to the limitations of the cognitive approach, or both). Such clients may understand on an intellectual level that their thoughts are irrational, distorted, or overgeneralized, but they find themselves believing in them with great conviction nonetheless.

To overcome such deeply held core beliefs, the therapeutic process sometimes needs to draw on some fundamental aspect of the therapeutic *relationship* that cannot be termed a "technical intervention." The relationship itself becomes the therapeutic vehicle that is restorative for the client, enabling a slow but sure modification of dysfunctional core beliefs. I do not think that this aspect of treatment is normally described by cognitive therapists as an element in the therapeutic process—perhaps because it is not amenable to empirical evaluation. In personal communication with Judith Beck, she agreed that cognitive therapists tend not to address this topic as a technical aspect of cognitive therapy (personal communication, 2004).

When explicating this aspect of the therapeutic relationship, I like to use the metaphor of "the gift." Of course, by "gift" I am not referring to any sort of object or commodity or present. Instead I am intending some sort of sustained aspect of the therapeutic relationship that serves to counter and replace core beliefs about helplessness or unlovability, or both. The gift consists of those positive life-sustaining features or characteristics that the therapist can share and pass over to the client during the therapeutic process. The gift involves the therapist affirming, in some fundamental, subtle, sustained way, that the client is both lovable and competent. This message must be conveyed in a caring, professional manner that is entirely within the boundaries of an appropriate therapeutic relationship.

For example, one client of mine was a severe trauma survivor. Her father had inflicted sexual intercourse on her for a 10-year period from ages 5 to 15. Not only did she endure this trauma, but in addition, she lived daily with the knowledge that her mother was aware of the abuse and did nothing to intervene. The client's core beliefs were that she was ugly, despicable, unlovable, and expendable. By age 20 she was overweight, self-loathing, substance abusing, chronically self-injuring, and occasionally self-mutilating (i.e., beyond self-injuring). Early in treatment she would often sit on the floor in my office rocking back and forth, saying how ugly and disgusting she was. From time to time, in response to all this suffering and incapacitation, I said to this client, despite all the challenges, "I have faith in you." Several years later, after a successfully concluded treatment, she reported that these words had had a restorative effect for her, that she repeated them in her mind over and over again and eventually took them to be her own. For this client, the words "I have faith in you" were "the gift." I find it difficult to describe this "intervention" in technical terms used by cognitive therapists.

Another example of "the gift" concerned the client referenced above as self-flagellating. She too had an extensive trauma history at the hands of a grandfather and next-door neighbor. Her preferred form of self-injury was striking herself with a wire until deep welts appeared on her back, after which she felt better. Her core beliefs included the ideas that she was invisible, unimportant, and homely. The gift for this client involved a transaction. Midway through the treatment, she encountered some significant financial troubles and had to declare bankruptcy to clear her debts. She told me she would have to drop out of treatment because she had no means to pay me. As an alternative, I arranged that she pay me in artwork. She was an accomplished painter. At the time I had moved into a new office and needed new decorations for various walls. I honestly appreciated her talent and wanted to support it. Not only was she able to continue treatment, but she saw her art prominently displayed in common areas of my office space. No more was she invisible, insignificant, and homely. The beauty of her talent was everywhere for others to see and appreciate.

I realize for some readers the notion of "the gift" may be much too "soft" and nonempirical. If they are able to point to ways in which the cognitive approach stipulates restorative aspects of the therapeutic relationship, as described here, I will gladly acknowledge them. Until then, I will persist in believing that some key curative aspects of therapy go beyond technique into the murky territories of inspirational intersubjectivity.

CONCLUSION

In summary, in the cognitive therapy of self-injury it is generally most helpful if clinicians and others:

- Explain the cognitive model to clients regarding automatic thoughts, intermediate beliefs, and core beliefs.
- First identify with the client the automatic thoughts that immediately precede self-injury.
- Use collaborative empiricism to evaluate the accuracy of these thoughts.
- Over time, identify the core beliefs that support the intermediate beliefs and automatic thoughts that precede self-injury.
- Gently challenge any core beliefs about unlovability and/or incompetence.
- Consistently convey, within the professional relationship, the client's considerable strengths and capabilities.
- Transform persistent negative thoughts into positive cognitions that are held with conviction.
- Use homework between sessions to consolidate progress and ensure generalization to the natural environment.

CHAPTER 11

Body Image Work

As noted, Beck (1995) has suggested that the negative core beliefs of individuals fall into two basic categories: incompetence and unlovability. I believe a third type of core belief is often centrally important for self-injurers: negative body image. It may seem intuitively obvious that many self-injuring individuals have compromised relationships with their bodies. Why else would they cut, burn, punch, pierce, pick, excoriate, or otherwise assault their bodies? It seems unlikely that people who hold their bodies in high esteem would subject themselves to such attacks. But understanding the relationship between self-injury and body image problems is complex. Applying this understanding in providing effective treatment is especially important and the subject of this chapter.

Body image has been a productive area of research since the 1930s (e.g., Schilder, 1935; Secord & Jourard, 1953; Fisher, 1970; Tucker, 1981, 1983, 1985; Cash & Pruzinsky, 1990, 2002). Some authors have emphasized broad psychodynamic formulations (Schilder, 1935; Fisher, 1970); others have concentrated on narrower, more behavior-specific topics such as body-size estimation (Thompson, Berland, Linton, & Weinsier, 1987), satisfaction with body parts or areas (Secord & Jourard, 1953; Tucker, 1985), or physical self-efficacy (Ryckman, Robbins, Thornton, & Cantrell, 1982). More recently, Cash and Pruzinsky (2002) have argued that body image is a multidimensional construct that is influenced by myriad biological, cognitive, affective, developmental, and contextual factors. A thorough review of the extensive body image literature is beyond the scope of this book; Cash and Pruzinsky's (2002) recent edited volume is highly recommended.

For present purposes, body image is defined as *a complex set of thoughts, feelings, and behaviors related to the physical experience, size estimation, appraisal of, and satisfaction with one's own body.* Based on the body image literature cited above and my own research regarding the body image of self-injurers (Walsh, 1987; Walsh & Rosen, 1988; Walsh & Frost, 2005), I have found it useful to consider six dimensions of body self-concept:

- Attractiveness
- Effectiveness
- Health
- Sexual characteristics
- Sexual behavior
- Body integrity

These six dimensions are defined in the sections that follow.

ATTRACTIVENESS

Attractiveness refers to whether or not an individual feels attractive and receives feedback from others regarding being attractive. This is a very subjective body image dimension. Many individuals who self-injure are objectively attractive people who consider themselves to be unappealing. Some go so far as to refer to themselves, quite unjustifiably as "ugly," "disgusting," even "deformed."

Attractiveness is an important feature of one's life. Particularly during adolescence, but also thereafter, attractiveness has been found to be associated with popularity, self-confidence, social competence, and academic achievement (Ashford et al., 2001). Individuals need to feel reasonably attractive to operate comfortably in social environments. For those who feel patently unappealing, the result can be avoidance of social encounters and withdrawal. Those who believe that others recoil at their appearance may choose to avoid "inflicting this pain" on the environment. Other individuals who feel profoundly unattractive may allow others to exploit them, feeling fortunate to receive any attention at all, even if it is exploitive.

EFFECTIVENESS

Effectiveness is an entirely different dimension of body image. It pertains to coordination, athleticism, and stamina (see Ryckman et al., 1982). Obviously, one can feel very competent athletically while also feeling very unattractive, or vice versa. For example, I worked with a chronic self-injurer who was an accomplished athlete but was extremely pejorative about her attractiveness. Although she was objectively quite pleasant looking, she frequently referred to herself as "a fat, ugly, disgusting-looking pig." However, she felt quite competent regarding her physical effectiveness. In high school and college she had been an accomplished athlete. There seemed to be a link for this individual between her athletic achievements and her self-injury. She reported that "when the physical pain of exercise kicked in," she almost always "got off on it." She was an example of an "endorphin addicted" self-injurer who sought the endogenous opioid release associated with sustained physical exertion. Effectiveness was an isolated area of body image satisfaction for this woman. In all other areas, she presented with extremely negative, self-critical thoughts and beliefs about her body.

HEALTH

The body image dimension of health involves both subjective and objective aspects. The objective aspect concerns whether or not the individual has any medically diagnosed conditions or illnesses. Persons with a serious or chronic physical illness can have a very compromised sense of body image (Geist, 1979; Hughes, 1982; Cash & Pruzinsky, 2002). Illness can cause considerable physical discomfort; it may also result in intrusive and/or painful medical procedures. Sustained illness may lead to isolation from family and peers and interruption of school or work, recreational activities, etc. For people with chronic illnesses such as diabetes, asthma, arthritis, or other problems, the body can be experienced as a major inconvenience or even as "an enemy." For such persons, the body seems to be rarely working in their best interests; instead, it is experienced as an impediment or obstacle to the life they want to live.

Although such illnesses are sometimes present in self-injurers, the far more common situation appears to be individuals who feel unhealthy *subjectively*. These are people who have no diagnosed physical conditions or illnesses but who nonetheless frequently experience their bodies as unwell. We are all familiar with clients who seem to have an unending series of physical complaints that migrate from one body area to another. These are people who are in frequent, almost daily, discomfort, reporting such problems as headaches, nausea, backache, muscle cramps, intestinal ailments, etc. Although it is tempting to refer to such people countertransferentially as "hypochondriacs," a more compassionate and insightful attitude is to view them as body alienated. Frequent complaints of physical discomfort are one way clients communicate their persistent negative attitudes regarding their bodies. Once physical illness has been ruled out by a physician, the clinician can begin to investigate the sources of body alienation in "the chronically ill but physically well" self-injurer.

SEXUAL CHARACTERISTICS

The dimension of sexual characteristics refers to comfort/discomfort with the physical changes in the body associated with puberty. Most individuals are comfortable passing into physical maturity and acquiring an adult body. Others, particularly trauma survivors or eating-disordered individuals, may experience considerable discomfort related to physical maturation. Trauma survivors may feel that their bodies are "betraying" them as primary and secondary sex characteristics emerge. Their adult bodies may remind them all too much of the bodies of their perpetrators. Other trauma survivors may be especially concerned that having a physically mature body may result in others approaching them sexually.

Eating-disordered individuals may be horrified in a different way by the growth in the size of their bodies; females, especially, may view the normal physical growth in hips, abdomen, and breasts as evidence of out-of-control weight gain and imminent obesity.

SEXUAL BEHAVIOR

The dimension of sexual behavior refers to comfort/discomfort with sexual activity with oneself and/or with others. As individuals move through adolescence, a normative part of development is becoming sexually active. Optimally, this behavior is one that people pursue with a sense of personal safety, self-respect, and reciprocal intimacy with others. Many self-injurers report the body image dimension of sexual behavior to be problematic. Discomfort related to sexual behavior can range from inhibited, phobic attitudes about sexuality to behavior that is hypersexual. Some individuals, usually trauma survivors, are entirely sexually avoidant. They may find the prospect of sexual intimacy in the present to be too fraught with associations to abuse from the past. Until these individuals have dealt with their trauma histories, the prospect of engaging in sexual behavior with others is intolerable.

Other self-injurers, who may also be trauma survivors, engage in behavior that is the opposite of avoidance. They may be unconcerned with safe sex practices and have multiple partners within very short periods of time. For these individuals the briefest of sexual encounters may be the only type of intimacy they can tolerate. Unsafe sexual encounters may also be reinforcing because the sex acts are simultaneously self-demeaning and potentially self-destructive. For those who are "addicted" to self-defeating forms of behavior, sexual risk taking can be as exhilarating as self-injury itself. Being exploited by others may be congruent with an overall diminished sense of self-esteem.

BODY INTEGRITY

Body integrity is a particularly intriguing and complex dimension of body image. To discuss the concept adequately requires the use of some rather odd language. Body integrity refers to whether or not individuals feel as if they "own" or "occupy" their own bodies. To have a sense of body integrity means to feel comfortable within one's body, to feel that it is of one piece and whole. A sense of body integrity requires freedom from prolonged states of dissociation or feelings of disconnectedness from one's body.

For clients who are fortunate enough to have a strong sense of body integrity, queries that involve the above language may seem strange. They may respond to questions about body integrity with, "Of course I feel that I 'own' my body. Without it I don't exist!" For a substantial proportion of self-injurers, however, a sense of body integrity is not self-evident or automatic at all.

For example, in responding to questions regarding body integrity on the Body Attitudes Scale (BAS) (Walsh & Frost, 2005; a copy is provided in Appendix B), many self-injuring clients indicate that they "strongly agree" with such statements as:

"Sometimes I feel disconnected from my body."
"Sometimes my body feels out of control."
"Sometimes my body feels like an enemy."
"I would prefer to live without a body."
"I often feel at war with my body."

Strong endorsement of such items suggests the opposite of body integrity; that is, *body alienation*. Many self-injurers seem to be body alienated in complex ways, and it is important to target body alienation over the course of treatment.

BODY IMAGE AS A FOCUS IN THERAPY

Asking self-injuring clients about the six dimensions of body image is often an extremely useful activity, productive for at least the following reasons:

1. Most clients have not been asked extensive questions about body image and it therefore represents new, uncharted territory; for clients who are therapy veterans, the topic of body image can open up useful new directions in treatment.
2. The presence or absence of negative attitudes regarding the body often serves to differentiate more disturbed from less impaired self-injurers.

3. The presence of negative attitudes regarding the body may have prognostic implications for the length of treatment and the course of self-injury.

4. The presence of profound body alienation often points to histories of sexual and/or physical abuse trauma that need to be explored and resolved.

5. Identifying which of the six dimensions are problematic for an individual allows the dimensions to be targeted quite specifically in treatment.

BODY IMAGE AS UNCHARTED TERRITORY

A portion of clients who self-injure are therapy veterans. They have seen a number of therapists over several years and have become somewhat jaded about the process. They may hold some modest hope that this new treatment will be different, but it is often no more than a glimmer. One reason for their jaded attitude is that too many therapists in hospitals and outpatient clinics have asked the same list of tired questions. One function of exploring body image with clients is to open a fresh topic for discussion. I find that many clients are surprised when first asked about their relationships with their bodies. Introducing an important new theme intrigues clients and fosters some hope that this treatment will be more effective than past attempts. Creating hope and optimism is basic to starting any new treatment.

Why is body image raised so infrequently by therapists, in general? Body image appears to be a neglected theme in therapy because it is rarely part of graduate school education. Clinicians are taught to focus on the general topics of thoughts, feelings, and behaviors (cognitive behaviorism) or fantasies, drives, and conflicts (psychodynamic treatment), but rarely on the specialized topic of the body. The contention here is that body image is a fundamental building block of self-efficacy and self-esteem (Schilder, 1935; Secord & Jourard, 1953; Cash & Pruzinksy, 2002) and should be given appropriate prominence in the course of treating the self-injuring client.

BODY IMAGE AS A PROGNOSTIC INDICATOR

Although I do not have extensive empirical data to support this contention, my clinical impression is that the presence of very negative body image attitudes in clients tends to be a negative prognostic indicator. In general, the more profound the body alienation, the more extended the course of self-injury and the more prolonged the treatment response.

Chapter 3 has discussed self-injury in clinical groups versus the general population. I have found anecdotally that self-injurers from the general population who are functioning adequately tend *not* have profoundly negative attitudes regarding their bodies. When such clients are asked about their attractiveness, effectiveness, health, sexuality, and body integrity, they usually do not report extensive negative thoughts or beliefs. Whereas adolescent and young adult self-injurers (from the general population) may report some age-appropriate self-consciousness about body image, they generally do not cite self-loathing or other extreme attitudes. Moreover, when asked questions about body integrity, such as "feeling disconnected from your body" or "experiencing the body as an enemy," they tend to looked perplexed and deny any such thoughts or beliefs.

In contrast, clinical populations of self-injurers tend to present with high rates of negative body image attitudes (Walsh & Rosen, 1988; Alderman, 1997; Conterio & Lader, 1998; Walsh & Frost, 2005). These attitudes often show evidence of gross distortions, such as:

- "I'm ugly, disgusting looking. I can't even look in a mirror." [attractiveness]
- "I have no athletic ability whatsoever. I have no interest in exercise or sports." [effectiveness]
- "My body is always breaking down. I'm sick of the headaches, nausea, and menstrual cramps." [health]
- "I'd rather have the body I had as a child. To me these breasts are disgusting and my stomach and butt are way too fat!" [sexual characteristics]
- "I hate it when anyone touches me. I just want everyone to stay away!" [sexual behavior]
- "I'd rather not have a body. All it causes me is pain and shame" [body integrity]

BODY ALIENATION AND THE LINK WITH TRAUMA

Many authors have found associations between self-injury and sexual abuse trauma (Walsh & Rosen, 1988; Darche, 1990; Shapiro & Dominiak, 1992; Miller, 1994; van der Kolk et al., 1996; Alderman, 1997; Favazza, 1998; Briere & Gil, 1998; Turell & Armsworth, 2000; Rodriquez-Srednicki, 2001; Paul et al. 2002). Self-injury has also been linked to physical abuse (van der Kolk et al., 1991, 1996; Briere & Gil, 1998; Low et al., 2000).

When clients report attitudes of profound body alienation in response to questions regarding the six body image dimensions, the possibility of trauma histories must be considered. The question to be addressed is: How did they become body alienated? Often the primary suspect is a history of abuse.

In trying to discuss trauma histories with clients, two very different types of problems tend to emerge. Some individuals are unwilling or unable to discuss their abuse histories. The topic is just too painful and retraumatizing to approach. Others present with the opposite problem. They have talked about their trauma histories so often in treatment that they have become desensitized to the content. They discuss physical or sexual abuse as if they were recounting a grocery list.

The topic of body image often provides an alternative avenue to open up productive exploration of abuse history. Body image is frequently a less threatening, more indirect route. An example of how body image discussion may lead to disclosure of trauma is provided below. For this client, previous direct questions about abuse history had not been helpful.

THERAPIST: How has your self-injury been lately?

CLIENT: Pretty low. Twice in the last week.

THERAPIST: That seems like progress. Six months ago it was about once a day, wasn't it?

CLIENT: Yes. It was *every* day.

THERAPIST: Congratulations!

CLIENT: Thank you (*smiling*).

THERAPIST: Reflecting back on your past self-injury, how do you think you got in the habit of cutting your body?

CLIENT: Well, I've always hated my body.

THERAPIST: That's strong language. Why do you "hate" your own body?

CLIENT: Oh, it is so complicated . . . (*looking away, clearly uneasy*)

THERAPIST: I can tell this topic is making you uncomfortable, but it may be important. Let's go a little further and if it's too much, you'll stop me, okay?

CLIENT: Okay.

THERAPIST: Why do you hate your body?

CLIENT: I've always hated my body. I've always felt it was dirty, disgusting . . . (*voice trails off*)

THERAPIST: Are there parts of your body you hate more than others?

CLIENT: (*with great intensity*) Oh, yes!

THERAPIST: May I ask what those are?

CLIENT: Anything to do with sex . . . (*evident shame and discomfort*)

THERAPIST: You're being very brave to pursue this. Can we go a bit further in our discussion?

CLIENT: I guess.

THERAPIST: Is there some part of your personal history that has caused you to hate the parts of your body that have to do with sexuality?

CLIENT: Yes . . . (*long sigh*) . . . I guess I need to talk about it. It has to do with my father . . .

THERAPIST: This is a topic we haven't talked about before, have we?

CLIENT: No (*starting to cry*).

THERAPIST: Do you think it's time we started to deal with it so that you can put it behind you (*conveying hope*)?

CLIENT: Probably . . .

THERAPIST: Good. We'll go at a pace that you can handle, but it's important to resolve so that you can go on with your life (*balancing risk with the need for hope and change*).

CLIENT: Yes. I know you're right. (*wiping her eyes*) . . . It's time now.

This type of dialogue emerges in the therapeutic relationship when a climate of trust and safety has been established. Very often the topic of body image provides access to the trauma history. The topic of the body is intensely personal and intimate. Discussing the body grounds the client in the more visceral, physical aspects of his or her experience. Opening the door via body image allows the work of resolving abuse trauma to proceed. This work, known as exposure treatment, is the focus of the next chapter.

ON THE SPECIFIC LINK BETWEEN SEXUAL ABUSE TRAUMA AND SELF-INJURY

For self-injurers with sexual abuse histories, the link between trauma and bodily harm is not an abstract concept but rather a concrete experience. The psychological wounds of such trauma often lead quite directly to the bodily wounds of self-injury. Over the years clients have taught me a great deal about the links between sexual abuse and their recurrent self-harm. Their instruction occurred not via didactic discussion but by sharing their anguished life stories in which sexual abuse played a central role. What these clients revealed over time were the specific links between their trauma history and their recurrent self-injury.

As discussed in Chapter 7, treatment with these clients began with a thorough behavioral analysis of their self-injury sequence. What these clients disclosed in discussing the sequence can be depicted schematically in Figure 11.1. The *upper* section of the figure refers to the self-injury sequence as discussed by the clients. Although clients have varied considerably in their use of language, the content has been very similar across individuals.

Over the course of treatment, the disclosures of clients shifted from the self-injury sequence to revealing their abuse histories. The sexual abuse sequences they described are depicted schematically in the *lower* section of Figure 11.1. First I describe the upper sequence, as clients have presented it, and then explicate the lower section with an emphasis on the links between the two.

As the upper portion of the diagram indicates, many clients identify their self-injury as being triggered by some form of loss. For some, the loss involves a blatant rejection in a relationship, a full breakup, or even a death. For others it can be far subtler, consisting of an almost imperceptible slight from a peer, colleague, or family member. Still others experience loss as related to performance problems in such areas as school, work, or athletic competition. Many individuals are reactive to *all* these types of losses.

In Figure 11.1 loss is followed by mounting intolerable affective tension—the escalating emotional discomfort that most self-injurers describe as preceding their self-injury. The type of affect varies widely and may include anxiety, sadness, depression, loneliness, anger, shame, or contempt. Regardless of the specific feeling reported, it is experienced as profoundly uncomfortable and requiring immediate relief.

The next step—and it is a key one—is that of dissociation. Many clients report dissociating in response to their escalating affect. They may use very different forms of language to describe the dissociation, such as "I feel like I'm outside my own body," or "It's as if I'm watching myself in a movie," or "I feel disconnected from everyone and everything." Although the specific terminology varies from person to person, the overall experience is generally the same: People report feeling some form of psychological disconnection from their bodies and their immediate experience.

The next step in the sequence is the irresistible urge to cut, burn, or otherwise injure the body. Once recurrent self-injurers reach this point in the sequence, they are unlikely to resist the impulse to self-harm.

Then comes the act of self-injury itself. Of note is that many self-injurers report an absence of pain at the time of the act. This anesthesia is probably due to the dissociation experience. There is some sort of profound mind–body disconnection in operation that causes the self-injurer to feel no pain. Most self-injurers state that they experience pain or discomfort only several hours or even a day after the act.

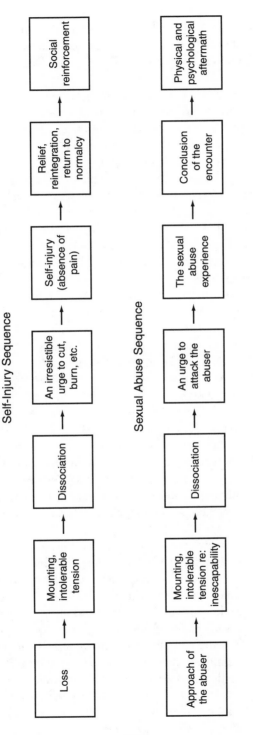

Self-Injury Sequence

Loss → Mounting, intolerable tension → Dissociation → An irresistible urge to cut, burn, etc. → Self-injury (absence of pain) → Relief, reintegration, return to normalcy → Social reinforcement

Sexual Abuse Sequence

Approach of the abuser → Mounting, intolerable tension re: inescapability → Dissociation → An urge to attack the abuser → The sexual abuse experience → Conclusion of the encounter → Physical and psychological aftermath

FIGURE 11.1. The parallel sequence for self-injury and recurrent sexual abuse.

177

The next step is the relief from discomfort. The intense affective distress is reduced and the dissociation experience terminated. There is a sense of reintegration and a return to normality—whatever that may be for the individual.

The final step in the self-injury sequence is the response of others in the environment, if any are present. These reactions vary greatly, ranging from outpourings of effusive support to bitter condemnations of the self-injury. Either way, the self-injurer may find the responses of others to be gratifying (or reinforcing), as is explained below.

The lower sequence in Figure 11.1 depicts the experience of recurrent sexual abuse. It is shown beneath the self-injury sequence because it is postulated here that it serves as *the foundation* for the self-abuse.

The first step in the sequence is the approach of the abuser. In several ways, this action is very much connected to the subsequent experience of loss. Most individuals are abused by someone they know (and trust). The abuser may be a grandparent or parent, the partner of a parent, an older sibling, an uncle or aunt, a babysitter, teacher, or clergyman. As soon as the abuse begins, this relationship is forever contaminated—in a word, *lost*.

Another form of loss related to abuse is the destruction of an emerging sense of body integrity. During childhood, a normative developmental task is learning to control one's body and achieve a sense of physical mastery (Ashford et al., 2001). The fragility of achieving this task is easily observed in young children. Whenever they receive a slight scratch or contusion, they invariably become quite upset by their "boo-boo." Their response of alarm and even panic points to how partial a sense of body wholeness and mastery is for young people. Imagine if instead of a scratch or contusion, the assault on the child's emerging sense of body integrity were genital violation or penetration. It is easy to imagine how disorganizing this would be for children in terms of their relationships with their own bodies.

A third type of loss that clients often report is a retroactive loss of self-esteem. Many young individuals who are sexually abused do not realize at the time that it is wrong or abusive. As many clients have told me, "I thought it was normal to have sex with my abuser until X told me it wasn't." This recognition is shocking to the abused and often results in a profound loss of self-esteem and related shame and guilt.

The next step in the sexual abuse sequence is the mounting, intolerable tension. Once children know what is coming, they experience intense affective arousal as the cues preceding the abuse emerge. The emotions commonly involve fear, anger, shame, and guilt—an amalgam of emotions not easily managed by a young child. How do they learn to survive this affect and the related physical discomfort associated with the abuse? The next step in the sequence is dissociation, which is the individual's adaptive response to an impossible, terrifying situation. Dissociation enables the individual simultaneously to escape the emotional distress and the physical pain connected to the abuse. However, one problem with this "solution" is that survivors tend to overlearn this response. In future years they may dissociate in response to other forms of affective distress that have nothing to do with abusive situations.

The next step is a key one. The individual being abused is inclined to tell others what is occurring, to fight back, and to say "no" to or even attack the abuser. However, abusers are adept at compelling their victims to stay silent and do nothing. Clients have reported such threats as "If you tell anyone, I'll kill you" or "If you say anything, I'll kill your dog." Other abusers are somewhat subtler. They control their victims by using manipulative tactics such as, "It would kill your mother if she knew our special secret," or "If you tell anyone, I'll go to jail and the family will be broken up."

The effect of these threats—whether subtle or bludgeoning—is that the survivor is compelled to remain silent. A key psychological shift is associated with this silence. Often, the survivor comes to *blame the body* for the abuse or at least to view it as a "collaborator" and thereby permanently contaminated. Some speak of the body with disgust, citing it as the "lure" or "attraction" for the abuser. Others blame the body for physiologically responding to the sexual stimulation and feel immense shame. All such self-blame is irrational, but it plagues the sexually abused survivors until they explore it in treatment and resolve it.

The next step in the abusive sequence is the sexual contact and abuse itself. Note that it is positioned directly beneath the self-injury. The two events are often inextricably linked in the minds of self-injurers. They disclose such judgments as "I hurt my body because I hate it," or "It is dirty, contaminated, evil, and not really me." They may say, "I can hurt it all I want because it's not me and I don't care what happens to it." The extent of their body alienation and tendency to dissociate is reflected in such statements.

The conclusion of the sexual abuse encounter signals the end of the particular episode. The abused child returns to whatever normality may be for him or her. The final step in the sequence is the physical and psychological aftermath. Note that it parallels the experience of social reinforcement in the self-injury sequence. During the sexually abusive sequence, survivors are forced to endure an aftermath of physical pain and psychological discomfort in silence. This may make the reaction of others to their self-injury all the more reinforcing to receive. After years of enduring abuse in private, at last they can suffer and have someone notice. It does not matter whether the response is nurturing or punitive. Either way, the silence is broken and a gratifying reaction from others is obtained.

OTHER SOURCES OF BODY ALIENATION

It cannot necessarily be assumed that a history of sexual abuse trauma exists whenever clients present with negative attitudes regarding their bodies. There are many other ways for people to become body alienated. For example:

- Individuals with a history of physical (nonsexual) abuse
- Individuals with a history of serious childhood illness
- Gay, lesbian, bisexual, or transgender individuals who are not yet comfortable with their sexuality
- Persons with other idiosyncratic circumstances

As noted by numerous authors (van der Kolk et al., 1991, 1996; Briere & Gil, 1998; Low et al., 2000), self-injury has also been found to be linked to physical abuse. The factors that produce body alienation in those who have been physically abused can be similar to those that emerge from sexual mistreatment. Survivors of physical attacks may come to blame their bodies for the assaults. Some seem to internalize the loathing that the abuser manifests for them and conclude that they deserve the physical punishment. This internalization can pave the way for subsequent self-assault. Such children often endure parents or other caregivers who rarely hold or physically comfort them. These children may conclude that the "unattractive" or "unappealing" body is at fault or to blame.

Sustained or serious childhood illness can also produce body alienation. Those with histories of physical illness such as asthma, diabetes, arthritis, eczema, psoriasis, or other abnormalities can develop very compromised, negative attitudes regarding their bodies. If the body frequently causes one physical pain, limited mobility, social embarrassment, isolation, or other adverse repercussions, it is no wonder that negative attitudes develop.

One example I encountered was a 13-year-old boy with diabetes. Although he occasionally self-injured, he came into treatment primarily because of his serious mismanagement of his diabetic illness. He refused to do his blood levels consistently, frequently delayed or missed doses of insulin, and ate an unhealthy diet of candy bars, snow cones, and soft drinks. His scores on the BAS were exceptionally negative, especially on the effectiveness, health, and body integrity subscales. In treatment, he said quite directly that he hated his body because it interfered with his desire to play basketball, made him different from his friends, and was a nuisance to manage. This boy was an excellent example of a client who was body alienated due to the considerable repercussions of his physical illness rather than any trauma history.

Another group of self-injuring individuals who have body image problems are gay, lesbian, bisexual, or transgender (GLBT) youth and young adults. In a sample of disturbed adolescents described in Walsh and Frost (2005), there was a substantially higher proportion of GLBT youth in the self-destructive group. My clinical experience is that the GLBT youth most at risk for body image problems are those who are not "out of the closet." Those who *are* out of the closet and have a supportive social network appear to do much better. An example of a gay client with considerable negative body image attitudes follows:

James was a 14-year-old struggling with his homosexuality. He frequently cut himself when in a rage or feeling anxious. He generally socialized with girls his age and sometimes stated he was "dating" one or more of them. Later he would reverse himself and say to his therapist, "Who am I kidding? I'm gay, but I don't want to be." James often presented with anguish about his gayness. He feared his parents' reaction to his coming out. He was convinced, perhaps accurately, that they would kick him out of the house. James frequently ranted, "Why can't I be like everyone else?" Early in treatment, his scores on the BAS were very negative on the sexual characteristics and behavior subscales. Only when James came out to his two most trusted female friends did he begin to feel better. They were supportive and did not abandon him, as he had feared.

Some extensive family work enabled James to come out to his family. They were upset but James continued to live at home. With this accomplished, his attitudes toward his body and life, in general, improved. His self-injury also markedly declined.

A fourth group of body alienated self-injurers can only be referred to as "idiosyncratic." Their problems with body image emerge from their own unique, or at least unusual, circumstances. Some examples of such clients include:

- A young woman (described elsewhere) who had cystic acne on her face and body that caused her considerable social embarrassment. She frequently pierced these pimples with pins or needles.
- An adopted Asian adolescent who was rejecting of her race, in part, because she was raised in an all-white suburb. She viewed her race as alien and faceless. She stated she "hated her eyes" and thought she was ugly. This client pulled out her hair when frustrated.
- An adolescent male who was self-conscious about his short height and slender build. He frequently burned himself after school, particularly when a peer had ridiculed his height or build.

- An overweight 13-year-old female who had been teased for years about her size. She was pervasively self-loathing about her body. After episodes of binge eating, she frequently cut her abdomen.

As these examples suggest, people can become body alienated for myriad reasons. The task for the therapist is to identify whether body alienation is a problem for the client and, if so, to design treatment strategies to address it.

TARGETING SPECIFIC BODY IMAGE DIMENSIONS FOR TREATMENT

Focusing on body image in treatment allows the therapist and client to identify specific dimensions that demand attention. This process can involve asking informally about the six dimensions or using the 36-item BAS provided in Appendix B. The strategy selected depends on individual clients and their receptivity to completing questionnaires. I generally use the more informal approach with adolescents and other clients who are wary or distrustful. However, it is better to use the questionnaire when possible because it provides more specific, detailed information about all six dimensions. It is also useful to administer the questionnaire recurrently so that change can be tracked.

For argument's sake, let us say that a client completes the BAS during a session and agrees to share it with the therapist. Suppose that the results identify problems with the dimensions of attractiveness, health, and body integrity. These three dimensions can then be explored at length in treatment. One approach will be a cognitive-behavioral one that focuses on identifying the automatic thoughts, intermediate beliefs, and core beliefs that support the negative attitudes. The goal over the course of treatment is to use cognitive techniques to gently challenge distorted cognitions, identify more accurate thoughts, and practice them in and out of therapy. Details of the cognitive therapy approach have been recounted in Chapter 10.

Another strategy in working with negative body image attitudes involves building positive body experiences *in vivo*. If the client reports feeling chronically unattractive, he or she may be asked to complete assignments outside of therapy designed to enhance feelings of attractiveness. These assignments may involve placing greater emphasis on grooming, obtaining a new haircut or clothes, or going for a complete "makeover." The strategy in negotiating such homework with the client is to make it both fun and adventurous. Chronic negative cognitions about being unattractive or ugly and related behaviors must be challenged with a combination of humor and compassion. The following is an example of such an exchange.

THERAPIST: How are you coming on your attractiveness homework?

CLIENT: Oh, God, not this again!

THERAPIST: 'Fraid so, this again!

CLIENT: Well, I didn't get that haircut . . . (laughing nervously)

THERAPIST: I didn't think so. I can be very observant and this appears to be the same exact haircut as last week.

CLIENT: Well, maybe I'll go this week!

THERAPIST: What's holding you back?

CLIENT: Only 25 years of negative thoughts about being an ugly eyesore (laughing)!

THERAPIST: Well, at least you're laughing about those absurdly inaccurate judgments!

CLIENT: If only I believed it!

THERAPIST: Well, you are getting there, aren't you?

CLIENT: I guess so. I promise next week you'll see a brand new me . . . or at least a new haircut. I really do want to change my hair.

THERAPIST: Great!

Other examples of homework that clients have used to deal *in vivo* with body image dysfunction are provided in Table 11.1. Many of these were suggested by the clients themselves. Although any one of these attempts is likely to produce only modest improvements in body image, the use of several in combination can effect considerable, positive change over time.

As with any new skill, the acquisition of these more positive bodily experiences involves extensive, recurrent practice. The therapist needs to monitor follow-through and reinforce the most modest of efforts. Making it fun for the client is important. The strategy is to identify a hierarchy of targets for the appropriate dimensions of body image and proceed cautiously but emphatically. Readministering the BAS over time usually reveals substantial improvements in the selected body image dimensions.

CONCLUSION

In summary, in providing body image work with self-injurers, it is important that clinicians and others:

- Understand and work with the six dimensions of body image comprised of attractiveness, effectiveness, health, sexual characteristics, sexual behavior, and body integrity.
- Assess clients in terms of the six dimensions either informally or using the BAS.
- Determine if body alienation is present.
- Ascertain if the client has experienced sexual abuse, physical abuse, serious physical illness, or other negative aspects linked to body alienation.
- Target specific dimensions of body image for treatment.
- Identify body-related activities that the client can pursue in order to improve body image attitudes and experiences.

TABLE 11.1. Examples of Homework to Improve Body Image

Attractiveness

Going to a skin salon

Charting weight loss associated with a diet

Obtaining electrolysis or derma-abrasion

Consulting a dermatologist

Having orthodontic work done or teeth whitened

Identifying "my top ten most attractive body parts or features"

Effectiveness

Joining a gym

Pursuing a new exercise activity, such as walking, volley ball, racquet ball, tennis lessons, dancing

Engaging in a new activity that involves dexterity, such as playing a musical instrument, painting, sculpting, croquet

Health

Charting physical discomfort by body area and linking these areas to an assessment of cognitive, affective, or behavioral antecedents

Initiating a diet or healthier eating

Reducing caffeine or alcohol intake

Asking for a modification of medication regimen

Taking up yoga, tai chi, kayaking

(continued)

TABLE 11.1 *continued*

Obtaining a physical and, if the results are good, ignoring future ailments as much as possible

Accepting that physical discomfort is the body's way of expressing feelings and working on modifying those feelings more effectively

Sexual characteristics

Identifying all the positives of having an adult body

Acquiring a variable wardrobe that includes both concealing and revealing clothing

Celebrating an adult body by going to a spa or having a massage

Becoming comfortable with androgyny as a mode of dress and appearance

Acquiring stylish but nonrevealing clothes

Wearing sexually revealing clothing alone in the privacy of one's home

Sexual behavior

Accepting that sexual activity is entirely within one's control; one can be sexually active frequently, occasionally, rarely, or not at all

Accepting masturbation

Accepting celibacy

Ensuring safe sex with multiple partners

Working on trauma in order to reclaim one's sexuality

Joining a dating service

Body integrity

Practicing looking into a mirror, extending the time limits

Practicing a body scan meditation with emphasis on wholeness (see Appendix A)

Taking a bubble bath

Walking mindfully, concentrating on the rhythm of breath

Making a snow or sand angel

Relaxing in pleasantly warm water at the beach

Floating on a raft

Having a massage

Doing visual imagery of floating, flying, or rocking

Engaging in any activity that conveys a sense of rhythm, full body coordination, and fluidity, such as washing dishes, raking leaves, shoveling snow, and chopping wood

CHAPTER 12

Exposure Treatment and Resolution of Trauma

A story from the Zen tradition serves as an appropriate introduction to exposure treatment:

Never Mind That

A professional dancer, who'd been forced to abandon her career after being pushed in front of a subway train and injuring one of her feet, attended a retreat with Maezumi Roshi (founder of the Zen Center of Los Angeles). Self-conscious about her injured foot, she always kept it covered with a sock.

In her first interview she asked Maezumi a question about her Zen practice, but he answered, "Never mind that. Tell me about your foot."

"Oh, it's nothing, Roshi," the student answered, trying to turn the conversation back to her practice. "I just had an accident."

Maezumi persisted. Finally she not only told him the story but, weeping, took off her sock to show him. At this Maezumi placed his hand silently on her foot. She looked up to find that he was crying too.

Their exchanges went on like this for some time. Every time she asked the roshi about her practice, he'd ask about her foot instead, and they'd cry together. "You might think you have suffered terrible karma," Maezumi told her, "but this is not the right way to think about it. Practice is about learning to turn disadvantage to great advantage." Finally the day came when the student walked into the interview room and began to tell her teacher about her injury, but it summoned no tears from her.

"Never mind about that," Maezumi told her. "Let's talk about your practice." (Murphy, 2002, p. 74)

This chapter focuses on exposure treatment for self-injurers who have histories of trauma. Favazza (1998) has estimated that between 40 and 65% of self-injurers have been sexually abused. However, as the new subset of self-injurers from the general population has emerged, this estimate is probably much too high.

As noted by Walser and Hayes:

> The etymology of the word [trauma] gives us a clue about how to approach the issue. "Trauma" comes from the Latin root meaning "wound." Unlike mere pain, wounds involve injury and bodily harm. They produce scars. They take time—perhaps a long time—to heal. (1998, p. 256)

For self-injurers, these scars are both internal (psychological) and external (visible on the body).

THE SYMPTOMS OF POSTTRAUMATIC STRESS DISORDER

The diagnosis most commonly associated with trauma is, of course, post-traumatic stress disorder (PTSD). Many self-injurers diagnosed with PTSD have also received other diagnoses, such as depression, anxiety, panic, and/ or borderline personality disorder. According to Meadows and Foa (1998), the symptoms of PTSD fall into three basic clusters: (1) intrusion, (2) avoidance, and (3) arousal. Self-injury can often be linked to all three of these clusters. More specifically:

1. The "intrusion" cluster includes flashbacks, nightmares, recurrent thoughts and images, and reactions to reminders of trauma (Meadows & Foa, 1998). Self-injurers who have survived trauma often report all of these forms of intrusive phenomena. In fact, it is not uncommon for these clients to state that they self-injure in order to *terminate* these experiences. For example, a client may say that if a flashback appears and he cuts or burns, "it goes away." This "success" can render self-injury a preferred method for handling intrusive trauma-related experiences.

2. The "avoidance" cluster includes deliberate efforts to avoid thoughts, feelings, behaviors, and environmental cues of trauma. Other symptoms within this cluster are emotional numbing, detachment from others, loss of interest in previous activities, and restricted range of affect (Meadows & Foa, 1998). For many individuals, self-injury is the ultimate, preferred avoidance behavior. It can terminate unwanted thoughts (e.g., "I started thinking of my abuser's face"), feelings (e.g., "I feel such shame

when I'm naked") and behaviors (e.g., "I can't possibly wear that close-fitting clothing"). It shifts attention away from the psychological pain of trauma to the intensely preoccupying sequence of self-harm. Some clients say, "For me, self-injury is an escape. Whatever is bothering me is canceled out. Cutting or burning obliterates whatever else is going on at that moment."

3. The "arousal" cluster refers to diverse problems, including sleep disturbance, interrupted concentration, hypervigilance, and frequent intense states of emotional arousal (Meadows & Foa, 1998). Rothbaum and colleagues have suggested that the emotional arousal of trauma survivors includes the *primary* emotions of fear, sadness, and anger and the *secondary* emotions of guilt and shame (Rothbaum et al., 2000). Note that these are the very emotions that most self-injurers cite as preceding their acts of self-harm. A predominant reason that self-injurers hurt their bodies is to obtain relief from the arousal states associated with PTSD.

The other arousal problems of recurrent sleep disturbance, poor concentration, and hypervigilance are commonly reported by self-injuring clients. These states often exacerbate the emotional distress of self-injurers. Sleep disturbance increases emotional vulnerability. Hypervigilance is exhausting in a different way, depleting the attentional abilities of the already overtaxed self-injuring person.

Thus all three PTSD symptom clusters play a central role in the onset and maintenance of self-injury. For traumatized clients to give up self-injury, they need to achieve mastery over these three symptom clusters via comprehensive treatment.

TREATING TRAUMA

Many forms of therapy have been employed to treat PTSD and its related symptoms. Foa, Keane, and Friedman (2000) have provided a thorough review of these diverse treatment methods. Their book discusses cognitive-behavioral therapy, pharmacotherapy, eye movement desensitization and reprocessing (EMDR), group therapy, psychodynamic treatment, inpatient care, hypnosis, psychosocial rehabilitation, creative therapies, and several others. In this review Foa and colleagues identify cognitive-behavioral treatment as having, by far, the most empirical support as to treatment effectiveness (Foa et al., 2000). For this reason I have chosen to feature this form of treatment in this chapter.

Under the rubric of cognitive-behavioral treatment of trauma, Foa and colleagues cite three main types of therapy as having been found to be effective in controlled studies: (1) cognitive therapy, (2) stress inoculation training (SIT), and (3) exposure treatment (Foa et al., 2000). Cognitive therapy has already been discussed in Chapter 10. SIT, which is essentially a combination of cognitive strategies and replacement skills training (the latter of which was covered in Chapter 9), involves teaching clients such techniques as muscle relaxation, breathing retraining, role playing, and guided self-dialogue. Therefore, the remaining modality that requires extensive discussion is exposure treatment.

EXPOSURE TREATMENT OF TRAUMA

Exposure treatment consists of systematic methods that help clients deal with the three symptom clusters. There are five components included in exposure treatment, as presented by various clinicians and researchers (e.g., Foa & Rothbaum, 1998; Meadows & Foa, 1998; Rothbaum et al., 2000). These five components are addressed in step-by-step fashion using well-established protocols (e.g., Foa & Rothbaum, 1998; Meadows & Foa, 1998). I find that it is sometimes necessary to modify these protocols because of client preferences and reactivity. These modifications are noted in my discussion of the five steps in treatment.

Step 1: Information Gathering

The first step in conducting exposure treatment of trauma is information gathering (Meadows & Foa, 1998). The recommendation of Foa and colleagues is to use a standardized instrument (e.g., the Standardized Assault Interview) to collect information, when possible. Whereas this first step may be ideal, I have found that most survivors of childhood abuse are not ready to complete a standardized trauma questionnaire early in treatment. Rather, they need to proceed cautiously and episodically in disclosing their trauma experiences. Only when considerable trust has been established do they reveal even *bits* of trauma material.

I prefer to collect information informally in a manner that allows me to zoom in when a client feels able to discuss the trauma and zoom back out as discomfort or dissociation escalates. Meadows and Foa state that "most clients do not have difficulties during the information-gathering stage" (1998, p. 108). This has not been my experience. I suspect that the reason why Foa and colleagues make this statement is that much of their work has been with rape victims for whom the trauma is very recent. In contrast, my work with self-injurers has involved individuals who were abused in the distant past. For these clients, the details of the trauma may have been out of consciousness for many years. Retrieval of this content is no small challenge.

I find that such clients have considerable difficulty the first time they disclose information about traumatic experiences. The discussion itself, when the clinician attempts to obtain this information, is often potentially retraumatizing. Thus the information gathering is its own "mini" form of exposure that requires the client to experience multiple trials in order to endure it. In working with self-injuring trauma survivors, the process of acquiring information about childhood abuse is often extremely hit or miss; at times it even feels chaotic. For example:

After several months in treatment, a client disclosed an intrusive traumatic dream in which her father was having intercourse with her. The client then became extremely distressed with this content, stated it was a nightmare, and denied that any similar experience had ever happened in the real world. Three weeks later the client revisited the content (of her own initiative) and offered that the experience was, in fact, true and had happened repeatedly. Immediately thereafter, the client retracted the statement, saying that she should not say such awful things about her father. Only a week later did the client remain steadfast, saying that the abuse had happened recurrently, exactly as she had first described it. This remained her position from that point on, and it was supported by an older sibling who had been similarly abused.

The therapist has to allow clients to weave in and out of such content until they have reached firm conclusions as to what has happened and who did what to whom. This process can take weeks or months and clearly cannot be rushed.

Step 2: Breathing Retraining

The second step in exposure treatment is breathing retraining (Foa & Rothbaum, 1998; Meadows & Foa, 1998). Similar versions of this skill have been discussed at length in Chapter 9 of this book and in the Breathing Manual provided in Appendix A. In treating PTSD, Meadows and Foa (1998) recommend a very specific form of breathing practice:

> Breathing retraining is taught by having the client inhale to a count of four, then exhale slowly while saying "Calm" to herself. A 4-second pause is then placed between the breaths, further slowing the breathing process. Initially, the therapist should count and say "Calm" for the client, until a rhythm is established, after which the client may take over. Once the method is learned,

clients are instructed to practice breathing for homework, at least twice daily for 10–20 minutes each time. (p. 109)

This technique is designed to help manage anxiety, calm the body physiologically, and teach mastery over unpleasant emotions. I find that this breathing technique is a very useful one and recommend it to, and practice it with, clients. However, it should be noted that early in treatment, not many clients are up to twice daily practice for 10–20 minutes. They need a great deal of coaching and "shaping" to achieve this level of participation over time.

Another suggestion I would make is to teach the client breathing retraining *before* information gathering is attempted. The breathing techniques can be very useful for clients as they attempt to provide information about their trauma histories. Mindful breathing allows clients to sit with the painful emotions and alarming imagery (or other sensations) for more extended periods of time. This increased capacity enables the treatment to progress with a greater sense of control for the client.

Step 3: Explanation of Common Reactions to Assault

This aspect of exposure treatment involves explaining and normalizing the reactions of clients to discussing their trauma (Meadows & Foa, 1998). The therapist needs to explain the three symptom clusters of trauma and ask the client which ones apply. Often there is evidence of all three. As clients begin to deal with trauma material, it is common for them to feel they are "going crazy." Their intrusive flashbacks and tactile memories may feel like hallucinations. Their terrifying nightmares may make them feel as if they have no control over their own minds and sleep patterns. The intense emotions of rage and shame often feel out of control.

The flood of emotions (or the opposite, of emotional numbing) may result in a temporary increase in the frequency or severity of the self-injury behavior. At this point in treatment, clients may feel they are getting worse rather than better. During this challenging phase, the therapist must first ensure that the client is safe. Ascertaining the degree of current safety entails conducting a thorough *reassessment* of their forms of direct and indirect self-harm (as described in Chapters 2 and 7). Once the therapist is confident that there is no risk of suicide or major self-injury, the task is to reassure the client that this period will pass and progress will resume. Sharing stories about previously successful clients can be reassuring.

Explaining the symptom clusters of PTSD and even predicting relapses of self-injury can be quite helpful to clients during this phase. Clients learn that their distress is normal, that they are not becoming mentally ill, and that their increased self-injury (if any) is time-limited—especially if they use the replacement skills they have learned.

Step 4: Imaginal Exposure

The fourth step in exposure treatment is imaginal exposure, in which the client describes the trauma experiences in great detail while working to achieve emotional relaxation and calm (Meadows & Foa, 1998). The goal is to experience the trauma memories repeatedly and to gradually master them while defusing their power. Recurrent discussion of the experiences has been found to lower anxiety and to assist clients in differentiating the traumatic experiences from other neutral or positive events (Foa & Rothbaum, 1998). Meadows and Foa recommend providing the following introduction regarding imaginal exposure to clients:

> " . . . Some of the symptoms of PTSD, like nightmares, intrusive thoughts, and flashbacks, are signals that you haven't yet dealt with the memories. So in imaginal exposure, you will deliberately confront the thoughts and memories without pushing them away. Reliving the assault in your memory lets you process the experience, so that you can file it away in your mind like any other bad memory, rather than have it be so real for you. . . . " (1998, p. 111)

The process of imaginal exposure involves multiple steps:

1. The first is to construct a hierarchy or rank ordering of trauma experiences ranging from the least to the most upsetting. In constructing the hierarchy, Meadows and Foa (1998) recommend using a subjective units of distress scale (or SUDs) ranging from 0, indicating no distress at all, to 100, reflecting the maximum distress imaginable. An example of a hierarchy that I constructed with a client is provided in Figure 12.1. Some of the content may seem beyond belief, but I assure the reader that it comes from an actual, credible individual. Note that the items on the client's hierarchy are from her past (about 20 years before). This hierarchy is by no means complete, but it is meant to be representative.

It took weeks to construct this hierarchy with the client. She was able to work on this task only after considerable trust had been established. It was important to explain the purpose of the imaginal exposure to her and to assure her that it would help her with her nightmares, flashbacks, deep sadness, rage, and self-injury.

2. Once the hierarchy has been constructed, the treatment proceeds by selecting an item in the middle of the hierarchy. Items from the middle

Experience	SUDs rating
Seeing my brother at the breakfast table	20
Passing my father in the kitchen when others are present	40
Answering the phone and hearing my father's voice	50
Having my brother grope me over my clothes	60
Having my brother molest me in the barn	70
Having sex with my father in the barn	80
Having sex with my father upstairs while others were in the house	90
Having sex with my father while my mother was "asleep" in the same bed	100

FIGURE 12.1. Imaginal exposure hierarchy of trauma experiences.

are usually chosen first because the content is reasonably challenging without being too overwhelming.

3. The client is then asked to describe the specific item in the hierarchy in complete detail. The therapist needs to be attuned to aspects of the experience that the client may want to skip over or avoid altogether. The client needs to be gently brought back to these aspects so that they can be explored and defused.

4. Any specific incident may have to be discussed multiple times in order to markedly reduce (and hopefully eliminate) the three symptom clusters.

5. Meadows and Foa (1998) suggest that clients should be asked about their SUDs level every 5 minutes or so during imaginal exposure. As the distress mounts, breathing is employed to manage and reduce the SUDs. I find that when clients report anything above 50–60 SUDs, breathing exercises are indicated. Clients find it supportive when the therapist practices the breathing along with them. As one person said, "It makes therapy feel like a joint enterprise."

6. It is generally a good idea to employ the breathing until the SUDs level drops to 30 or below. If the client reports being stuck at a high level of distress, it may be necessary to take a break. However, doing so runs the risk of further reinforcing the pattern of avoidance. It is best to "hang in there" until the effectiveness of the breathing emerges and the repetition of the discussion results in habituation.

7. Foa and colleagues also recommend having the client talk in the *present tense* during imaginal exposure (Foa & Rothbaum, 1998; Meadows & Foa, 1998). I tend not to follow this recommendation because of adverse reactions from clients. When clients begin talking about their trauma histories, I take great pains to emphasize that *discussing* the experiences is very different from *living* them. I frequently reassure clients that they are safe and in no danger in the present. I find that having clients use the present

tense to describe their traumas tends to blur this distinction. Clients seem more likely to feel retraumatized and unsafe. I am in no way claiming that my approach is superior to Foa's. On the contrary, hers is the one with empirical support. Nonetheless, I have had to modify my approach in response to recurrent feedback from clients.

8. Another suggestion from Foa and colleagues is to ask clients to close their eyes during the imaginal exposure (Meadows & Foa, 1998). The intent of this suggestion is to encourage clients to retrieve memories vividly without outside distractions. I have found that many trauma-surviving self-injurers do not feel safe closing their eyes in the presence of others. I therefore offer this suggestion without emphasizing it, and am struck by the very high percentage of self-injurers who choose to keep their eyes open.

9. The process of imaginal exposure moves through the hierarchy until all items have been dealt with and mastered. The pace of this work varies greatly from client to client. Sometimes a single item can take weeks; other times several items from the hierarchy can be handled in a single session.

10. In doing imaginal exposure I find it helpful to use replacement skills in addition to breathing. Thus, clients working on an item from the hierarchy may opt to listen to soothing music, have a cup of herbal tea, or do walking meditation in the office. It is important to emphasize that the replacement skills are used to reduce the SUDs level in the sessions rather than to escape the discomfort of the traumatic memory or related experiences.

11. It must be stated that some clients resist overly structured approaches to treatment. This can be particularly true for late-adolescent and young-adult clients. For those who complain that working with a hierarchy is too formulaic, I am quite willing to proceed informally. Hierarchies can be constructed and worked on without ever writing them down with the client. The risk of using an informal approach is that it can fail to be sufficiently thorough. As a result, key trauma experiences may not be addressed. However, with persistence and acumen, the clinician can avoid this risk as a detailed hierarchy emerges in his or her mind but remains off-line for the client.

Step 5: *In Vivo* Exposure

The fifth and final step in exposure treatment is *in vivo* exposure. This technique is essentially the same process as imaginal exposure, but it brings the treatment into the real world (Foa & Rothbaum, 1998; Meadows & Foa, 1998). I find that many clients need to do imaginal exposure work regarding their trauma memories before they can attempt major changes in their daily living environments. *In vivo* exposure focuses on activities in the client's present life that have been negatively affected by associations with trauma. These are activities that trigger the symptom clusters of intrusion, avoidance, and arousal. As with imaginal exposure, the therapist and client begin by constructing a hierarchy. Clients then progressively expose themselves to these situations *in vivo* in order to achieve mastery. An example of an *in vivo* exposure hierarchy is provided in Figure 12.2. This hierarchy was developed with the same client whose imaginal hierarchy was presented in Figure 12.1. Note that all of the experiences identified were problematic for the client in the present.

As indicated by the SUDs ratings, the items in this hierarchy triggered varying degrees of emotional arousal and avoidance behaviors. For example, if the client saw a photo of a man who resembled her father in the paper, she felt noticeably uncomfortable but could continue reading. However, if she saw a man who resembled her father or a policeman on the street, she would immediately experience intense fear. Generally she would cross the street or enter a building in order to distance herself from the approaching man. In a similar vein, if this woman were waiting for an elevator and a solo man approached, she would not enter the elevator but wait for another. Obviously, these avoidance behaviors caused the client considerable inconvenience.

The *in vivo* exposure treatment for this client progressed through several steps. First she brought photos of persons who resembled her father to my office. We practiced looking at these photos until she felt little or no discomfort. She then did the same practice at home. Next she began to practice *in vivo* exposure on the way to my office. She would intentionally walk by men on the street in situations that would normally be distressing for her. When such men approached, she used her breathing *in vivo* and forced herself not to alter course. She then would discuss the results (including her SUDs levels) in the sessions immediately thereafter. Over time this cli-

Experience	SUDs rating
Seeing a photo of a man in the newspaper who resembles my father	20
Walking past a police officer on the street	30
Walking past a man on the street who resembles my father	40
Entering an elevator alone with a strange man	50
Seeing a photograph of my father	50
Having my brother call on the phone	60
Seeing my mother or father at our family home	80
Having my husband approach me sexually "at the wrong time"	90

FIGURE 12.2. *In vivo* exposure hierarchy of trauma experiences.

ent took great satisfaction in her progress. These avoidance behaviors had plagued her for many years and she was glad to be rid of them.

Next the client progressed to looking at photos of her father. She did this first in my office and subsequently at home. With practice, she was able to reduce her SUDs to close to 0. Then she took on the challenge of managing her emotions more effectively when her brother called on the phone, and ultimately, when she visited her mother and father at the old family home. The sexual issues with her husband were more complicated and required couple treatment later on.

One other issue that deserves comment is that the therapist needs to assess for circumstances in the real world that are *legitimately* dangerous. Although my client may have practiced walking by men in the city during daylight hours, her homework would never have included this activity at night. Some clients have very poor judgment in distinguishing the truly dangerous from the irrationally frightening. They may need considerable help in learning to make this distinction and to self-protect.

INTEGRATING EXPOSURE TREATMENT WITH OTHER TECHNIQUES

The five steps of exposure therapy do not occur in isolation from the other modes of treatment. For example, as clients retrieve traumatic memories and learn to "sit with them," thoughts and judgments about these memories inevitably emerge. Frequently, after clients experience the primary emotions of fear, sadness, and rage, they have to endure the secondary emotions of shame and guilt (Rothbaum et al., 2000). These latter emotions can be as overwhelming and problematic as the primary states. Trauma survivors often start asking themselves accusatory questions such as, "How did I allow this to happen?" or "Why didn't I do something to stop it?" or "How could this have gone on for so long?" or "Did I somehow *want* this to continue?"

At these moments in treatment the therapist needs to shift from the exposure treatment to cognitive therapy to address the survivor's *attitudes* and *interpretations* about the abuse, not just exposure to the memories or images of the abuse. Kubany (1998) has presented a comprehensive cognitive therapy approach to treating trauma-related guilt and other interconnected problems. He states that "guilt and guilt-related beliefs play an important causal role in the maintenance and perpetuation of posttraumatic stress, depression, and low self-esteem" (Kubany, 1998, p. 125). He has written extensively about four types of faulty conclusions presented by trauma survivors:

1. *Hindsight bias*, which refers to survivors incorrectly concluding after the fact that they "should have" told someone or "could have" escaped or stopped the abuse (Kubany, 1998, p. 127).

2. *Justification distortion*, which refers to clients concluding that decisions they made were not justified, despite ample evidence to the contrary. For example, a client may contend, "I did not pursue options that would have stopped the abuse," discounting the reality that the abuser had absolute power and control over the individual.

3. *Responsibility distortion*, which refers to clients inappropriately placing responsibility for their abuse on themselves. For example, as one client said to me, "I must have done something wrong for my father, who loved me, to have abused me like that." The faulty thought process is: "I was treated badly; therefore I must have behaved badly and deserved it."

4. *Wrongdoing distortion*, which refers to survivors concluding that they have "participated in" and thereby "committed" immoral acts. As noted by Kubany, "Some incest and rape survivors feel 'betrayed' by their bodies for being paralyzed with fear or by experiencing sexual arousal during the abuse" (Kubany, 1998, p. 130). Consistent with Kubany's comments, I sometimes say to clients: "The fact that your body experienced physical sexual arousal does not mean that *you* did anything wrong." "If you're force fed, digestion still happens. It doesn't mean you wanted food shoved down your throat."

Kubany's list of cognitive distortions highlights how survivors can hold many thoughts and beliefs that are profoundly irrational and self-denigrating. The types of negative cognitions that survivors report range from automatic thoughts (e.g., "I deserve whatever mistreatment I receive on a daily basis") to rules (e.g., "All men will exploit me") to core beliefs (e.g., "I'm completely unlovable and incompetent—why shouldn't people abuse me?"). Integrative treatment involves moving forward with imaginal and *in vivo* exposure while simultaneously addressing cognitive distortions as they arise.

At some point in treatment it can be helpful for the therapist to take an active stance regarding the abuse. I sometimes ask clients if they would like to hear my opinion. If they say "yes," I tell them, "I think you were exploited and abused in a most dehumanizing, horrific, and destructive way for which you bear absolutely *no* responsibility." I find that many clients need the therapist to model for them expressing justifiable outrage and placing blame where it belongs. After such pronouncements—and they are intentionally rather dramatic—clients may feel more empowered and as if they "have received permission" to vent their full rage about their abusers. In some instances, clients move on to confronting their abusers directly.

AN EXAMPLE OF INTEGRATIVE TREATMENT OF TRAUMA

When Penny began therapy at age 22, she was one of the more severe self-injurers I had treated. She had cut her arms and legs hundreds of times and her extremities had extensive scarring. She had also burned herself occasionally, pulled out her hair, and episodically engaged in bulimia. Penny was an intelligent young woman who was attending college. However, she was already in her eighth semester and was nowhere near graduation due to a pattern of missed classes, exams, and papers. She was a very capable individual who was nonetheless self-defeating, self-loathing, and self-destructive.

Early in treatment Penny was very distrustful. She rarely made eye contact and refused to let me see the wounds on her arms. Her responses to questions were often defensive, such as, "Why do you want to know that?" or "What business is that of yours?" or "How could that possibly be of interest to you?" Although these questions sound abrupt and off-putting, they were often delivered with a wry, sarcastic sense of humor. Due to her intelligence and wit, I sensed there was considerable reason to be hopeful.

After several months of gradually conducting a behavioral analysis, a clearer picture of her self-harm emerged. Penny cut herself in response to three main situations: (1) academic deadlines and pressure, (2) conflicts with peers, and (3) some as-yet-to-be articulated discomfort with body image. Early in treatment the topic of her relationship with her body was clearly too much for her, so we concentrated on academics and peer issues. We worked on identifying a number of replacement skills. She particularly liked mindful breathing, expressive artwork that included drawing and clay sculpting, and walking meditation. We also practiced breaking down her academic assignments into very small steps so that they were not so overwhelming.

As Penny began to use these replacement skills consistently, her academic performance improved. She used the skills to avoid panic as she was writing a paper or preparing for an exam. She also employed her breathing skills in social situations when she felt herself starting to "tighten up." The result was that over the first 6 months of treatment her self-injury declined from multiple times per week to a few times per month.

Although all this work was fine and good, therapy had yet to address the heart of the matter: her relationship with her body. Her dislike for her physical self manifested in several ways beyond her self-injury. She said quite explicitly that she "hated" her body; she frequently mocked her appearance with statements such as "Being ugly is not a social asset," "I wish Quasimodo were still alive, I might get a date once in a while," and "I only purchase stainless steel mirrors"); and she also scored very low on all six subscales of the BAS (see Appendix B).

When the timing seemed right, I asked her how she had come to hate her body so much and why she assaulted it so frequently. These questions opened the floodgates. For many minutes Penny just wept and could not speak. I listened as calmly as I could and assured her it was good that she could "finally let it out." She then began to tell her tale of abuse and exploitation—which took months to complete.

Penny's story recounted 10 years of abuse. She had been abused from ages 6–16, first by her father and then by her older brother. The father's abuse involved full intercourse; the brother's, genital touching. Once her history of abuse was on the table, we began full exposure work. First we started with imaginal exposure, followed by in vivo exposure. Excerpts from the hierarchies we used in her treatment have been provided above in this chapter.

In doing imaginal exposure with this client, it was not possible to include every situation of abuse that she had endured. Because of the duration and frequency of the abuse, the sheer number of experiences was in the thousands. During the 10-year period it was not unusual for the client to have intercourse with her father two to four times per week. Therefore, the hierarchy could not identify every experience but concentrated on <u>categories</u> of abuse, such as "being groped by my brother over my clothes," "having sex with my father in the barn" or "having sex with my father upstairs when others were present in the house."

Not surprisingly, the retrieval of this material produced incredibly powerful emotions in Penny. She expressed rage, sadness, emptiness, and an overgeneralized fear for many weeks. Over time she also added great shame and a sense of guilt to the mix. She asked herself a myriad of questions about how the abuse could have gone on for 10 years without discovery or respite. She attacked herself with questions about "complicity" and "passive acceptance." This portion of treatment required me to respectfully challenge her irrational, self-blaming cognitions. The facts were that her father was an alcoholic with a vicious temper. He had beaten his wife frequently over the years and had been known to kill family cats when in a rage. He had also threatened Penny that if she ever told anyone, "the police will come and take you away"—which explained why Penny was so avoidant of police later in life. Many times I actively sided with Penny during this phase in treatment, emphasizing that she was in a totally powerless situation and bore absolutely no blame.

The most challenging period in Penny's therapy was not the exposure work regarding the sexual abuse. It occurred when Penny realized that her mother had known about the abuse and had done nothing to intervene and protect her. The most flagrant example of this situation was the incident when Penny had been forced to have sex with her father while her mother was "asleep" in the same bed. Retrieving this memory was the cruelest blow for Penny, and it produced a marked short-term deterioration. Although Penny had not self-injured for over 6 months, when she began talking about her mother's role, the self-harm came back with a flourish. She cut herself repeatedly and even burned herself—something she had not done in years. She also became briefly suicidal, stating that she was "thinking of taking pills to end it all." As she worded it at the time, "I always knew my father and brother were bastards, but it's just too much to accept that my mother was too!" During this period, hospitalization was considered but not utilized. We increased the number of sessions and added frequent phone and e-mail contact.

Penny was able to meet this challenge. She eventually directly confronted all three family members regarding their abuse. Penny started with her father and chose to have the conversation in my office with me present. This allowed her to feel safe and not worry about violent retaliation. (I also made sure there were colleagues close by.) Later on she also met with her mother and brother privately.

Penny moved beyond her self-injury and trauma. In fact, she turned great misfortune into a vocation as she eventually became a social worker doing protective interventions with abused children.

CONCLUSION

In summary, in providing exposure treatment for self-injurers, it is important for clinicians and others to:

- Know the symptom clusters of PTSD (intrusion, arousal, and avoidance).
- Understand how self-injury may be directly linked to these three clusters.
- Employ the five steps of exposure treatment, including (1) gathering information, (2) teaching breathing retraining, (3) explaining common reactions to trauma, (4) conducting imaginal exposure, and (5) providing *in vivo* exposure.
- Modify the formal aspects of exposure treatment, as needed, in order to meet the needs of diverse clients.

CHAPTER 13

Family Treatment

Relatively little has been written about the family treatment of self-injury. The sole book-length contribution is Selekman's (2002), which focuses on adolescents and their families. He employs a "solution-oriented brief family therapy" approach. His assessment uses a "multi-systemic . . . framework that takes into consideration the complex interplay between the adolescent, family, peer-group, larger-system, cultural, gender, community, and societal factors in the development and maintenance of self-harming behavior" (Selekman, 2002, p. 27). As this description suggests, his multisystemic framework is very inclusive as to the scope of its targets.

Selekman's treatment approach is highly eclectic. His recommended therapeutic interventions range from cognitive restructuring, relaxation training, mindfulness, and visualization to "family sculpting and choreography," "Native American storytelling," and "shamanic healing methods." He also employs such diverse techniques as "family vision quests," "the imaginary feelings x-ray machine," and the "family collage mural" (Selekman, 2002). For therapists looking for flexible, creative, expressive methods of treating families with self-injuring adolescents, Selekman's book can be a helpful resource.

Miller and colleagues have described an intriguing modification of dialectical behavior therapy (DBT) in working with self-destructive adolescents and their families (Miller et al., 1997; Miller & Glinksi, 2000). Their version of DBT shrinks the length of treatment from 1 year (standard DBT) to 12 weeks, reduces the number of skills taught, simplifies the language of the skills, and provides an optional 12-week follow-up consultation group (Miller et al., 1997). Most importantly, the DBT skills training involves both the adolescent and the family in the same groups. This approach would seem to be especially helpful in ensuring generalization from the treatment setting to the home environment.

Initial outcome data appear promising. Rathus and Miller (2002) reported that their version of family DBT provided significantly better results than treatment as usual in terms of rates of psychiatric hospitalization for adolescents. In addition, pre- and posttreatment measures within the DBT group showed reductions in suicidal ideation and in DSM-IV Axis I and II symptomatology. To date, no randomized clinical trials of this family DBT approach have been conducted (Miller & Glinski, 2000), nor have studies focused on the specific problem of self-injury.

One limitation of using the DBT approach with individuals and/or families is that it is very complex to learn. Conducting DBT according to protocol requires the provision of (1) individual DBT treatment using daily diary cards, (2) group skills training using the DBT manual, (3) coaching in crises between sessions, as needed, and (4) the establishment of an ongoing staff consultation team. Learning this model requires intensive and expensive training that may not be feasible for some professionals. Nonetheless, DBT is a treatment of choice for self-injurers and their families.

A COGNITIVE-BEHAVIORAL APPROACH
TO THE FAMILY TREATMENT OF SELF-INJURY

My own approach in working with families of self-injurers is cognitive-behavioral. I use a step-by-step cognitive-behavioral model that works collaboratively with family members. There are three phases in the treatment: (1) educating family members about self-injury; (2) including family members in the assessment of self-injury; and (3) using family members as skills practice allies. Much of the content of these phases will be familiar to anyone who has read the previous chapters in this book.

Educating Family Members about Self-Injury

The first step in working with families with a self-injuring member is to assess the severity of the self-injury. When the behavior falls within the "common" range of self-injury, the family treatment can begin with education about the nature of self-injury. When the damage is major, the client must first be protected and stabilized before the psychoeducational family work can begin.

Educating families about self-injury involves teaching them the concepts presented in Parts I and II of this book. Family members learn to:

• Understand the full range of self-destructive behaviors, including direct and indirect self-harm (as presented in Chapter 2). The family assists in identifying which forms of self-harm are a problem for their loved one. They may come to recognize that self-destructive behavior is a problem for other family members as well. Many families have more than one member with a history of self-harm, such as suicide talk or attempts, substance abuse, eating disorders, and risk-taking behaviors. Identifying such patterns in a family tree can point to biological vulnerabilities of which all family members need to be aware. In the process of identifying family self-harm patterns, self-injurers may come to feel less stigmatized and "unique" within the family system.

• Understand how self-injury and suicide differ (as presented in Chapter 1). This step is crucial in assisting families to become allies in the treatment. Reframing self-injury as nonsuicidal allows families to avoid panic and to move forward helpfully and strategically. Families are often greatly relieved to learn that self-inflicted cutting, burning, hitting, and excoriation are unlikely to result in death. However, the therapist has to walk a careful path with families on this topic. It is crucial that they recognize that the behavior is indicative of serious distress that requires treatment. Families should not minimize the behavior by referring to it as "not really suicidal," "just attention seeking," or "a fad among kids these days."

• Understand which behaviors *should be* considered suicidal; namely, the use of a gun, overdose, hanging, jumping from a height, and ingestion of poison (as presented in Chapter 1). Family members need to understand which forms of self-harm represent an immediate crisis and which do not. Whenever they are unclear regarding this distinction, they should always rely on mental health professionals to make the determination.

• Understand that certain types of self-injury require immediate assessment by a psychiatric emergency service; namely, those that involve significant tissue damage requiring medical treatment or those that involve face, eyes, breasts, or genitals (as presented in Chapter 7).

• Understand that body modification (e.g., tattoos, body piercings obtained from professionals, etc.) is not the same thing as self-injury (as presented in Chapter 4).

• Understand that the best way to respond to common self-injury is with a "low-key, dispassionate demeanor" (as presented in Chapter 6).

• Understand that the problem of self-injury is complex and that biological, environmental, and psychological factors combine to produce the behavior and must be addressed to eliminate the behavior (as presented in Chapter 5).

Including Family Members in the Assessment of Self-Injury

Family members can be a major ally in the assessment phase of self-injury. They know the self-injurer far better than the therapist ever will. With the client's permission (especially when the client is an adult), the therapist can share the Self-Injury Log (Figure 7.1, p. 81) with family members and ask for their assistance in completing it. Family members can be immensely helpful in identifying the antecedents to self-injury; they can also provide information about the frequency and details of self-injury when the client is unable or unwilling.

Of course, family members often play a role in the occurrence of self-injury. Their behaviors may be key antecedents in triggering self-harm. In such instances, the therapist identifies, in a nonblaming way, the interactions within the family that seem to be followed by self-injury. These interactions become targets for family interventions that may play a major role in reducing the incidence of self-harm. For example:

Natasha is a 16-year-old whose parents are divorced and have joint custody. She lives with each parent on alternate weeks. A baseline assessment of Natasha's self-injury reveals that she is far more prone to self-injure when she is living at her father's house. Natasha would prefer to spend the majority of time at her mother's because they are much closer and better able to communicate. However, Natasha is also loyal to her father and is afraid to express her preference out of concern that she will hurt his feelings. The therapist negotiated an agreement between Natasha and her father that she spend more overnights at her mother's but the same number of evenings and weekend days at her father's. Subsequently, Natasha reported substantially fewer urges to self-injure because she feels less lonely and more supported in her mother's home. (It should be noted that the possibility of paternal abuse had been ruled out in this family.)

Sometimes the antecedents within a family that trigger self-injury are more *indirect*:

James is a 22-year-old mechanic who lives at home. He frequently burns himself with cigarettes and excoriates his wounds. Family treatment reveals that James hates it when his father drinks excessively and argues with his mother. Loud voices trigger sadness and anger in James. At such times, James "feels like a loser for still living at home and having to listen to all their crap!" As a result, he retreats to his room and burns away his feelings on his arms and legs.

James's parents are concerned about his self-harm. They were not aware of how reactive he has been to their arguments. They agree to engage in their disagreements more privately or to suggest to James that he "take a walk" when "things get hot" between them. As James's rate of self-injury declines, he shifts to learning to become more self-sufficient so that he can move out. The father's substance abuse is a more long-term challenge, beyond the scope of James's treatment.

In other situations, the family does not play a significant role in triggering the self-injury. Family members can nonetheless be very helpful in defining antecedents of which even the self-injurer is unaware. For example:

Family work with 14-year-old Denise and her mother identifies that the teenager generally self-injures shortly before going to bed. No pattern of events in the family environment seems to play a role. Denise herself is unable to explain the timing of her self-injury. Her mother proposes a link between Denise's computer use and her cutting. Toward the end of each evening, Denise tends to log onto a teen chat room. Not uncommonly her peers in the chat room make fun of Denise for her "uncool attitudes" and even her spelling errors. Her so-called friends often refer to her as "out of it" and "intensely dense." Trying to fit in, Denise even takes the latter as her chat room name. Although Denise enjoys the contact with peers because she has few friends at school, she ultimately ends up feeling sad and rejected by the end of her chat room exchanges. Her mother's insight into these triggers resulted in Denise voluntarily reducing her use of the computer immediately prior to bedtime. Denise's self-injury declined moderately thereafter, although she still required extensive skills training and cognitive therapy.

Using Family Members as Skills Practice Allies

Once assessment of self-injury has been accomplished, family members can then become very helpful allies in assisting self-injurers to learn replacement skills. They often assume three roles in providing such assistance:

1. Noticing triggers and reminding self-injurers when these cues have occurred.
2. Prompting self-injurers to practice their skills and helping them monitor whether the skills are effective.
3. Actively practicing skills *with* the self-injurer.

Family members can be treatment's greatest asset in terms of generalization to the real world. Whereas a therapist can only *urge* a client to practice skills at home, a family member can all but *ensure* it. Families can be very helpful both in prompting routine skills practice and in assisting clients in using skills in a crisis. Family members can also assist the self-injurer in completing their Brief Skills Practice Log (Figure 9.2, p. 146).

Not uncommonly, self-injurers become flooded with emotions when they experience particularly provocative cues. When family members observe these cues, they can say reassuringly, "You know you tend to get triggered when this happens—how about if you practice one of your skills right now?"

In order for families to assume such an active stance, they need to have learned which skills are effective for their self-injuring family member. This requires teaching families replacement skills at the same time the self-injurers are learning them. (An extended discussion of replacement skills is provided in Chapter 9 of this book.) Teaching skills to family members can occur with the self-injurer present or in parallel fashion. Some clients require individual attention and prefer to learn skills with no one else in the room. They may feel self-conscious practicing skills with family members present or may be distracted by ongoing family issues. Other self-injurers are quite receptive to learning skills with their family members, which is the most efficient way to proceed when possible.

Learning how to prompt skills practice varies greatly from family to family. Some self-injurers require a very directive approach, such as, "Please go practice visualization right now; you know it will really help!" For others, the coaching needs to be much subtler and low-key, such as, "You look really stressed in reaction to that phone call. What might help you stay calm right now?" Generally, coming across as a lecturing expert or an impatient bystander will not work—especially with adolescents. Knowing how best to approach the family member is key to advancing skills training. In some cases, it is very helpful if the family member offers to practice the skill *along with* the self-injurer. Then the skills practice becomes a collaborative effort in which both family members are equal partners. For example,

Twenty-five-year-old Ann lived with her 26-year-old boyfriend, Sam. Sam found Ann's frequent cutting to be upsetting, and he was instrumental in convincing her to go into treatment. Ann seemed unlikely to continue in therapy unless Sam came to the sessions, so he arranged to make the meetings. Sam was very helpful in identifying Ann's triggers. She was most prone to cut when she had had a dream or flashback related to childhood abuse or after sexual contact with Sam.

Early in therapy, Ann and Sam learned a number of mindful breathing techniques. Sam especially liked them because he had a high-stress job that

overwhelmed him at times. He began to practice breathing regularly at home, and he encouraged Ann to practice with him. Subsequently, when Ann was triggered by sexual content, he would hold her hand and they would practice breathing together. Ann began to learn that not all touch was sexual and that some touch could be comforting. Pairing this simple form of physical contact with breathing helped them both. Without Sam's assistance, this treatment was unlikely to have been successful.

As shown in the above example, family members can be crucially important in encouraging skills practice in self-injurers. A parent or partner may say, "You know, you look like you're getting pretty upset right now, and I'm feeling the same way. How about if you and I do X together in order to calm down?" (i.e., taking a walk, making dinner, visualizing, breathing, cleaning the house, grooming the dog, etc.). Defining emotional distress as a common and shared predicament is empathic and empowering. Instead of the self-injuring client being identified as the "sole dysfunctional one," both family members acknowledge their reactivity and strive to manage their emotions collaboratively.

An interesting turnabout is to have self-injurers teach family members skills in sessions. In these situations the self-injurer has learned and mastered skills and assumes the role of trainer with family members. Teaching others skills shifts the role of the self-injurer from identified patient to instructor and caregiver. For example:

Effie is an 18-year-old high school senior who frequently cuts her arms. Her major affective antecedent to self-injury is anxiety. In individual therapy she learned a number of breathing and visualization techniques that she finds very helpful. She has quickly learned to practice her new-found skills when her anxiety starts to rise.

Effie is close to her father. He also has had problems with anxiety over the years related to social situations and making presentations at work. In a series of family meetings, Effie taught her father both breathing and visualization skills. He finds them to be effective, which is very gratifying for both father and daughter.

WORKING WITH SEVERELY TROUBLED FAMILIES

The three-phase approach described above assumes that the families in treatment are basically well-intended and reasonably competent. Of course, as any experienced therapist knows, there are some families that are neither. Some families are so dysfunctional that self-injury is relatively modest in the overall scope of their problems. For example, many chronic self-injurers come from families in which they have been extensively physically and/or sexually abused (see Chapters 11 and 12). When a therapist encounters such families, launching into an assessment of self-injury and teaching replacement skills are beside the point. The priority is always to ensure the safety of the individual self-injurer (and, in some instances, other family members). Sometimes, removing a self-injurer from a toxic family environment may result in an immediate reduction in self-harm behaviors.

However, all too often, clients who have endured years of physical and/ or sexual abuse have also internalized the negative thoughts, feelings, and behaviors of their abusers. Their self-injury is now internally triggered. Such clients may require extensive cognitive therapy to deal with their dysfunctional core beliefs regarding their unlovability and helplessness (as presented in Chapter 10). They may also need extensive help with their dysfunctional body image (Chapter 11) and with trauma resolution (Chapter 12).

As an example of this type of predicament is provided in the following vignette:

I provided a consultation regarding a 22-year-old female self-injurer. Her history consisted of frequently cutting her arms and legs and, occasionally, her genitals. In the process of interviewing this young woman, I asked her a series of questions about body image. In response to the dimension of sexual behavior, she began to speak at some length about her sexual experiences. She disclosed that she had been abused by her mother's live-in boyfriend for a 10-year period (from ages 5 to 15). The abuse had consisted of the boyfriend touching her genitals on scores of occasions.

I was then surprised to learn that this young woman still lived with this abuser and that her mother was, as the client said, "in denial that the abuse ever happened." This was alarming enough, in that the client had never been validated regarding the horror and unacceptability of her long-term abuse. Making the situation even worse was that the mother's boyfriend still occasionally "touched her on the butt" when he passed her in the kitchen.

Because this woman was deemed to be "emotionally disturbed," state law required that a complaint be filed against this boyfriend (who qualified as an "abusive caregiver"). An investigation ensued that held the boyfriend accountable for his behavior. The client's therapist also assisted the young woman in finding alternative living arrangements.

In this case, as with many others, the priority was on providing protective intervention in the family rather than on proceeding with family treatment in an already out-of-control situation.

DEALING WITH IDIOSYNCRATIC
FAMILY SITUATIONS

In the course of conducting family treatment with self-injurers, myriad situations are discovered that are intimately related to the self-harm. Families generate idiosyncratic problems that need to be identified and resolved in order for the self-injury to improve. Time and again I have encountered family situations that have been entirely unique. In such situations, there are often few guideposts, only a clinical attunement and "respectful curiosity." For example:

A 16-year-old boy was all but dragged into treatment by his mother and father. The boy was 5 feet 3 inches tall and a sophomore in high school. Although he was a competent football player, he was otherwise struggling in school. His parents described him as increasingly angry. The boy had cut himself on a number of occasions and had inflicted two crudely executed tattoos on his forearms.

In the course of the first interview, the three family members were asked about the boy's possible sources of distress. They were unable to generate much in the way of hypotheses until the end of the hour. At this point the parents mentioned that their son was concerned about "how big he would grow," given his interest in football. I commented that this didn't seem to be a long-term concern in that his father was well over 6-feet tall. Mother then disclosed that "their" son's biological father was not her husband—a detail she had oddly omitted during the earlier discussion of family history.

Sensing that the mother was extremely emotional about this topic, I offered to have the next session with the parents alone. In this meeting the mother revealed that her son was the product of a long-term live-in relationship that had dissolved when she became pregnant. It was clear that this time in her life was extremely painful to recall. She had seldom, if ever, discussed the situation with her son, although he did know that his "father" had adopted him.

A version of informal exposure treatment (Chapter 12) allowed this mother to discuss her ex-boyfriend and the father of her son with greater comfort and control. With this accomplished, the mother was able to talk with her son about his biological father. The boy was eager to learn more about this man. He asked his mother many questions he had always wanted to pose. He disclosed that he had secretly worried that his father might have been "crazy" or "a drug addict." He was especially relieved to learn his father was 5 feet 11 inches tall. After several sessions, the adolescent became noticeably less angry and his self-injury disappeared. Unmasking the family secret and establishing open communication made all the difference.

Another case example illustrates a very different type of family dilemma related to self-injury:

A family from Thailand came into treatment. The parents had emigrated to the United States when they were in their teens. Their children had been born in the United States. Their daughter, now age 15, was a high achiever who excelled at everything. As a reward for her accomplishments, the parents gave her a trip to Thailand, her first, where she was to visit relatives. On the trip the teen became very lonely and depressed. She missed her family and was disoriented by losing her normal daily routine. Secretly, she began cutting her forearms on the trip. When the daughter returned, the parents discovered the cutting—to their horror.

The daughter's self-injury brought the family into treatment. The parents were reserved people, uneasy with emotional expression or displays. Once the daughter felt comfortable, she poured out her feelings about the disastrous trip. She had felt isolated and alone. Although her relatives were kind and generous to her, she was unable to really communicate with them. And then there was the matter of "her eyes." The daughter explained that the relatives had asked her many times if she planned to have cosmetic surgery on her eyelids. She discovered that it was commonplace among wealthy Thais to have their eyelids modified for "aesthetic reasons." The daughter was utterly confused by this persistent questioning. Up to this point in her life, she had never considered her eyelids to be "deformed." As with many adolescents, she was exquisitely sensitive to negative comments about her appearance.

The girl's parents explained that such surgery was a status symbol in Thailand and, in their opinion, represented some irrational discomfort with Asian physiognomy. They urged her to forget her relatives' advice and to return to her normal life.

Family treatment also focused on the perfectionistic expectations of this family. The parents agreed to make "straight A's" less of a demand in the family. The child's level of distress diminished and she ceased hurting her body. She abandoned any thoughts of cosmetic surgery.

CONCLUSION

In summary, for those who provide treatment to self-injurers and their families, it is often helpful for professionals and others to:

- Educate family members about the nature of self-injury and its difference from suicide.

- Educate family members as to which forms of self-injury represent a psychiatric crisis.
- Encourage family members to respond to self-injury with a low-key, dispassionate demeanor.
- Engage family members in assisting with the assessment process, especially in identifying triggers.
- Train family members in replacement skills so that they can prompt practice for their self-injuring members.
- Ask family members to practice skills along with self-injurers; such practice is both empathic and empowering.
- In working with seriously dysfunctional families, ensuring safety from abuse takes priority over treatment of self-injury.
- Resolution of idiosyncratic family dilemmas often can alleviate self-injury in younger family members.

CHAPTER 14

Psychopharmacological Treatment

GORDON HARPER

Pharmacotherapy can help many individuals with self-injurious or self-mutilative behavior. However, symptoms, by themselves, do not lead directly to choice of agent or class of agents. Clinical pharmacotherapy, although informed by experience with other patients, individually and in clinical trials, consists of focused assessment, hypothesis generation, and empirical trial.

THE BIOLOGY OF SELF-INJURY

How Do We Understand What Is Wrong?

All efforts to help individuals with self-injury are directed ultimately at the brain, the source of all thinking and behavior. Because pharmacotherapy, unlike psychosocial interventions, is directed at the mediating neurological structures, it is useful to put self-injury in a biological perspective.

All animals, not just humans, protect the self. Self-protective behavior—that is, turning away from harmful stimuli—can be seen in nonhuman primates, in other mammals, and in other vertebrates (birds, reptiles, fish). Even invertebrates protect the self: Worms withdraw from heat or dryness,

Gordon Harper, MD, is Associate Professor of Psychiatry at Harvard Medical School and Medical Director, Child and Adolescent Services, Massachusetts Department of Health.

and cockroaches scuttle away from the light. "Higher" animals such as mammals visibly care for the body, grooming and licking. Harming or mutilating the body represents an overriding of deeply preserved evolutionary behavior—a derangement of developmental biology.

In culturally prescribed body modification, as described in Chapter 4, culture modifies the biological program. But the psychosocial context of these body modification practices differentiates such behavior from what is called self-destructive. Some even argue that culturally prescribed body modification can enhance the self (Favazza, 1996). On the other hand, pathological self-injury differs from culturally prescribed modification in that it occurs without the sanction of the group. Such behavior cannot be said to affirm the self. Indeed, it violates a powerful self-protective biological imperative.

The emergence of self-protection in higher mammals is highly contingent. Clinical experience and animal experimentation indicate that it does not emerge "automatically," as it does in birds or fish, but only when facilitated by the caretaking environment.

Several domains of development are implicated. For example, children normally identify with caretaking adults and grow up to care for themselves. But such identification is distorted in many survivors of abuse or neglect. Similarly, reciprocal caretaking relationships normally develop in humans and other primates, but they can be distorted in both human and in nonhuman primates who have been deprived of expectable nurturance. Stimulus seeking occurs normally in development, but it can be prolonged or take malignant form in individuals with cognitive or perceptual deficiencies, in survivors of trauma, and in those who grow up in isolation. Distorted self-care behavior can be seen even in nonhuman mammals, for instance, in the canine "acral lick syndrome" (Rapaport, Ryland, & Kriete, 1992). Self-injury also occurs in individuals with distorted mood, especially depression, or delusional thinking, as in psychosis. Furthermore, the emergence of self-care and self-protective behaviors can be blocked by dysfunctional environments—that is, when self-harm is inadvertently reinforced (cf. Mace, Blum, Sierp, Delaney, & Mauk, 2001).

Mediating Mechanisms

Inquiry into biological models of self-injury is motivated both by the wish to understand behavior physiologically and by the wish to develop effective pharmacotherapy. In some disorders, the neurological mechanisms are well worked out. For instance, Parkinson's disease arises from the death or dysfunction of dopaminergic cells in the nigrostriatal pathway, and supplementation with dopaminergic* agents enhances function (Cookson, 2003). In self-injury the pathways are less clear; remediation is largely empirical.

A review of the current evidence implicating biological systems is beyond the scope of this chapter but is available elsewhere (Pies & Popli, 1995; Villalba & Harrington, 2000; Gerson & Stanley, 2002; Tiefenbacher, Novak, Lutz, & Meyer, 2005).

For current purposes, it suffices to note:

1. Several different systems play a role in self-injury: the limbic system (a subcortical brain system regulating mood, affect, and pain); dopaminergic systems leading to and within the cortex; serotonergic systems; and the endocrine system that leads from hypothalamus to pituitary to adrenal and other secretory organs (the so-called HPA axis; Tiefenbacher et al., 2005).

2. Several different kinds of evidence are relevant: the physiology of normal individuals and of those with major developmental disorders, in whom self-injury is much more common than in the general population; results of inducing lesions, surgical or pharmacological, in animals; and responses to pharmacological trials.

3. Some of the evidence is intriguing—for instance, that self-injury is directed to body sites that are biologically different, such as, sites with altered skin temperature (Symons, Sutton, & Bodfish, 2001) or with acupuncture analgesia (Symons & Thompson, 1997).

4. Biological studies, like clinical observations, make clear that self-injury arises not from dysfunction in a single pathway or mechanism but is a heterogeneous phenomenon.

5. Correspondingly, not one but a range of pharmacological agents has been shown to have some role in treating self-injury: antidepressants, antipsychotics, mood stabilizers (Cassano et al., 2001; Shapira, Lessig, Murphy, Driscoll, & Goodman, 2002), anxiolytics, opiate antagonists (Sandman et al., 2000), even alpha-agonists (Blew, Luiselli, & Thibadeau, 1999; Macy, Beattie, Morgenstern, & Arnsten, 2000).

---

*The suffix "-ergic," as in "dopaminergic" or "serotonergic," designates neural pathways in which a neurotransmitter acts. For instance, in a dopaminergic pathway, dopamine is released from one nerve, crosses a short space (the synaptic cleft) and activates the next nerve. Agents that enhance the availability or activity of a transmitter are called "agonists," and those that limit availability or activity are called "antagonists." Thus medicines such as fluoxetine (Prozac and others) and sertraline (Zoloft and others) are called serotonin agonists. Because they act by blocking the reuptake of serotonin from the synaptic cleft, they are called selective serotonin reuptake inhibitors, or SSRIs.

6. Published studies vary in methodology—from uncontrolled single-case reports to well-controlled clinical trials—and caution is indicated in interpreting their results; a Cochrane Controlled Trials Register review (Hawton et al., 2000) ranked no intervention as well established.

7. Clinical epidemiology and animal studies suggest that self-injury must be understood in terms of long-term vulnerability (associated with developmental disorders or arising from life experiences such as neglect or abuse) and in terms of current conditions that act upon such a background.

As an example, consider the role in self-injury of serotonin (also known as 5-hydroxytryptamine), a neurotransmitter that is critical to the maintenance of mood and a feeling of well-being. Drugs that enhance serotonin availability include, in addition to fluoxetine (Prozac and others) and sertraline (Zoloft and others), paroxetine (Paxil and others), fluvoxamine (Luvox and others), citalopram (Celexa), and descitalopram (Lexapro). In the last 15 years serotonin has been shown to be effective in treating clinical depression. The evidence for such efficacy is well established in adults; controversy attends the use of SSRIs in children and adolescents (see up-to-date statement at www.nimh.nih.gov/press/stmntantidepmeds.cfm).

A role for serotonergic pathways in self-care as well as a role for serotonin deficiency in self-injury are suggested by several kinds of evidence. For instance, controlled clinical trials in people with disorders in the obsessive–compulsive spectrum show that serotonergic agents reduced the frequency of self-injury, especially hair pulling or other damage to the skin and its appendages. Some individual case reports document striking responses, even life-saving, to SSRIs, in patients with severe skin-picking behavior (O'Sullivan, Phillips, Keuthen, & Wilhelm, 1999; Velazquez, Ward-Chene, & Loosigian, 2000). As mentioned above, the same effect is seen in dogs with a syndrome in which excessive licking leads to erosion of the skin (Rapaport et al., 1992).

But data have also raised the possibility that some SSRIs may increase problem behavior, especially in the young. Case reports document *emergent* skin-picking behavior when patients begin SSRIs (Denys, van Megan, & Westenberg, 2003; Weintrob, 2001). Such reports indicate how incomplete is our knowledge of the biology of skin-picking and other self-injurious behaviors. They also mandate close attention to individual patients whenever a pharmacological trial is initiated—no matter how impressive may be published results for groups of patients.

FOCUSED ASSESSMENT

Pharmacotherapy must be guided by a focused assessment. Drugs must not be prescribed as "magic-bullet" therapy just because a patient engages in self-injury.

Current Behavior

The behavior to be treated must be characterized. The following questions can guide assessment:

> What does the behavior consist of?
> What is the pattern of the behavior?
> When does it occur?
> Does it occur when the patient is frustrated? Anxious? Angry? Sad?
> How long has it been present?
> Does it occur in a predictable sequence? In response to identifiable triggers or precipitants?
> Are certain caretakers repeatedly present?

Associated Clinical Syndromes

What diagnoses does the individual have? Both lifelong developmental syndromes and acute psychiatric disorders must be considered. The developmental disorder itself may be undertreated. With regard to depression and other acute psychiatric disorders, Haw, Houston, Townsend, and Hawton (2002) found a high prevalence of depression in patients with self-injury. Tsiouris, Cohen, Patti, and Korosh (2003) showed decreased self-injury with treatment of depression and other disorders. Psychotic disorders must also be considered, including presentations in which frank psychotic symptoms may not be apparent but the patient shows severe mental disorganization.

Current Context

Which elements of the patient's current context are relevant to the self-injury? Are caretaker responses unintentionally reinforcing self-injury? Does caretaker fatigue, therapeutic uncertainty, or unacknowledged anger at the patient play a part?

In response to disruptive behavior, an adolescent hospitalized on a psychiatric unit was restricted from peers and unit activities. She inserted small objects under her skin and into body orifices, necessitating trips to emergency medical facilities. Efforts to "keep her safe" included one-on-one staffing, "small-obs restrictions" (limited access to small objects), and trials of antipsychotics, antidepressants, mood stabilizers, and opiate antagonists. The behavior continued. Only when the unacknowledged staff reaction to her (fear, anger, helplessness, and hopelessness) was explored, the pattern of responding to self-insertion with visits to the other hospital altered, and a more hopeful relationship established with the patient did the behavior decrease. In an adverse and pathologically reinforcing environment, pharmacological interventions were of no avail.

Mace et al. (2001) also reported greater short-term efficacy of behavioral interventions in reducing self-injury, compared to pharmacological intervention.

Life Context

What is the patient's life situation? What are his or her future prospects? Lack, or loss, of a "future vision" may constitute part of the existential trap in which despair and regression occur. Who, among caretakers, family members, in- and outpatient team members, holds that future vision?

Adaptive Perspective

To implement the future vision, one must define the best level of functioning that can be anticipated for the patient. Have educational, vocational, and family assessments defined how the patient, while self-injurious symptoms continue or abate, can best be expected to function?

Hypothesis Generation

On the basis of a focused assessment, factors that may be contributing to the self-injury can be identified. These factors should be stated in language that points to possible intervention. They should also be stated in terms that specify the degree to which the factor has been recognized or treated. Such factors comprise a formulation or set of hypotheses, put in operational terms. For instance, one might cite such factors as:

- Poor frustration tolerance, longstanding, associated with developmental disorder, possibly undertreated
- Possible undertreated depression

- Severe cognitive and affective disorganization, without frank psychosis, but possibly responsive to antipsychotic medication
- Mix of competencies and vulnerabilities, presently underevaluated
- Patient's clinical team and family are at an early stage of finding a way to talk about the patient's strengths and challenges and the adaptive implications
- Unrecognized dysfunctional responses by caretakers, with unintended reinforcement of self-injury (cf. Mace et al., 2001)

Listing all possible contributing factors explicitly makes it easy to see whether important domains—such as developmental, existential, or social—have been omitted.

From such a list of possible contributing factors, the clinician chooses for intervention those most susceptible to influence and most likely to make a difference in the target symptom.

EMPIRICAL TRIALS

One of the advantages of stating factors in the form of testable hypotheses lies in not having to "commit" to a particular formulation ("It's this . . . "). Rather, such a list leads to empirical trials of possibly useful agents.

When depression is a possibility, either because of significant depressive symptoms or because the patient might be suffering from despair that is difficult to articulate, a trial of antidepressant medication is indicated. Both newer antidepressants (the SSRIs and others) and first-generation antidepressants (amitriptyline or nortriptyline, imipramine or desipramine) may be considered. Although side effects complicate treatment with first-generation agents more than with SSRIs, side effects of the SSRIs are increasingly recognized, both during treatment and on withdrawal. With all antidepressants emergent activation must be watched for, whether or not patients have a diagnosis of bipolar disorder.

Anxiety in self-injury is sometimes manifest, sometimes only inferred. Treatment with anxiolytic agents, especially benzodiazepines such as lorazepam (Ativan and others) or diazepam (Valium and others), is sometimes useful but in some patients exacerbates target symptoms. Clinical observation of such disinhibition on benzodiazepines is consistent with evidence from the treatment of self-injury in monkeys, in which 50% showed decreased self-injury and 50% showed worsened self-injury in response to diazepam (Tiefenbacher et al., 2005).

In patients with delusional self-injury, trials of antipsychotic agents are indicated. In addition, second-generation antipsychotic agents such as risperidone (Risperdal and others) and clozapine (Clozaril and others) have an increasingly well-defined role in the treatment of self-injury, especially in the developmentally disabled. This role goes beyond the treatment of psychotic disorders. Well-designed placebo-controlled clinical trials have shown that risperidone reduces a number of symptoms, including self-harm behavior and symptoms prioritized by parents, in developmentally disabled children (RUPP, 2002; Arnold et al., 2003). Individual case reports have shown clozapine to be effective in patients with borderline disorder, psychosis, and self-injury (Chengappa, Ebeling, Kang, Levine, & Parepally, 1999), and in patients with retardation whose self-injury had not responded to risperidone (Hammock, Levine, & Schroeder, 2001). Treatment with second-generation antipsychotic agents may be complicated by weight gain and other metabolic side effects; treatment with first-generation agents may be complicated by movement disorders. The risk of bone marrow suppression with clozapine requires regular monitoring of white blood counts throughout treatment.

Mood stabilizers include valproate (Depakote and others), carbamazepine (Tegretol and others), lithium carbonate, and topiramate (Topamax). Although mood stabilizers have not been shown to be effective in treating self-injury in controlled trials, individual case reports have indicated some benefit (Cassano et al., 2001). Mood stabilizers may be considered as second-line agents in self-injury, particularly when affective instability is prominent, whether or not the patient has a diagnosis of bipolar disorder. Side effects of mood stabilizers are diverse and potentially serious, varying with the choice of agent.

The role of endogenous opioids in pain regulation has led to interest in a possible role for opiate antagonists, especially naltrexone (ReVia and others), in self-injury (Sandman & Hetrick, 1995). The hypothesis is that self-injury serves as a behavioral opiate equivalent in tension or pain regulation and that the "relief" experienced with self-injury could be blocked by blocking the opiate receptor. Both clinical experience and the published literature (e.g., Modesto-Lowe & Van Kirk, 2002) suggest that this benefit occurs infrequently.

The medications called alpha-agonists include clonidine (Catapres and others) and guanfacine (Tenex and others). Compared to other psychoactive medications, they have benign side effect profiles. Their role in treating attention-deficit/hyperactivity disorder, tics, and posttraumatic symptoms has been well established. Some case reports suggest a role in treating self-injury (Blew et al., 1999; Macy et al., 2000).

CONCLUSION

In summary, efforts to help those with self-injury behavior pharmacologically should be guided by the following considerations:

- Self-injury represents a derangement of basic biology, namely self-protection by the individual.
- Present knowledge of the development and neurobiology of self-injury implicates *several* likely mechanisms and points to *several* classes of possibly useful agents; there is no single magic bullet.
- Care of the individual patient should be guided by the literature, focused assessment, generation of hypotheses regarding possible contributing factors, analysis of context, and empirical trials.
- Antidepressants, anxiolytics, neuroleptics, mood stabilizers, alpha-agonists, and (occasionally) opiate antagonists may all be considered. Attention must be given simultaneously to several dimensions of context:
  - Developmental context
  - Psychiatric disorders
  - Existential–adaptive context
  - Social context, including both caretakers and family

CHAPTER 15

Managing the Reactions of Therapists and Other Caregivers to Self-Injury

Favazza has written that the treatment literature on self-injury "is basically one of countertransference" (1998, p. 265). Although this statement is hopefully somewhat of an exaggeration, there is little doubt that self-injury can produce extreme reactions in caregivers. Many authors have discussed the negative responses of treatment professionals to self-injuring clients, including Linehan (1993a), Alderman (1997), Conterio and Lader (1998), Hyman (1999), Farber (2000) and Shaw (2002). As an example of such a reaction, Alderman vividly described her experience of working with her first self-injuring client.

> Although I had been studying in the area of self-injury for some time, seeing the fresh jagged wounds on [the client's] arms had a major impact on me. I felt as if *I* had been wounded. I imagined the great amount of pain this girl must have felt in order to cut herself, and I felt quite sad. I wanted her to talk to me about the pain, to tell me about what she was going through when she hurt herself. I wanted her to promise me she would never injure herself again. I wanted to make her stop. And, as commonly experienced in any therapeutic relationship, what I wanted and what the client wanted were two different things. She continued to injure herself. I continued to want her to stop. Eventually, I became discouraged and frustrated because she wouldn't do what I wanted. (1997, p. 192)

Alderman's remarks are an appropriate introduction to this topic. This chapter reviews the considerable range of negative reactions of caregivers to self-injury. It also offers some suggestions as to how to manage these responses. Although this chapter is written primarily for professionals, the concepts presented may also be relevant for family members and significant others.

Consistent with the theoretical framework of this book (see Chapter 5), the reactions of caregivers to self-injury can be conceptualized as bio-psychosocial phenomena. Therapists, nurses, physicians, residential counselors, case managers, educators, and other professionals respond to self-injury physically, psychologically, and interpersonally. Of greatest concern are the responses that threaten to harm clients and derail the treatment. As noted by Linehan, "Therapy-interfering behaviors on the part of the therapist include any that are iatrogenic; as well as any that unnecessarily cause the patient distress or make progress difficult" (Linehan, 1993a, p. 139).

Some of the negative reactions that I have encountered in professionals working with self-injuring clients include the following:

- *Biological responses.* Therapists report increased heart and respiration rate, nausea, lightheadedness, physical arousal and agitation, episodic insomnia, or other psychosomatic symptoms in response to self-injury.
- *Psychological responses.* Comprised of three elements:
    - *Cognitive.* Therapists present with confusion, disorientation, indecisiveness; pejorative judgments regarding self-injurers; pessimism regarding the treatment; self-doubt regarding professional competence; exaggerated "savior" fantasies.
    - *Affective.* Therapists experience anxiety, fear, shock, disgust, panic; or anger, frustration, bitterness, rage; or sadness, discouragement, hopelessness, helplessness.
    - *Behavioral.* Therapists present with excessively sympathetic, emotionally charged, or agitated responses; employ pejorative language (both technical and slang) to refer to clients; attempt to coerce, control, and extinguish the behavior via the use of demanding safety contracts; withdraw, avoid, transfer, or terminate treatment of clients; abandon normal professional boundaries by becoming overly involved with clients or preoccupied with their self-injury.
- *Social–environmental responses.* Professionals punish clients for their self-injuring behavior by withdrawing privileges, suspending them from school or treatment settings, etc.; intervene inappropriately in a client's life outside of treatment, such as imposing unnecessary psychiatric hospitalizations; violate confidentiality by contacting

adult clients' significant others or employers without permission; warn other clients to "avoid" the self-injurer.

And these biopsychosocial phenomena represent only a partial list.

Why does self-injury produce such intense reactions in professionals trained to help those in distress? Therapists and other caregivers are human beings who have the same adverse reactions as anyone else to self-inflicted bodily harm. Self-injury violates the expectation that all people naturally seek to avoid pain and seek pleasure. Most forms of self-injury cause immediate tissue damage that is shocking to see. Blood, wounds, scabs, scars, and sutures are violations of normal human bodily form. Blood and related bodily fluids present some risk to others of acquiring serious and even fatal diseases.

Encountering the wounds of self-injury often produces a visceral, automatic recoiling in others. To withdraw from or avoid those who have intentionally damaged their own bodies may be "wired into" the human organism. The impulse to escape may be especially intense when the behavior is at the level of major self-injury or self-mutilation. When people disfigure their eyes, face, breasts, or genitals, or cause themselves extensive physical damage that requires medical attention, almost any human being is likely to be shocked and want to withdraw, at least temporarily.

How then should caregivers learn to manage and overcome such understandably negative responses? They need to "unlearn" normal reactivity in each of the biopsychosocial realms in order to manage their own distress and to fulfill their roles as caregivers. Clients have every right to expect that professionals will respond compassionately and therapeutically to their self-destructive behavior. In order to become effective caregivers in response to self-injury, professionals need to acquire and employ at least the following set of skills.

PHYSICAL SELF-SOOTHING

Professionals need to be able to calm themselves when they find themselves reacting physiologically to self-injury. A basic way to achieve this calming state is to practice and employ the breathing skills (and other self-soothing techniques) presented in Chapter 9. Breathing skills are well documented to be useful in slowing respiration and heart rate and fostering a sense of physical calmness (Foa & Rothbaum, 1998). It is very difficult for a therapist to feel anxious or agitated when his or her body is in a state of relaxation. In other words, professionals treating self-injurers need to use the very same replacement skills in managing their emotions as their clients are learning over the course of treatment.

COGNITIVE RESTRUCTURING

The main way in which professionals can manage their negative reactions to self-injury is by cognitive self-monitoring and restructuring. Intense biological, affective, behavioral, and social/environmental reactions begin with thought processes. If the professional interprets routine low-lethality self-injury to be a "suicidal crisis," he or she is likely to overreact to the situation. Therapists who require of themselves that their clients "get better" rapidly will inevitably find themselves frustrated when the self-injury persists for months. Professionals who question their own competence because a client recurrently self-injures need to modify unrealistic expectations. Clinicians who think they should be able to control the behavior of adolescents and adults and "make them get better" are only setting themselves up for needless conflicts and power struggles. A dispassionate, patient attitude is crucial in conducting therapy with self-injurers.

Many authors have written about the challenges of dealing with negative judgments and behavior toward self-injurers (Alderman, 1997; Favazza, 1998; Farber, 2000; Linehan, 1993a) Unfortunately, it is not unusual to hear professionals use pejorative language when referring to self-injurers. I have often heard caregivers refer to self-injurers, or their behavior, as:

- "Manipulative"
- "Attention seeking"
- "Just a suicide gesture"
- "Just behavioral" (i.e., the client is not truly upset, just using the behavior strategically)
- "Gamey" or "game-playing"
- A "bad" borderline (i.e., insulting the client with an unflattering psychiatric diagnosis)
- "Faking"
- "Contrived"
- "Exploitive"
- "Beating the system"
- "Con man/woman"

When caregivers employ such terminology in referring to their clients, they are well on the way to having lost a helpful perspective. Professionals who make such statements are usually suffering from serious "compassion fatigue." Peer supervision or a regularly scheduled staff consultation team (Linehan, 1993a) can be helpful in reducing the frustration of therapists and getting them back on track. Therapists should assume that they will occasionally have adverse reactions to self-injuring clients. That is to say, counterproductive thoughts and feelings are all but unavoidable. It is no disgrace to experience such negative responses unless they go unacknowledged and unaddressed. The rule-of-thumb is that clinicians should deal with negative reactions when they are still *at cognitive and affective levels*, before they emerge *behaviorally* in the therapeutic relationship itself.

REGULATING AFFECTIVE RESPONSES

In my opinion there are three main categories of negative emotions that therapists experience in relation to self-injury in clients:

1. Anxiety, fear, and related avoidant emotions
2. Frustration, anger and related aggressive emotions
3. Sadness, discouragement, and related hopeless/helpless emotions

The task of the therapist is to recognize the occurrence of such emotions and to "turn them" into therapeutic responses. For example, anxiety and fear can be transformed into positive attentiveness. Avoidant feelings such as anxiety and fear suggest that the clinician is on alert for danger. Therapists can use such "alarm responses" productively by becoming finely attuned in assessing and monitoring the self-injury. Hypervigilance can be a strength when it is used to understand all the details and nuances of the self-injurious behavior.

Anger can also be a useful response if it is transformed into a commitment to assist the client and strategically "fight" the problem. The primary utility of aggressive feelings is the energy they provide the therapist in committing to help the client acquire and employ useful replacement behaviors. A certain amount of fierceness can also be useful in challenging the self-denigrating cognitions and self-loathing emotions of clients. This is particularly true for trauma survivors who suffer from irrational self-blame and need the therapist to model appropriate indignation directed at abusers.

Sadness and discouragement on the part of therapists have no place in the treatment of self-injury. Clients quickly discern any pessimistic attitudes in the minds of their treaters. The negativism of a therapist instantaneously becomes the hopelessness of the client. The way to transform discouragement into proactivity is to return to the wealth of techniques available in the psychotherapeutic repertoire. The spectrum of therapeutic interventions, including psychopharmacology, cognitive therapy, replacement skills training, body image work, and exposure treatment, offers the therapist an extensive range of options. It is very rare that all these methods can be exhausted without some measure of therapeutic success.

MANAGING NEGATIVE BEHAVIORS

Alderman has presented an extensive list of counterproductive therapist behaviors that may emerge in relation to self-injury (Alderman, 1997, p. 196):

- Being late for, or forgetting, sessions
- Being inattentive during sessions
- Refusing to discuss self-injury in sessions
- Being argumentative with clients
- Making judgmental statements to clients
- Using self-injury contracts coercively
- Threatening the client with hospitalization
- Raising fees inappropriately

Hopefully such behaviors are rare among treaters of self-injurers. I believe that if caregivers become aware of their pejorative judgments (listed in the cognitive structuring section above) early enough, their behavior with clients will never deteriorate to such an extent. In order for therapists to manage their behavior appropriately in sessions, the following basic "rules to live by" are helpful to keep in mind:

- Self-injury is not about suicide and should not be treated as a suicidal crisis. If therapists remind themselves that self-injury is an alarming behavior but not a life-threatening crisis, they are more likely to remain calm, strategic, and helpful.
- The best interpersonal approach in responding initially to self-injury is to employ a low-key, dispassionate demeanor in combination with respectful curiosity (see Chapter 6).
- Clients are slow to give up self-injury because they rely on it for affect regulation. Therapists should be patient in their expectations for change.

- To give up self-injury, clients need to learn replacement skills that are at least as effective as self-injury.
- The emphasis in treatment should be on learning new skills rather than on giving up self-injury. Addition is easier than subtraction.

INTERVENING APPROPRIATELY IN CLIENTS' ENVIRONMENTS

Interventions in the living environments of self-injuring clients should generally be positive and nonintrusive. Clients should not be punished for self-injuring. Self-injury is the problem for which they seek or require treatment. The behavior should not be viewed as a form of noncompliance, defiance, or provocation. Coercive interventions in the client's living environment should generally be few and far between. If self-injury is properly viewed as nonsuicidal, then immediate protective interventions in the environment are usually not necessary. Arranging outpatient intervention is generally the more appropriate course. Whenever possible, interventions in clients' living environments should involve their consent. Thus, if a therapist wants to speak with a spouse, partner, or close friend, explicit written permission from the client should be obtained. However, there are some exceptions to this rule, including the following:

- *Self-injury in minors.* When children or adolescent minors self-injure, their parents or guardians should be notified immediately. A detailed protocol for dealing with self-injury in minors in school settings is presented in Chapter 17.
- *Circumstances when the behavior has passed beyond self-injury into self-mutilation.* When clients self-injure their eyes, face, breasts (in females), or genitals, or if they inflict damage requiring medical intervention, they sacrifice their right to direct their own treatment (at least, temporarily). In such cases, protective interventions such as psychiatric evaluation and/or hospitalization should be pursued for the clients' own safety.
- *Circumstances when the self-injury is worsening and may shift to suicidal behavior.* These circumstances are even more alarming than the previous. In some situations, persons who are frequent self-injurers discover that the behavior is "no longer working." Such clients may attempt to gain relief by increasing the level of physical damage or by shifting to hurting other areas of the body. If these methods still fail to provide relief, the individuals can become actively suicidal—at which point, protective interventions are required.

CONCLUSION

By and large, therapists are able to treat self-injurers with equal measures of compassion, optimism, and technical skill. The entire professional identity of caregivers is based on their desire to help and relieve distress. Self-injury can tax the best intentions of clinicians, but with proper self-monitoring and the use of skills, professionals can avoid the pitfalls. Becoming actively aware of the risks of negative thoughts, feelings, and behaviors can serve to inoculate professionals against acting counterproductively in the treatment. Clients deserve care that is fresh, positive, and technically proficient.

In summary, it is helpful in providing treatment to self-injurers if professionals and other caregivers:

- Are aware of the inevitable risk of negative responses to self-injury.
- Learn to carefully monitor their cognitive, affective, and behavioral responses to self-injury.
- Remain alert to pejorative language regarding self-injuring clients as a tip-off to negative reactivity.
- Manage and diffuse pejorative judgments and negative emotions regarding self-injury before they are acted on in the treatment.
- Practice the same skills that clients learn in order to deal effectively with negative responses to self-injury.

PART III

Specialized Topics

CHAPTER 16

Contagion and Self-Injury

The topic of self-injury contagion has a long history that has been reviewed in Ross and McKay (1979), Walsh and Rosen, (1988), Favazza (1996), Taiminen, Kallio-Soukainen, Nokso-Koivisto, Kaljonen, and Helenius (1998), and Farber (2000). Rosen and I have defined self-injury contagion in two ways: (1) when acts of self-injury occur in two or more persons within the same group within a 24-hour period (Rosen & Walsh, 1989), and (2) when acts of self-injury occur within a group in statistically significant clusters or bursts (Walsh & Rosen, 1985). These two definitions have different emphases and are not incompatible.

Contagion episodes have generally been reported in children, adolescents, or young adults living in institutional or treatment settings such as orphanages (Holdin-Davis, 1914), inpatient units (Offer & Barglow, 1960; Crabtree & Grossman, 1974; Kroll, 1978; Taiminen et al., 1998), prisons (Virkkunen, 1976), juvenile detention facilities (Ross & McKay, 1979), group homes (Walsh & Rosen, 1985), or special education schools (Rosen & Walsh, 1989). Self-injury contagion has yet to be studied extensively in normative settings such as public schools, universities, and the community at large. Only a few informal reports exist regarding contagion in these locales (e.g., Walsh & Rosen, 1988; Farber, 2000).

Although the phenomenon has been reported anecdotally for almost 100 years, Rosen and I were the first to provide some empirical evidence of self-injury contagion (Walsh & Rosen, 1985). We studied a group of 25 adolescents in a community-based treatment program over a 1-year period. We found that self-injury occurred in statistically significant clusters or bursts, whereas other problems such as aggression, substance abuse, suicidal talk, and psychiatric hospitalizations did not.

Taiminen and colleagues (1998) replicated our findings in Finland. They studied a group of 51 adolescent psychiatric inpatients over a 1-year period. They also found that self-injury occurred in statistically significant clusters. Of particular interest in their report was that two subjects self-injured for the first time while on the psychiatric unit. Taiminen and colleagues concluded that a majority of self-injury events in closed adolescent units may be triggered by contagion, and that *self-injury can spread to adolescents previously naive to self-injury* (Taiminen et al., 1998). Thus treatment programs can be hotbeds of contagion where iatrogenic effects emerge. Clients who go to such settings to receive help may instead acquire new problematic behaviors such as self-injury. Such risks make the need to understand, manage, and prevent contagion all the more important.

MOTIVATIONS REGARDING SELF-INJURY AND CONTAGION

When individuals are asked why they self-injure, they usually cite intrapersonal (internal psychological) reasons as being most important. This internal explanation would seem to be counter to an interpersonal or "contagion explanation" for self-injury. For example, Osuch, Noll, and Putnam (1999) studied a sample of 75 adult inpatient self-injurers. They collected self-report data and employed a factor analysis to explore the motivations for self-injuring. Six factors emerged in the order of (1) affect modulation, (2) desolation (desire to escape feelings of isolation or emptiness), (3) self-punishment and other motivations, (4) influencing others, (5) magical control of others, and (6) self-stimulation. The first three and the last involve intrapersonal dimensions, whereas the fourth and fifth factors concerned more interpersonal arenas. For this sample, the interpersonal factors appear to have been less important.

In a similar vein, Nock and Prinstein (2004) found intrapersonal motivations to be more powerful than interpersonal in predicting self-injury. They proposed and evaluated four primary functions of self-injurious behavior: (1) automatic–negative reinforcement (e.g., removal of unpleasant affect), (2) automatic–positive reinforcement (e.g., to feel something better, even if it were a different form of pain), (3) social–negative reinforcement (e.g., to avoid punishment from others), and (4) social–positive reinforcement (e.g., to gain attention from others or communicate unhappiness).

Their sample consisted of 108 adolescents admitted to an inpatient psychiatric unit. The group yielded a sample of 89 individuals who had self-injured at least once. The authors performed a factor analysis on patient self-report data and found that "scores on the automatic–positive reinforcement subscale were significantly higher than both social reinforcement subscales." More than half of the self-injurers reported engaging in the behavior "to stop bad feelings." Items on the automatic reinforcement subscales were endorsed by 24–53% of the subjects, whereas items on the social reinforcement subscales were endorsed by only 6–24% of the subjects. They concluded that the subjects "reported engaging [in self-injury] in order to regulate emotions much more frequently than to influence the behavior of others" (p. 14).

Rodham, Hawton, and Evans (2004) reported similar results in their study of adolescents who performed deliberate self-harm. Their sample included 220 15- and 16-year-old self-cutters from school settings in England. The most frequently selected reasons for cutting (from a list of eight options) were intrapersonal in nature. These included such items as "I wanted to get relief from a terrible state of mind" and "I wanted to punish myself." Interpersonal items such as "I wanted to find out if someone really loved me," or "I wanted to get some attention," or "I wanted to frighten someone" were cited much less frequently (Rodham et al., 2004, p. 82). The authors concluded that youth who self-cut were more likely to cite depression, escalating affective pressure, or a need to take one's mind off problems than interpersonal items such as reacting to arguments with others or seeking attention (Rodham et al., 2004).

These findings would appear to suggest that interpersonal issues are generally of lesser importance in supporting self-injury. However, these results seem to contradict much of the current anecdotal information emanating from U.S. public schools and universities, where self-injury is now rampant. A number of explanations can be proposed to explain the discrepancy between the empirical reports cited above and the anecdotal information emerging from community settings regarding self-injury contagion.

One explanation is that for the studies cited above, contagion elements may not have been operative in the samples employed. The samples may have been comprised of people who were not intensely engaged with each other and therefore interpersonal factors were not salient. (Proximity alone in inpatient units or schools does not necessarily produce engagement.)

Another explanation as to why self-injurers emphasized intrapersonal motivations over interpersonal aspects may be related to the limitations of self-report data. Individuals may be loath to admit two types of motivations for self-injuring. First of all, most human beings are unlikely to concede that they deliberately *imitate* the behavior of others. This is especially true for behavior that is viewed as negative or pathological. Imitation is generally viewed as a weak, low-status behavior. From an early age, children are socialized to avoid being "copy cats."

In addition, people are unlikely to admit that their self-injury is *strategic* or *instrumental*. They are disinclined to acknowledge that their acts are intended to "manipulate" others. Such behavior is likely to be condemned as devious and exploitive. A much more acceptable reason to self-injure is a desire to reduce psychological pain. Affect regulation is a preferable rationale to being viewed as a "copyist" or a "schemer." Citing pain generates compassion; citing imitation or manipulation generates disdain or resentment.

INTERPERSONAL DIMENSIONS SUPPORTING CONTAGION

Interpersonal aspects play a central role in contagion episodes. These interpersonal factors include at least four categories of behavior: (1) limited communication skills, (2) attempts to change the behavior of others, (3) response to caregivers, family members, or significant others, and (4) additional peer-group influences.

Limited Communication Skills

Desire for Acknowledgment

One reason that multiple people self-injure within a group is that they lack effective communication skills. Many individuals say that they self-injure in order to let others know that they are angry, sad, anxious, or depressed. When asked why they do not use words to communicate this discomfort, they are dismissive of verbal communication, saying it is not powerful enough to convey the intensity of their message. They believe that for others to really understand their distress, the communication must be concrete, visible, and dramatic. They fear that otherwise, their distress will be viewed as insignificant and will be ignored or not taken seriously.

Desire to Punish

Sometimes self-injury is intended as an attack or an accusation. It can be a dramatic expression of "Look what you've done to me!" The feelings that tend to accompany this form of self-injury are rage and vengefulness. The assumption of this type of motivation is that the others in the immediate environment will react to the self-harm with fear or guilt. If the response of others is dismissive or even neutral, the communication will have failed.

Attempts to Change the Behavior of Others

Desire to Produce Withdrawal

In many cases self-injury within a group is intended to do more than communicate; it is designed to change the behavior of others. In some instances the goal is to shock and offend in order to provoke withdrawal. For example, a peer group consisting of five boys in a high school shared an interest in gothic clothing, alternative music, and violent video games. On the periphery of this group were other males and females who wanted to be included, in part because of access to marijuana. The original five members began burning each other with cigarettes. This scared off the hangers-on, which is exactly what the core group intended.

Desire to Coerce

Self-injury can be an effective means to coerce others to behave as desired. The term "coercion" is used here as presented by Patterson (1975), meaning "to control others by inflicting pain." When parents or significant others become aware of self-injury in a loved one, they often experience intense pain such as fear and panic. Parents may become hysterical when they first learn that their child is cutting or burning. They may feel desperate to do whatever it takes to stop the behavior. Small groups of youth may choose to exploit this reactivity. This is not to say that they do this in an entirely conscious or deliberate way. Rather, it is a primitive type of coercive communication, an ultimatum taking the form of "Give me what I want *or else!*"

Response to Caregivers, Family Members, or Significant Others

Competition for Caregiver Resources

A third category of influences that inadvertently reinforces self-injury contagion involves behavior directed specifically at caregivers. In treatment settings caregivers include direct-care staff, therapists, and administrators; in schools, teachers, coaches, counselors, and administrators; and in families, any significant other.

Self-injury is sometimes inadvertently reinforced in such settings by the competition for scarce resources among caregivers. Both professionals and family members have to attend to many competing demands. Self-injury can be a very effective means of gaining extra attention within a milieu, because it is hard to ignore and it places caregivers in a difficult position. To attend to the behavior in a solicitous, supportive fashion runs the risk of reinforcing it. To ignore it is ethically questionable and has been found to escalate the severity of self-injury acts in some instances (Offer & Barglow, 1960; Lester, 1972).

Self-injurers are generally aware of the dilemma facing caregivers. Some choose or feel compelled to exploit the situation by relying on self-injury to dominate a milieu. Other non-self-injuring individuals observe that self-injury results in the person receiving medical assessment, therapy appointments, skills training practice, extra medication, and the like. The temptation becomes considerable to follow suit and obtain the benefits offered by self-injury. When a contagion episode erupts, the rate of self-injury may skyrocket as individuals perceive the availability of caregivers to be declining. They become motivated to be the most recent or most severe in order to have the solicitous attention shifted to them.

Anticipation of Aversive Consequences

In some settings such as treatment programs, clients learn to differentiate desirable from aversive consequences. They recognize that violence or substance abuse may get them suspended or even expelled from a program. In contrast, they realize that self-injury tends to result in less radical and punitive consequences. Self-injury may therefore be differentially reinforced. If clients feel a need to express intense emotion, they may learn to inhibit violence because of legal consequences or physical restraint within the program. Self-injury can be a more advantageous and strategic act. The emotions get expressed, but the consequences are modest and may even be inadvertently positive, as discussed above.

Additional Peer-Group Influences

Direct Modeling Influences

Bandura (1977) established long ago that some behavior is markedly influenced by direct modeling influences. Human beings often imitate the behavior of others even when no external contingencies apply. An example would be a youth imitating the self-injury of a peer even when no emotional relief or social reinforcement was expected or forthcoming.

Berman and Walley (2003) conducted an interesting experiment to test the contagion hypothesis regarding self-inflicted aggressive behavior. They examined the influence of a self-aggressive model on self-aggressive behavior in others under controlled laboratory conditions. A sample of 94 adults was given the opportunity to self-administer shock while competing with a fictitious opponent in a reaction time task. Participants observed the opponent self-administer either increasingly intense shock (a self-aggressive model) or constant low shocks (a non-self-aggressive model). Results suggested that social information influenced the expression of self-aggressive behavior. Berman and Walley found that participants attended to the opponent's shock choices in both model conditions and chose shocks consistent with those of the observed model.

One reason that people self-injure within a group is the influence of direct modeling effects. Several youth have said to me, "I saw my friend do it, so I said, 'What the heck, I might as well try it.'" These adolescents seemed unmindful of contingencies when they performed the self-harm.

Disinhibition

A second group effect that plays a role in producing contagion is disinhibition. In these circumstances the self-injuring behavior of one person reduces or eliminates the inhibitions of another regarding self-injury. Sometimes this sequence happens quite explicitly, as when one person says to another, "Come on, try it, you may like it." Or it can happen via more distant observation, such as the individual who stated, "I saw the scars on her arms and figured if she could do it, so could I. It's not like she's particularly tough or anything."

Competition

In some groups of self-injurers, a competition develops. Individuals may try to outdo each other in terms of the type of weapon employed, extent of physical damage, level of disfigurement, number of wounds, or the body area assaulted. In such cases the normal human instinct for self-protection is turned upside down and outrageousness rules. The most common example are youth who "play chicken" by burning each other with cigarettes. The "winner" is the one who tolerates the most pain and refuses to "give up." The victor achieves a certain brief status by being deemed the toughest or most courageous.

THE ROLE OF PEER HIERARCHIES

Another way to understand contagion is to identify peer hierarchies that influence the behavior. Matthews (1968), Ross and McKay (1979), and Walsh and Rosen (1988) have all noted that "high status instigators" may play a role in the spread of self-injury through a group. One way to assess whether peer influences of this type are operational within a group is to

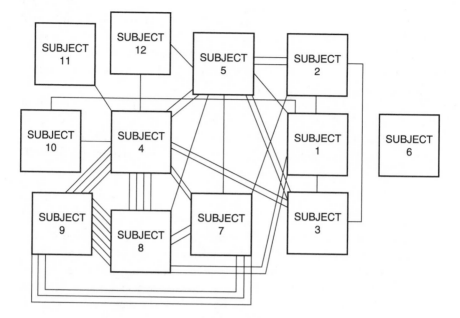

FIGURE 16.1. Schematic representation of self-injury contagion over a 10-month period.

create a sociogram, such as the one provided in Figure 16.1. As discussed in Rosen and Walsh (1989), each box in the figure represents a student who self-injured over a 10-month period while enrolled in a special education school. For this study an "episode of contagion" was defined as any occasion when two or more individuals self-injured within a 24-hour period. Such episodes are represented in the sociogram as a line connecting two subjects. As shown in Figure 16.1, subjects 8 and 9 shared the most contagion episodes: six during the 10-month period.

Although some co-occurrences of self-injury could have been coincidental, we believe that if they happened recurrently, interpersonal factors were in play. This conclusion was supported by comments from the students themselves when they were interviewed by us. For example, subjects 4 and 7 stated that subjects 8 and 9 were individuals they looked up to and liked to "hang out with." They reported enjoying the "action" that subjects 8 and 9 created in the milieu, saying, "It's never boring when they're around. They drive the staff crazy!" Subjects 4 and 7 also said they liked the attention they received from 8 and 9 when they self-injured. During these periods students 4 and 7 felt more accepted and more important in the overall peer group.

By constructing a sociogram and debriefing self-injuring individuals, it is possible to determine the highest-status and most influential members. This determination enables caregivers to target those individuals for intervention in order to manage and reduce contagion. Taiminen and colleagues (1998) employed the same sociogram technique in their study of adolescent inpatients.

Ross and McKay (1979) used a similar strategy in attempting to diffuse what was perhaps the most extensive contagion phenomenon in history. Their study of a Canadian training school for girls revealed that 86% of those incarcerated (117 of 136) had carved their bodies at least once. Ross and McKay reported that the administrators at the school tried various methods to diffuse the contagion, such as manipulation of contingencies. Dispensing more attractive awards or more severe punishments did not work; in fact, the contagion only got worse. Only when the school staff decided to "co-opt" the high-status leaders in the peer group did their interventions lead to success. With the peer leaders on board, the contagion episodes markedly declined.

DESIRE FOR GROUP COHESIVENESS

Another major reason that momentum toward self-injury develops within a group is a desire for cohesion. Many self-injurers state that "there is a special bond between people who cut or burn themselves." The source of the cohesiveness appears to be both inclusive and exclusive. Those who share the problem of self-injury have taken a step most are unwilling to take. Once that club has been joined, the members feel they share a unique experience that is intensive and intimate. They may choose to share details of how it feels to lacerate the skin, or what they do with the blood, or how they clean the wounds. These are conversations that foster a rather exclusive intimacy; those who have not self-injured cannot participate. Self-injurers who are part of a contagion episode often believe that they understand each other's pain at a visceral level. They may state that no one "understands a cutter like another cutter," and that no one else can provide such empathic forms of support.

When a contagion episode is unfolding, a sense of escalating excitement often develops. People within the group may feel a sense of intimacy and exhilaration that they are unable to achieve through other means. Contagion episodes can be intensely invigorating until the inevitable "crash" happens. Self-injury contagion cannot really provide sustained and stable intimacy within a group.

A CASE EXAMPLE OF SELF-INJURY CONTAGION

The following case example demonstrates many of the interpersonal dynamics discussed above.

Several years ago I worked with a woman who was the captain of her college lacrosse team. At the same time I shared on-call duties with a colleague who was the therapist for another member of the team. As a result I came to know about the second client's situation because I was her "backup" when my colleague was unavailable. Through these clients I learned about a sustained contagion phenomenon that involved five women on the lacrosse team. These women tended to have very stormy relationships ranging from those involving sexual intimacy, to close personal friendships, to vehement disagreements, and relationship breakups.

One of the major measures of psychological distress in this group was the frequency and intensity of their self-injury. All five had self-injured at some point in their college careers. My client had done so hundreds of times. She was by far the "leader" in terms of self-destructive behavior within the group. The rate of self-injury for the others in the group ranged from 2 or 3 times to 50 (for my colleague's client).

Early in the treatment of my client, whom I will call Ms. O, a contagion episode developed for this group. The cluster of self-injury began after the lacrosse team lost a game. Going into the season, expectations had been high for this team because their record the previous year had been good and they had many returning athletes. Nonetheless, they lost three of their first four games. Particularly vexing was the third loss, which occurred despite a noticeably weaker opponent.

On the evening after the loss, Ms. O cut herself eight times on her forearm and several more times on her calf. Immediately after this action she walked down the hall of her dorm and entered the room of one of her teammates (modeling influence). The teammate gasped as she saw the blood running down her friend's extremities and said, "What have you done?!" Ms. O replied, "I'm sick of this shit! The team sucks, our record sucks, and most of all, I suck!" (This statement belied the fact that Ms. O was clearly the best player on the team.) She then burst into tears and as she told me later, "made a fool of myself crying for several minutes" (limited communication skills). The woman to whom Ms. O had vented was Ms. Z, the sec-

ond most experienced self-injurer in the group. After beginning treatment with my colleague, she had not self-injured for several months. However, that evening she cut herself about four times on her forearm. As she later explained to my colleague, "Seeing all that blood and hearing the crying was just too much for me. I couldn't contain myself any longer." (disinhibition).

Ms. Z then let Ms. O and another team member know that she had hurt herself. Ms. O felt guilty, believing that Ms. Z would not have relapsed but for her, so she cut herself several times again the next afternoon (limited communication skills; competition; desire for cohesion?). Ms. X, the other individual Ms. Z had informed, quickly told two other team members within their group "that Ms. O is cutting herself like crazy." Ms. X and the other two members of the group then rallied around Ms. O, expressing their concern in effusive ways. They brought Ms. O flowers and took her to lunch. With this level of support, Ms. O appeared to stabilize. She began spending inordinate amounts of time with the teammates who had supported her so intensively (cohesiveness achieved).

Before long, Ms. Z began to feel ignored. She felt "closed out" by this tight new group and wondered if she had done something wrong. In response to this feeling of isolation, Ms. Z cut herself several more times and made sure that Ms. X and the other two team members were aware of the incident (limited communication skills; competition for scarce resources). The attention of the group then shifted back to Ms. Z. One member of the team gave her a massage because she "seemed so stressed out." Another made a dinner for her so she "could stop all this cutting."

Eventually Ms. X and the two members of the team who had the least experience with self-injury (i.e., two or three times) decided to scratch their arms while together (disinhibition; limited communication skills; competition for scarce resources; desire for cohesion). They reported feeling overwhelmed by all the support provided to Ms. O and Ms. Z. Their behavior seemed to pay off as the attention of the group shifted briefly to meeting their needs—even though they tended to be lower-status members of the group (cohesiveness achieved).

The episode concluded as it had begun, with another incident from Ms. O. In response to all the uproar, she cut herself more deeply, resulting in 11 sutures on her left arm (disinhibition; competition). The level of damage for this self-injury seemed to shock the group and cause them to step back from the round of self-injurious acts. No further self-injury ensued for several weeks.

Oddly, the performance of the lacrosse team improved after this contagion episode. As one of the women stated, "the cutting wasn't a good thing, but it did bring us together. We were so close afterward that we played better as a team."

OTHER UNUSUAL ISSUES RELATED TO CONTAGION

Pseudocontagion Episodes

It should also be noted that "pseudocontagion" episodes sometimes occur (although rarely). In these circumstances, a burst of self-injury in a group may pertain less to interpersonal issues than to intrapersonal dilemmas experienced in parallel fashion. For example, a peer group may learn of the imminent departure of a favorite teacher or staff person. If the group is not cohesive, each member of the group may experience emotional pain independently in relation to the loss. In such groups little communication is exchanged about their common experience of loss. In a pseudoepisode, individuals start self-injuring at the same time due to the experience of a common trigger. The episode may look like an interactive contagion phenomenon, but it is not. Rather, it is a series of relatively independent events happening at the same time in parallel fashion.

Electronic Communication Contagion Episodes

Relatively recent phenomena are contagion episodes that involve people who have never met face-to-face. These have become possible because of electronic communications such as voice mail, chat rooms, instant messaging, and websites. I have treated multiple clients in psychotherapy who frequently participate in chat rooms devoted to self-injury. Most or all of the mechanisms described above related to contagion can influence behavior in such chat rooms. Members may use disclosures regarding self-injury to communicate intense feelings (e.g., "I can't believe you ignored my messages for two days! I ended up cutting myself"), coerce others ("Without your help, I would cut myself"), model for others ("I always use an X-acto knife; it's so precise"), compete with others ("That's nothing, I just cut myself 12 times . . . "), and disinhibit others ("Knowing that you cut yourself today means that I may have to"). Pecking orders also emerge in chat rooms whereby those who self-injure with the greatest "conviction" have the highest status. Some self-injurers go so far as to create their own self-injury websites. Most claim to have developed the websites to provide support and help others, but the content on the sites is often more triggering than therapeutic.

One of the anomalies of these electronic communication media is that contagion episodes emerge among people who have never met face-to-face.

Members seem to take on faith that the disclosures of self-injury are accurate and truthful. There is no way to know if the self-injuries described have really happened or are the creations of those with vivid self-injurious imaginations. This lack of validation was previously impossible in face-to-face groups.

CONCLUSION

The ultimate goal in trying to understand the complex factors related to contagion is to learn how to manage and prevent it. The next chapter presents a protocol used in public schools to respond to self-injury. One of the goals of this protocol is to prevent self-injury contagion in school settings. The principles presented in the next chapter can also be applied to other settings where groups of self-injurers comingle, such as inpatient units, residential schools, group homes, prisons, and day treatment programs.

CHAPTER 17

A Protocol for Managing Self-Injury in School Settings

Unfortunately, many middle schools and high schools in the United States are experiencing an explosion of self-injury among their students. This phenomenon often produces confusion and alarm in school staff who are not used to dealing with high rates of self-harm. Such reactions are entirely understandable; schools, after all, are institutions of learning, not mental health clinics.

In order for school personnel to respond effectively to self-injury, they need a systematic approach. This chapter presents a protocol that has been used successfully in several public schools in Massachusetts. In order for this protocol to work effectively, staff must first receive several hours of training. This training should include at least the following:

1. Staff begin by learning about the full range of self-destructive behaviors, including direct and indirect self-harm (as presented in Chapter 2). Personnel in schools who are responsible for the first line of assessment need to understand and ask about the entire spectrum of self-destructive behavior. This involves going beyond the presenting problem (e.g., self-injury, substance abuse, eating disorder) and asking about all forms of direct and indirect self-harm (see Figure 2.2). This enables staff to discern if a student has one or more self-destructive behaviors and to determine if he or she is in a crisis requiring immediate intervention. In many schools the role of providing a preliminary assessment is assumed by a social worker or psychologist, but in some cases the point person can be a guidance counselor, nurse, or even a vice principal or principal.

2. Next, staff should be trained in differentiating self-injury from suicide (as presented in Chapter 1). Staff need to learn which behaviors should be considered suicidal (i.e., the use of a gun, overdose, hanging, jumping from a height, and ingestion of poison) and which should be considered self-injurious (e.g., most forms of self-inflicted cutting, burning, abrading, hitting, biting, and excoriation). Staff need to be cognizant that the former behaviors may result in death but that the latter are unlikely to. Whenever school professionals are unclear about the distinction between self-injury and suicide, they should always rely on mental health professionals to make the determination.

3. Staff also need to understand that certain types of self-injury require immediate assessment by a psychiatric emergency service: namely, those that involve significant tissue damage requiring medical treatment (such as suturing) or those that involve face, eyes, breasts, and genitals (as presented in Chapter 7).

4. Staff should be aware that body modification (e.g., tattoos and body piercings obtained from professionals) is not the same thing as self-injury (as presented in Chapter 4).

5. Staff should learn that the best way to respond to common self-injury is with a "low-key, dispassionate demeanor" and "respectful curiosity" (as presented in Chapter 6). The behavior should not be responded to hysterically, but should also not be dismissed, minimized, or normalized.

6. Staff should understand that the problem of self-injury is complex and that biological, environmental, and psychological factors combine to produce the behavior. These various factors must be addressed to eliminate the behavior (as presented in Chapter 5). Treatment usually takes time and school staff should not expect rapid extinction of the behavior. Requiring that students return to school only after the self-injury is eliminated is completely unrealistic.

Once these various training topics have been addressed with staff, a school is in a position to implement a protocol to deal with self-injury. The advantage of having a written protocol is that staff know how to respond to self-injury systematically and strategically. An established protocol is comforting to staff, students, and parents alike.

The protocol presented below has been used effectively in multiple school settings. However, it does not represent a "boiler plate" solution that can implemented in every school. Each school needs to decide on the components of its own protocol. These should be tailored to meet the unique needs of each educational environment. The protocol that follows describes steps in assessing and responding to self-destructive behavior, including

self-injury. It describes staff responsibilities and expected interactions with
students and their families.

PROTOCOL FOR DEALING
WITH SELF-DESTRUCTIVE BEHAVIORS

1. All school staff should contact the designated point person (e.g., school
   social worker, guidance counselor, psychologist, nurse) *immediately*
   when a student presents with any of the following behaviors:
   • Any suicidal talk, threats, "joking," notes, poetry, other writings, art-
     work, or other communications that have suicidal themes.
   • Any instances of self-injury or self-mutilation, such as wrist, arm, or
     body cutting, self-scratching, self-burning, self-hitting, picking of
     wounds, crude self-inflicted tattoos, disfiguring hair pulling and
     removal, or excessive accident proneness.

   *Note: Self-injuries of this type are generally not suicidal in intent and
   are generally not likely to result in death. However, they do indicate serious
   psychological distress requiring professional assessment and treatment as
   soon as possible.*

   • Eating-disordered behavior, such as self-induced vomiting, sustained
     fasting, marked ongoing weight loss or gain, use of diet pills or laxa-
     tives.
   • Disclosures regarding risk-taking behaviors, such as:
     a. *Physical risks* (e.g., walking in high-speed traffic, walking on an
        elevated railroad bridge, straddling the edge of high roof)
     b. *Situational risks* (e.g., getting into a car with strangers, walking in
        a dangerous area of a city alone late at night)
     c. *Sexual risks* (e.g., having many sexual partners, having unpro-
        tected sex with strangers)
   • Substance use behavior that exceeds "normal" adolescent experimen-
     tation, suggestive of abuse or addiction (e.g., students who get high
     before school or who drink or smoke marijuana multiple times per
     week).
   • Students who discontinue prescribed medications without their doc-
     tor's permission.
   • Other behaviors that suggest serious emotional distress or dyscontrol,
     such as uncontrollable crying, explosive anger, frequent fights,
     extreme reactions to minor events, serious isolation, or extremely
     poor hygiene.

2. Once the school social worker, psychologist, or nurse receives information about any of the above behaviors, he or she will contact the student
discretely and confidentially investigate. *If requested, the social worker,
psychologist, or nurse may keep the identity of the referring school staff
person confidential.*

There are three possible outcomes based on the information obtained
from interviewing the student, peers, and school staff. These are:

a. *If the incident is deemed minor and/or already resolved,* there will
be no action beyond the interview with the student. The student
will be encouraged to contact the social worker, psychologist, or
nurse in the future, should he or she again become distressed.

*Note: The school staff person who contacted the social worker, psychol-
ogist, or nurse will be advised of this outcome as soon as is feasible within
the confines of confidentiality. This feedback loop is important so that the
referring staff person knows that his or her report resulted in an intervention.*

b. *If the incident is deemed important and requiring additional
intervention,* the child's parent or guardian will be called by the
social worker, psychologist, or nurse immediately and briefed
on the situation. Whenever possible, the student will be
advised in advance that the social worker, psychologist, or
nurse is calling the parent or guardian. The purpose of the call
will be explained as ensuring that the student has adequate
support, protection, and assistance. The social worker or nurse
will emphasize that the call has no disciplinary or punitive purposes. Also, whenever indicated, the call to the parent or
guardian will be made with the student present so that he or
she is aware of the specifics of the communication.

When a student presents with any of the above self-destructive behaviors, the parent or guardian will be asked to pursue a number of possible
options to assist the student. These include:

- Initiating outpatient counseling for the child and/or family.
- Seeking psychotropic medication for serious cognitive or emotional
disturbance such as depression, anxiety, obsessive–compulsive disorder, thought disorder, etc.
- Agreeing to the child's receiving enhanced academic and/or counseling supports within the school setting itself.

- Providing releases of information to the school so that the social worker or nurse may communicate with any outside professionals who are assisting the student.

Once the social worker, psychologist, or nurse has made the recommendation for professional help, he or she will recontact the parent or guardian within 1 week to ascertain whether or not the referral has been pursued. The social worker or nurse will emphasize the importance of this referral and the need for action, if none has been taken. Failing to take action repeatedly in support of the mental health needs of a child may be grounds for filing a neglect or abuse report on the parent or guardian, as mandated by the state's child protection agency.

Note: The school staff person who contacted the social worker, psychologist, or nurse will be advised of this outcome as soon as is feasible within the confines of confidentiality. This feedback loop is important so that the referring staff person knows that his or her report resulted in an intervention.

    c. *If the incident is deemed to be an emergency or crisis involving imminent risk*, the social worker, psychologist, or nurse will arrange for an immediate screening at the local psychiatric emergency service and/or police intervention. Examples would include a student disclosing a specific plan to overdose, shoot him- or herself, hang him- or herself, or jump from a dangerous height on that day. In such circumstances, parents or guardians will be informed of the situation as soon as the crisis is handled and stabilized.

Note: The school staff person who contacted the social worker, psychologist, or nurse will be advised of this outcome as soon as is feasible within the confines of confidentiality. This feedback loop is important so that the referring staff person knows that his or her report resulted in an intervention.

IMPLEMENTING AND USING THE PROTOCOL WITH SELF-INJURY

The protocol employs formal language designed to produce consistent responses in school staff to a variety of self-harm behaviors. In order to explain how the protocol works in the real world, it is useful to provide a case example:

Amy is a 14-year-old freshman in high school. One day her friend, Beth, tearfully discloses to the school social worker, James, that Amy has been cutting herself. Beth tells James that she feels guilty saying anything about Amy's cutting because she promised her friend that she wouldn't tell. However, Beth is afraid that her friend may die from her "suicide attempts" and so she "just can't keep it a secret anymore." The social worker reassures Beth that she has done the right thing. He tells Beth that cutting usually won't result in death, but that it is an indication of serious distress. He tells Beth that he will take over from here and see that Amy gets some help. He also assures Beth he will try not to reveal his source of information in order to protect her friendship with Amy.

Within an hour, James catches Amy between classes and asks to speak with her. He jokes, "Don't worry! You're not in trouble!" Amy looks relieved to hear she hasn't "done anything wrong." In his office, James tells Amy gently that he has learned that she has been cutting herself. Amy dissolves in tears and asks "Who told you that?" James says that is less important than learning more about her self-harm. He then begins to assess the nature of her cutting. He learns that she has been cutting her left forearm and left leg "for about 3 months." He asks to see the cuts on her arm and is relieved to see that the tissue damage is modest and that the number of cuts is under 10. Amy states that the cuts on her leg "are about the same as on my arm but not so many." James's preliminary assessment is that Amy's self-injury is of the common type and not a psychiatric emergency.

James then continues his informal assessment and learns from Amy that she has not hurt herself in other ways, has no suicidal plans or history, and is not a risk taker. She reports that she occasionally smokes marijuana or drinks a beer on weekends, but that her substance use is not frequent. Amy denies having an eating disorder and is not taking any psychotropic medication.

Based on this information, James is convinced that Amy is in no immediate risk but that she does require help on an outpatient basis for her self-injury. His next step is to call Amy's mother with Amy present in the office. He explains that he is going to call her mother in order to get Amy some help with her cutting behavior.

On the phone with the mother, James follows the school protocol. In speaking with the mother, he first explains that he is not calling because of any disciplinary problem. However, he's learned that Amy has been cutting her arm and leg with a razor for about 3 months. The mother expresses shock at this information and exclaims, "Why would my daughter want to kill herself?" James attempts to reassure the mother that self-injury usually doesn't have much to do with suicide, but is indicative of serious emotional distress. He explains that cutting unfortunately has become a relatively com-

mon problem among teens. He then asks if she would be willing to pursue outpatient counseling for her daughter to help with the problem. He also suggests that an assessment regarding medication might be indicated. Mother responds affirmatively, saying that she will follow up on both suggestions immediately. James then provides the names and numbers of three local counselors, all of whom have an affiliation with a psychiatrist. He asks that the mother call him back when the appointments have been scheduled. The mother agrees and the phone call ends.

Amy seems relieved that her "big secret is out" and that her "mother isn't mad." James sends Amy back to class and says he'll check on her tomorrow to see how she is doing. As a postscript, the mother called the next day to say that a therapy appointment had been scheduled in 3 days and that the therapist would arrange for a psychiatric consultation regarding medication. James promised to stay in touch with the mother to monitor Amy's progress.

Of course, not all situations proceed as smoothly as this example. The reactions of families are highly variable. Some families are dismissive and insist that their child is "just doing it for attention" or that the behavior is "part of some fad." These families need to be counseled to be more sympathetic and responsive. Other families may present with extreme reactions such as becoming enraged at the child for his or her "misbehavior" or for "embarrassing the family in the community." Such reactions are usually indicative of other family problems that may need to be addressed via outpatient family work. Usually, it is best for the school staff to gently but firmly suggest that such families obtain some "short-term counseling" in order to learn how to deal more effectively with their "challenging adolescent." Defining the problem as residing in the adolescent may be necessary initially to move a family past defensiveness and distrust of mental health professionals.

Some self-injuring youth have little or no family resources. They may be living in a short-term foster home, a respite program, or with a minimally involved, distant relative. In such cases, the school may need to take the initiative in obtaining mental health services for the child. Many schools have a mental health clinician on site who has been assigned by a local mental health clinic. Such services may be billable through third-party insurance. These resources can be an important source of support for students who do not have a family resource that will arrange follow-up care.

MANAGING AND PREVENTING CONTAGION

Another common problem that schools face is dealing with epidemics or contagion episodes of self-injury. In these situations multiple students who know each other self-injure within short periods of time. Such students often appear to be communicating frequently about self-injury, in effect, triggering the behavior in each other. In some situations the contagion is immediate and direct: Youth self-injure in each other's presence. Peers may share the same tools or implements or may even take turns injuring the body of the other.

As noted in Chapter 16 youth may trigger self-injury in each other because (1) the behavior produces feelings of cohesiveness (e.g., as one teen said, "There is a special bond among people who cut themselves"); (2) the behavior has powerful communication aspects (e.g., "My friend must really be upset to cut herself so many times"); (3) the behavior may be viewed as outrageous and provocative (e.g., "It really freaks out my parents when we do this"); and (4) the behavior may also be inadvertently reinforced by adults (e.g., "Finally, my parents believe I'm in a lot of pain").

School professionals should consider three main interventions in order to minimize the risk of contagion: (1) Reduce communication about self-injury among members of the peer group; (2) reduce the public exhibition of scars or wounds in the school milieu; and (3) treat the behavior using individual counseling methods and *not* group therapy, with a few exceptions.

Reducing Communication about Self-Injury

Students talking to each other about self-injury generally has a very triggering effect. Youth may compete with each other to produce more cuts or burns or use grislier methods of self-harm. Students may also take turns assuming the role of caregiver and victim. As one adolescent exclaimed to me, "My group of friends is so crazy! Someone is always cutting! There is always someone who needs help!"

A strategy that sometimes works to reduce contagion is for school staff to explain to individual students that talking (or e-mailing or instant messaging) about self-injury has a negative effect on peers by making self-harm much more likely. Many students injure themselves without remorse, but feel guilty about behaving in a way that may hurt their friends. Appealing to them to reduce or cease communications about self-injury can work with those who have a social conscience. As one adolescent said to me, "It's my business if I cut myself in the privacy of my own home, but I don't want to be responsible for others doing this stuff." Of course, some youth do not mind triggering the behavior in others and may even take delight in "playing uproar." When such youth deliberately and repeatedly trigger self-injury in others, disciplinary action may be needed to reduce the climate of contagion. On rare occasions students may have to be suspended for refusing to behave in nontriggering ways within the school milieu. Such students may need to agree in writing to reduce their contagion-generating behaviors in order to return to school.

Managing Students Who Exhibit Their Scars or Wounds

A related problem is students who openly show their scars or wounds while at school. Such individuals may wear short-sleeve shirts, pants, or skirts that place their scars in open view within the school community. Viewing these scars or wounds can be very triggering for vulnerable students. My recommendation regarding this problem is first to meet with the student alone. A direct request is made to the student that he or she cover the scars with clothing (or jewelry, a bandana, or some other means) when at school. Merely covering the wound with a large bandage is not acceptable (it is all too obvious that wounds are underneath). Many students are agreeable to covering their scars once an explanation is provided.

For students who are not responsive, the next step is to involve parents. A staff person explains to family members that visible wounds or scars are triggering to others in the school community. Parents are asked to assist in monitoring the student's choice of clothing. Most families are responsive to this request and the problem rapidly declines.

Some students and families are not helpful and a more limit-setting approach becomes necessary. Families may be asked to provide extra sets of clothing to be stored at school so that these can be used when a student's attire on a given day is ill-advised. In some cases, students may need to be sent home and directed to return only when they have changed into less scar-disclosing attire.

Treating Self-Injury Using Individualized Methods, Not Groups

A number of years ago I was asked to consult at a middle school that was experiencing an epidemic of self-injury. I learned that eight females in the seventh grade, all of whom knew each other, had been cutting for several months. The social worker who worked with the girls was convinced that they were influencing each other to cut. She attempted to deal with the situation by establishing a "cutters group." She told me she knew she "had a problem" when she was approached by a ninth-grade girl who asked, "How bad do I have to cut myself to get into the cutters group?"

The school social worker's assessment was correct. She did have a problem. Despite her best intentions, she had inadvertently contributed to a contagion episode. My recommendation to this staff person was that she disband the cutters group and refer the girls out for individual therapy. She proceeded to follow this suggestion, using the protocol described above. A year later she reported that none of the eight girls was still cutting.

This anecdote has a basic message. It is often exceedingly dangerous to treat self-injury in groups because open discussion of self-injury antecedents, behavior, and consequences runs the risk of being exceptionally triggering. A much more strategic course is to refer clients to individual therapy where they can focus on their specific needs for replacement skills, cognitive therapy, and resolution of trauma. A notable exception to this rule is to use groups for replacement skills training. Such groups should be governed by strict rules that prohibit discussion of the details of self-injury. Members are told, "It's very important that you discuss self-injury in great detail, but you should do this in individual therapy, *not* in group therapy."

The focus in these groups is on learning, practicing, and generalizing the use of skills in the real world. Replacement skills, as presented in Chapter 9, can be taught quite efficiently to groups of self-injurers as long as the focus remains consistently on skill acquisition. Maintaining this focus can often be quite challenging for therapists, because members find talking about self-injury so alluring. Quick redirection to the skills training topic of the day is important for the success of the group. A brief anecdote illustrates this process:

GROUP LEADER: Hello, everyone. Let's begin by reporting on last week's homework, which was mindful breathing. Who brought their mindful breathing tracking card?

MEMBER 1: I did. I had a good week in terms of using my breathing.

GROUP LEADER: Great! What happened?

MEMBER 1: Well, I practiced four times, which is good for me. And I even used it once when I felt like cutting.

GROUP LEADER: Great, it's good to be able to use breathing skills when you're distressed. Did it help?

MEMBER 1: Yes, I was able to calm myself down and not to cut.

MEMBER 2: (*breaking in*) Breathing doesn't usually work for me when I get an urge to cut. When I get really pissed, I go into my bedroom and just . . .

GROUP LEADER: (*quickly raising his hand in a stop gesture and interjecting gently but firmly*) Remember, we don't get into details about self-harm behaviors in group, but it is important for you to explore that in individual therapy.

MEMBER 2: Oh, yeah, I forgot.

GROUP LEADER: *(turning to look at member 1)* Okay, what were you saying about using your breathing?

Running skills training groups with multiple self-injurers generally
requires co-leaders. The primary leader can be responsible for the skills
training topic of the day and the secondary leader can focus on preventing
triggering behavior as well as other tasks (such as scanning the group for
anyone who looks distressed). Skills training can be effectively taught in
groups, but the leaders need to be focused on their mission and alert to
detours that may produce contagion. Examples of skills groups that have
been run effectively in schools include those focusing on self-soothing
skills, violence prevention, dating skills, and grief groups (for students who
have lost a parent through death). All of these groups have assisted self-
injurers in learning new skills that enable them to reduce the frequency of
self-harm.

CONCLUSION

This chapter has focused on managing self-injury in school settings. The
components of a thorough staff training sequence have been reviewed. A
protocol for responding to self-destructive behavior in students has also
been discussed. Finally, specific suggestions have been offered to prevent
and manage contagion in school populations. For a more extensive discussion of contagion, see Chapter 16.

CHAPTER 18

Treating Major Self-Injury

This chapter is the most disturbing to read in the book because it focuses on *major* self-injury. This is *not* a relevant chapter for those working in school or university settings or other locations where the clientele is high functioning. It can be useful for those employed in correctional facilities, psychiatric hospitals, group homes, supported housing programs, PACT teams, clubhouses, and other programs that serve the seriously mentally ill or those with severe personality disorders.

DEFINITION

Favazza stated that "major self-injury refers to infrequent acts—such as eye enucleation, castration, and limb amputation—that result in the destruction of significant body tissue" (Favazza, 1996, p. 233). This type of self-injury can properly be referred to as "self-mutilation" because it meets *Webster's* definition for the word "mutilate," meaning "to cut up or alter radically so as to make imperfect" and "to maim, cripple" (1995, p. 342). In this chapter the terms "major self-injury" and "self-mutilation" are used interchangeably.

INTENT

Although major self-injury, by definition, involves significant tissue damage, such behavior usually does not involve suicidal intent. Persons who perform major self-injury are generally in very acute distress and/or states of intoxication. The extreme behavior often indicates that they are trying to solve a major life problem, transform themselves, or are following perceived instructions from a powerful external force (e.g., God or the devil). Noticeably absent in the intent of these self-injurers is a desire to die (Menninger, 1938/1966; Walsh & Rosen, 1988; Favazza, 1996; Grossman, 2001). Case examples provided below describe the type of idiosyncratic intent that often accompanies major self-injury.

PREVALENCE

The overall prevalence of major self-injury is unknown. Fortunately, the behavior appears to be quite rare. For example, Grossman noted that only "115 cases of male genital self-mutilation have been reported in English, German, and Japanese literature since the end of the nineteenth century" (Grossman, 2001, p. 53). He also identified 90 cases of ocular self-mutilation in the modern literature during the same time period. Because it is a rare behavior, the literature on major self-injury consists almost entirely of individual case reports. I am not aware any empirical studies of major self-injury. Some authors (e.g., Greilsheimer & Grove, 1979; Kennedy & Feldman 1994; Grossman, 2001) have provided summative discussions of case reports for categories such as genital or ocular self-mutilation. These articles are the best available in terms of trying to generalize across the population of major self-injurers.

FORMS OF THE BEHAVIOR

Grossman (2001) noted that four main types of major self-injury have been reported in the literature:

- Genital (e.g., transection of the penis, castration, removal of the penis, female laceration of the urethra and vagina)
- Ocular (e.g., enucleation, puncture, laceration, self-blinding through self-hitting)
- Digit and limb amputation (e.g., finger and limb removal)
- Other especially rare forms (e.g., major self-injury to the nose, tongue, mouth, face, autocannibalism)

DIAGNOSTIC DIVERSITY

When people hear of such horrific acts, they understandably jump to the conclusion that the behaviors must be associated almost exclusively with psychosis. In actuality, the literature describes many examples of major self-injury from a startlingly wide range of psychiatric diagnoses. Favazza has stated that the major forms of self-injury are "most commonly associated with psychosis (acute psychotic episodes, schizophrenia, mania and depression)" (1996, p. 234). However, he also noted that major self-injury has been reported in states of "acute intoxication" and "carefully planned transsexual castration" in which psychosis played no part (Favazza, 1996, p. 234).

Based on his review of the literature, Grossman (2001) noted that approximately 80% of genital self-mutilators have been psychotic at the time of the act. He summarized the diversity of diagnoses and circumstances for genital self-mutilators, indicating that they fall into five generalized groups:

1. Young, acutely psychotic males
2. Violence-prone males during acute intoxication
3. Transgender males seeking a sex change
4. Older males with psychotic depression and somatic illness
5. Individuals with severe personality disorders acting out rageful feelings (Grossman, 2001, p. 53).

To this list I would add, from my own experience, adolescent and adult females who have been repeatedly sexually abused and are suffering from PTSD and related states of dissociation. A case example of this type is provided below.

Grossman (2001) indicated that 75% of ocular self-mutilators have been described as psychotic at the time of the act. The remaining 25% have had diagnoses such as depressive disorder, Munchausen syndrome, substance abuse, and obsessive–compulsive disorder (OCD) (Grossman, 2001; Kennedy & Feldman, 1994). Thus individuals who perform major self-injury come from a broad range of psychiatric diagnoses, including the psychoses, personality disorders, substance abuse disorders, PTSD, OCD, and even comorbid Tourette's disorder with (OCD) (Hood, Baptista-Neto, Beasley, Lobis, & Pravdova, 2004). For a thorough review of this diagnostic information, see Greilsheimer and Groves (1979), Kennedy and Feldman (1994), and Grossman (2001).

PREVENTION AND RISK ASSESSMENT

The primary goal in working with persons capable of major self-injury is to prevent the behavior from happening in the first place. Warning signs for major self-mutilation have not been precisely defined, in part, because the literature is based on case reports rather than empirical studies. The majority of work in performing risk assessments has focused on those with psychotic disorders rather than other diagnoses. As noted by Grossman, "It should be clearly acknowledged that accurate prediction of major SIB [self-injurious behavior] is not possible but that certain factors should heighten the clinician's level of concern with regard to the probability of such behavior occurring. In general, as positive symptoms of psychosis increase, so does the risk of SIB" (Grossman, 2001, p. 58).

Rosen and I presented a protocol (Walsh & Rosen, 1988) for assessing self-injury associated with psychosis. This protocol is similar to the list of risk factors presented by Grossman (2001), but is more extensive and inclusive. I have updated this protocol and present it below. The protocol is not empirically validated, but is informed by clinical experience and knowledge of the self-mutilation literature.

PROTOCOL FOR ASSESSING RISK
OF MAJOR SELF-INJURY

1. Key points of historical information
   - History of previous self-injury and major self-injury
   - History of impulsive violence directed at self and/or others
   - History of childhood deprivation, physical or sexual abuse
   - Recent interpersonal loss or major change in life circumstances
   - Recent self-imposed change in physical appearance (e.g., shaving one's head, donning military garb)
2. Assessment of mental status
   - Presence of auditory hallucinations with self-injurious content (e.g., hearing a voice stating, "You must hurt yourself because you deserve it, you are no good").
   - Belief in the credibility of the source of the hallucinations (e.g., "The voice comes from God and must be obeyed"; it could be the voice of a deceased parent, an angel, or some other figure perceived as powerful, omniscient).
   - Presence of delusions with self-injurious content (e.g., "My self-injury is part of the plan for the universe").
   - Presence of religious delusions, especially any regarding sinfulness, expiation of sins, unworthiness, etc. (e.g., "I must assault or remove this body part to atone for my sins").
   - Presence of persecutory delusions (e.g., "People are after me and will stop only if I remove my eye").

- Presence of somatic delusions (e.g., "My penis is rotting and must be removed"; "My vagina is dirty, disgusting, and must be cleansed and punished").
- Presence of delusions of grandiosity (e.g., "If I remove my eye, I will experience no pain and will sit at the right hand of God").
- Belief in the credibility of any of the above delusions (e.g., "The nature of reality has been revealed to me and only me"; "God must be obeyed"; "My father told me I was no good for so long, it must be true").
- Presence of self-destructive thoughts, ideation, plans, or preoccupations (e.g., "If I hurt myself, all my problems will be solved").
- Substance use or intoxication that exacerbates any of the above mental status conditions.
- Unauthorized discontinuance of psychotropic medication that triggers decompensation and exacerbation of any of the above symptoms.

3. Details related to major self-injury
  - Presence of rituals associated with self-injury
  - Preoccupation with any body areas or body parts
  - Preoccupation with any tools or methods of self-injury
  - Preoccupation with or quoting of Biblical passages with self-injury content (e.g., "And if thy right eye offend thee, pluck it out . . . and if thy right hand offend thee, cut it off"; Matthew 5: 29–30)
  - Preoccupation with any historical or mythological self-injurers (e.g., van Gogh, Bodhidharma, Oedipus)
  - Preoccupation with transgender issues (especially desire for a sex change)
  - Preoccupation and discomfort with unwanted sexual fantasies, impulses, behaviors
  - An absence of physical pain related to any previous self-injury

CASE EXAMPLE RELEVANT TO ASSESSMENT

I have previously described in detail a case of self-enucleation (Walsh & Rosen, 1988). I initially became aware of this individual when I was asked to conduct a critical incident investigation immediately after the act. Subsequently, this individual came into care at my agency, residing in a group home for seriously and persistently mentally ill adults. His residency in this program provided an unusual opportunity to follow a self-enucleator for many years after his major self-injury. I will discuss this case in two parts: (1) as an illustrative case example related to the protocol presented above,

and (2) by providing an update regarding the life (and death) of this
individual post enucleation.

*At the time of his self-enucleation (circa 1986), Mr. M was a single, 31-year-
old white male well known to the local mental health system. He had an
extended history of mental illness and had had many admissions to the local
state hospital. Mr. M's first psychiatric hospitalization had occurred at age
18. Since that time, he had lived at home with his aunt when he was not hospitalized. Mr. M's primary diagnosis was paranoid schizophrenia, although
he had acquired others over the years. During the previous 13 years, his pattern was to experience recurrent psychotic decompensations, chronic unem-
ployment, poor compliance with treatment programs and medication regimens, limited social relationships, and episodic poor self-care skills such as
money management and personal hygiene. His strengths included good
intelligence, a sense of humor, an interest in art, and a generally pleasant
demeanor.*

*During his most recent state hospital stay, plans had been made to place
Mr. M, upon discharge, in a community residential program with another
agency. The reason for the change was that he was becoming increasingly
difficult for his aunt to manage due to dangerous smoking behavior, inconsis-
tent sleeping habits, refusal to do chores, poor personal hygiene, and isolation. Thus, at the time of Mr. M's self-enucleation, he was living in a super-
vised community residence. Despite his participation in the program, his
mental status had deteriorated over the previous several months. As we
learned subsequently, he had periodically stopped taking his psychotropic
medication.*

*Two days before the act, his outreach worker perceived him to be "more
paranoid than usual." However, he did not present with any self-destructive
ideation or behavior. In fact, Mr. M had no history of self-destructive behavior whatsoever.*

*Staff were alerted to be attentive to his medication ingestion, because it
seemed likely that his deterioration was due, in part, to his "cheeking" his
medications. Record material indicated that Mr. M seemed depressed and
required reassurance that he was safe and that no one wanted to harm him
in the residence.*

*On the morning of his self-enucleation, an overnight counselor found
notes written by Mr. M that were puzzling, vague, but ominous in content.
The notes read: (1) "Julie forgive me"; (2) "Perhaps it was a good home . . . it
was the best"; (3) "Good bye Julie"; (4) "Always try to live in a good home . . .
I'm a coward." (Julie was an acquaintance from high school whom he had
not seen for over 10 years.)*

Mr. M left the residence unaccompanied that morning and went to a local psychiatric emergency room. When he arrived, he asked that he be given "a lethal dose of poison." At this point Mr. M was readmitted to the state hospital.

He arrived on the ward during the 3–11 P.M. shift and was given a low dose of prolixin for agitation. In a nursing assessment note Mr. M was described as saying, "I want something lethal—a lethal injection," and "I'm a dirty bastard." Due to his restlessness and preoccupation with death-oriented thoughts, he was given an additional low dose of prolixin, again without noticeable positive effect. Subsequent low doses of prolixin produced no improvement.

Throughout the night Mr. M talked in a rambling, deluded fashion. At one point he ran down the hall of the ward screaming, turned over a table, and had to be physically restrained. He spoke repeatedly about crucifying a girlfriend, said he was a murderer and rapist of young girls, and stated that he had fathered multiple illegitimate children. He also stated that he was soon to die and to be reincarnated as a "Jewish black prince." However, when he was asked if he planned to hurt himself, he emphatically said "No."

Mr. M remained psychotic and bizarre over the next 12 hours and was being watched closely by staff. However, at one point he slipped into a bathroom unaccompanied. The staff then heard Mr. M scream. Upon opening the door to the bathroom, the staff found Mr. M standing with one hand covering his right eye, which was bleeding profusely. Asked what he had done, Mr. M stated he had flushed the eye down the toilet. Mr. M was then transferred to an intensive care medical unit.

ASSESSING THE RISK OF MAJOR SELF-INJURY

The case of Mr. M provides a good example regarding the assessment of risk for major self-injury. Mr. M presented with many warning signs from the protocol, although there were also many other items that did not apply. For example, if we look at section 1 of the protocol (historical information), we see that Mr. M meets only two of the five criteria. He had no history of prior self-injury. He also had no history of abuse or deprivation, nor had he made any recent changes to physical appearance. He did present with some relatively modest physical violence on the ward prior to his self-injury, and he certainly had experienced a recent loss in being placed away from his aunt for the first time. Mr. M clearly seemed to be grieving this loss in his statements about the importance of "living in a good home" and perhaps referring to his aunt's home as "the best."

In terms of assessing Mr. M's mental status, as delineated in section 2 of the protocol, he presented with multiple problems indicative of serious risk. His rambling verbal content included religiosity (Jewish black prince, crucifying girls, condemnation of his immorality), sexual preoccupations (committing rape and fathering illegitimate children), and persecutory ideas (requiring reassurance at the group home as to his safety). He also presented with a variety of highly unusual self-destructive thoughts in that he requested a lethal dose of poison or medication on multiple occasions. Another warning sign was that he had discontinued his psychotropic medication surreptitiously. He had not used or abused any substances. Thus, in terms of the second category of the protocol, there were many "hits" that should have alarmed someone conducting a professional assessment. This portion of the protocol is the one that pointed most directly to the risk of major self-injury posed by Mr. M's mental status.

The third and final section of the protocol concerns details regarding the self-injury. This section would not have been especially helpful with Mr. M because he had no prior history of self-harm. Also, he did not present with any preoccupations with body parts, tools, or transgender issues. At one point Mr. M did quote the passage from the Bible regarding plucking out one's eye, but this was several days *after the fact*. He certainly did present with preoccupation about sexuality and seemed to be experiencing guilt about imagined sexual offenses.

Mr. M provided additional information about his motivations to remove his eye in the days following the act. For example, he described some homosexual fears and wishes related to having a roommate at his group home. He remained preoccupied with harming and impregnating young girls. In the end, he seemed to have struck some sort of "psychic bargain" by removing his eye to expiate his sins and being allowed to survive (Menninger, 1938/1966). He also disclosed some persecutory ideation, saying that he "needed to remove his eye or the bomber pilot would have gotten it." Much of his ideation was so floridly psychotic that others could not decipher its meaning. It is important to note that most of this content emerged only several days *after* the self-enucleation. Unless this ideation had been elicited prior to the act, it would not have helped in prevention.

In summary, the case of Mr. M demonstrates that the protocol for assessing major self-injury can be a useful tool in alerting clinicians to danger. However, it is far from being as precise as a thermometer measuring temperature. The protocol provides some useful guidelines, but only a very astute team of professionals might have been able to prevent Mr. M's self-enucleation. Identifying precise predictors of major self-injury is regrettably still a long way off.

UPDATE ON THE CASE OF MR. M

Shortly after his self-enucleation, Mr. M entered a residential program operated by my agency. His life postenucleation was generally stable. He continued to suffer from schizophrenia, but he became more compliant regarding his medication and treatment program participation. His compliance seemed to improve as his aunt became less involved in his day-to-day care. Mr. M gradually came to accept living away from his aunt and eventually took pride in his greater level of independence. He became active in a local clubhouse program for mentally ill people.

Occasionally, Mr. M presented with increased levels of agitation, anger, and restlessness. At these times, Mr. M sometimes stated that his "good eye hurt." He also made what seemed to be veiled self-threats, such as, "I hope nothing happens to my good eye." At these time staff in the residential program became appropriately alarmed and hypervigilant. They encouraged him to talk about whatever frustrations he might be experiencing. They also used the protocol presented above. In addition, without exception, a consultation regarding medication was immediately arranged. Increases were usually prescribed for relatively short periods. During the 10 years he lived in the program, Mr. M never presented with another self-harm behavior. He passed away from natural causes (heart attack) in the mid-1990s.

TREATMENT

Psychopharmacology

For individuals suffering from psychosis, the treatment of choice to prevent major self-injury is psychopharmacological. As noted in Chapter 14 by Dr. Harper, trials of antipsychotic agents are indicated for clients with delusional self-injury. He describes the possible benefits of using antipsychotic agents such as risperidone (Risperdal and others) and clozapine (Clozaril and others). Grossman (2001) has discussed the pharmacotherapy of major self-injury at length. He suggested that the basic principles of medication treatment in preventing self-injury are (1) rapid treatment of the psychosis, (2) establishment of a regimen that optimizes medication compliance, and (3) sedation during acute periods of agitation (Grossman, 2001, p. 61). (These are exactly the principles we followed in treating Mr. M in our residential program.) Grossman also discussed the use of benzodiazepines, mood stabilizers, and antidepressants in the treatment of major self-injury.

Psychological Therapies

Psychological therapies are designed both to prevent major self-injury and to manage it in those for whom it is ongoing. Some clients have extended histories of performing major self-injury. The psychological treatments provided to those at risk of novel or recurrent major self-injury, in part, depends on the diagnosis. As noted by Grossman (2001), in the majority of cases the diagnosis is one of the psychoses. For these individuals, the treatment of choice (in addition to medication) is often a symptom management skills training approach (e.g., Brenner et al., 1994, 1999). Liberman (1999) employs an empirically validated manualized treatment that teaches psychotic individuals symptom management and relapse prevention skills. He employs four skills modules that focus on (1) medication management, (2) recreation for leisure, (3) symptom management, and (4) conversational skills. If clients learn to manage their medication properly, to identify warning signs of decompensation, to cope with persistent symptoms, and to avoid alcohol and drugs (Liberman, 1999), they are far more likely to avoid relapse into psychosis. When psychotic decompensation is avoided, related risk of major self-injury is thereby reduced.

Cognitive-Behavioral Therapy

The symptom management approach is sometimes combined with cognitive-behavioral therapy. The basics of this treatment have been described in Chapter 10. As noted there, cognitive therapy (1) targets the automatic thoughts, intermediate beliefs, and core beliefs that support self-injury; (2) collects information about these types of cognitions; and (3) gently challenges and corrects inaccurate or dysfunctional cognitions that support the behavior. Prognosis in working with psychotic individuals may be linked to how firmly the individual believes in the delusions, how flexible the delusions are in accommodating new information, and how pervasive the delusions are in the person's daily experience (Kingdon & Turkington, 1994). Some basic modifications to the cognitive therapy approach often need to be made in working with people with psychosis (Kingdon & Turkington, 1994; Merlo, Perris, & Brenner, 2004). For example, Kingdon and Turkington (1994) have identified four steps in working with delusional material in schizophrenic clients:

1. Target the less strongly held beliefs first.
2. Avoid direct confrontation of the delusional material.
3. Focus on the evidence for the delusion, not the content of the delusion itself.

4. Encourage the client to voice his or her own doubts about, or arguments against, the beliefs.

An example of such therapy with a schizophrenic man with major self-injury is provided below.

Cognitive Therapy with Mr. Z

I first met Mr. Z, a 45-year-old Caucasian, as part of a consultation I provided to a residential treatment program. Mr. Z's self-harm behaviors included self-hitting of his legs, arms, and chest and, more alarmingly, punching of his eyes. The eye-punching behavior had resulted in significant loss of sight for Mr. Z over the years—to the extent that he was now legally blind. Mr. Z could still read but only when he held text within inches of his face.

When I interviewed Mr. Z as part of the consultation, I uncovered some important information. A standard part of my interview with recurrent or chronic self-mutilators is to ask them about the six dimensions of body image, as discussed in Chapter 11. I therefore asked him about the dimensions of (1) attractiveness, (2) effectiveness (athleticism), (3) health, (4) sexual characteristics, (5) sexual behavior, and (6) body integrity.

When I asked Mr. Z about sexual behavior, he shared information that his caregivers at the residential program had not heard before. Mr. Z stated that he had "consorted with prostitutes" a number of times when he was a college student and had also looked at pornographic magazines. He considered these to be grievous sins for which he was still being punished. When asked who was punishing him, Mr. Z replied, "the devils." The program staff was very familiar with this delusional material.

At the conclusion of this consultation, I made two recommendations. The first was that the staff should differentiate between two categories of self-harm for Mr. Z: (1) the self-hitting that caused little tissue damage, versus (2) the eye-punching that was blinding Mr. Z. The new plan was to call for evaluation for a respite placement outside his residential program whenever the eye punching occurred, whereas the other, less damaging self-harm behaviors would continue to be handled internally. This simple contingency management technique was designed to provide aversive consequences for Mr. Z for the major self-injury. We hoped this would shape his responses in the direction of less severe self-injury.

I also recommended that the staff collect data for the two categories of self-injury on a daily basis at the program and that his therapist pursue the sexual material and related guilt in therapy. The goal in therapy was to try to lessen his irrational thoughts and guilt about past "sins" and thereby reduce his motivation to self-injure.

About a year later I was asked to provide individual therapy with Mr. Z because his long-time therapist had left the program. Since then I have met with Mr. Z twice a month for several years. Sessions with Mr. Z have generally lasted about 30 minutes, which is as much time as he can tolerate. During the sessions Mr. Z is cooperative, sincerely tries to answer all my questions, and gives direct, honest, and thoughtful replies. The only time he is uncooperative is when I pursue information regarding his relationship with the devils too extensively. Then Mr. Z may say that he is "not supposed to talk about the devils so much," whereupon he changes the subject and will not return to it.

Of interest is that in my first therapy meeting with Mr. Z, he brought up the topic of the prostitutes to me, even though he had not seen me in about 14 months. A bit taken aback, I pursued the topic and learned that he continued to believe he was being punished for his sexual indiscretions from some 20 years previous. Since this behavior was causing Mr. Z considerable discomfort and it appeared to have a direct link with his self-harm behaviors, I decided to pursue it each session if possible.

Over time, Mr. Z continued to discuss the punishment he was receiving via the devils. More specifically, he indicated that the devils "took over [his] body and punished [him] for having had sex with prostitutes." At these times, Mr. Z said, the devils have complete control of his body, and he is powerless to resist them or the self-harming acts inflicted by them.

Intrigued by this content regarding devils, I explored his religious background with him and learned that Mr. Z had been raised a Roman Catholic. He indicated that he had practiced his religion quite faithfully throughout his childhood, but that his practice had lapsed since he had been in residential treatment.

The conversation regarding Mr. Z's religious background led to a treatment strategy, which I proposed to the residential program staff. I suggested that Mr. Z meet with a priest in order to confess his "sins." The speculation on my part was that if Mr. Z were willing to confess his sins and then to receive absolution, he might gain some much needed relief and reduce his motivation for self-injury.

When I shared this proposal with the treatment team, I emphasized that it was a speculative one, at best, and that I had no idea if it would work. My goal was to alter Mr. Z's core beliefs about his basic sinfulness and need for punishment. The team agreed to the plan, but it took months to locate a priest who was comfortable hearing the confession of a delusional psychotic man. Finally, Mr. Z and I located a local priest who was willing. At this meeting all three of us were present for the first part of the discussion. I explained to the priest (with previously obtained permission from Mr. Z) about his experiences with prostitutes and pornography. I also stated that Mr. Z believed that he is still being punished for these sins. With this introduction concluded, the priest spoke with Mr. Z directly. When Mr. Z referred to his behavior as adultery, "one of the worst sins," the priest corrected him, saying that it was not adultery since it seemed unlikely that any of the involved parties was married. The priest also clarified for Mr. Z that if he decided to confess his sins and did so in a sincere manner, his sins would be forgiven in the eyes of God forever. After some additional discussion, I left the room and the priest heard Mr. Z's confession and administered absolution.

When I met with Mr. Z a week later, he indicated that he was pleased with the meeting and the confession and that he felt it had done him some good. He also stated that he believed he was harming himself less since the confession. However, over the next several months, data collected at the program indicated (1) no decrease in the rate of self-harm, and (2) no decrease in the assaults to the head. It became clear that modifying Mr. Z's fixed delusions would be no easy task. His delusions were especially hard to change in that, as noted by Kingdon and Turkington (1994), they were characterized by great conviction, flexibility, and pervasiveness.

He also became agitated if pushed too much regarding his conviction in his "relationship with the devils." In fact, the only two times I have seen him assault himself was when I had pushed too long or too hard about his delusional material. In addition, he sometimes spoke positively about the devils, saying that they "granted [him] mercy and taught [him] positive things." The fact that the devils were sometimes "helpful" to him made challenging his belief system all the more difficult.

Another strategy I pursued with Mr. Z was exploring the "evidence for his beliefs," as recommended by Kingdon and Turkington (1994). Mr. Z had received training in the sciences as an undergraduate. He had a good understanding of biology and chemistry. I pursued a strategy in which we discussed the scientific explanations for schizophrenia and the symptom of delusions. Mr. Z participated actively in these discussions as long as they were general and not applied to himself. When the conversation got more personal, he simply changed the subject or asserted emphatically, "The devils cause my self-injury" and "brain chemistry has nothing to do with it." Thus my efforts at cognitive restructuring using this approach failed as well.

The most productive strategy in working with Mr. Z to date has focused on skills training. I decided to try some replacement skills training in that the cognitive strategies had not been productive. First, I attempted to teach him a couple of breathing techniques, as presented in Chapter 9. He was initially cooperative in learning these, but he failed to practice, and eventually refused to do them any longer, saying that the devils disapproved.

Next, I decided to pursue a visualization strategy—frankly, grasping at straws. In each session I would create for him a visualization that was relevant to his daily experience. For example, I would describe a day in which he was sitting in the living room of the residence, feeling peaceful, relaxed, and self-injury-free. Mr. Z reported that he liked hearing these visualizations and found them relaxing. However, he was not able or willing to practice them on his own. He relied on me for each "new chapter."

To my surprise, after several months of therapy that invariably involved a visualization, Mr. Z started to repeat back to me the language used in the exercises. For example, he reported feeling "more peaceful" in the residence, "more relaxed," and relatively self-injury-free. It appeared as if suggesting indirectly a different way of experiencing himself and the world was more productive than directly challenging his core delusional beliefs.

It is unclear at this point whether Mr. Z's improvement is temporary or will be sustained. What this case example is designed to demonstrate is that altering delusions that support major self-injury can be very difficult. Many different techniques may need to be tried until one is identified that is congruent with, and not too challenging of, the individual's highly idiosyncratic world view.

THERAPY WITH NONPSYCHOTIC CLIENTS

For self-mutilating clients who are not psychotic, the treatment strategies described in Part II of this book are generally appropriate without substantial modification. Clients with diagnoses such as borderline personality disorder, PTSD, antisocial personality, OCD, anxiety, or depression will usually benefit from some combination of contingency management, replacement skills training, cognitive therapy, and psychopharmacology. For those who have endured trauma, body image work and exposure treatment may also be important. This chapter concludes with one such case example of a self-mutilating individual who is not psychotic:

Rosa was a woman in her 30s who had had a very difficult life. Sexually abused for years as a child, she had learning problems and did not complete high school. She began using substances as a teen, including alcohol, marijuana, and cocaine. She became addicted to crack and began prostituting to support her habit. During her late teens and 20s, she had three children by three different men. All of the children were removed by state protective services.

Eventually, Rosa ended up in prison for cocaine possession, dealing, and prostitution. She did not adjust well to prison, frequently assaulting other inmates and harming herself. Her self-injury generally took the form of cutting her arms and thighs with sharp objects. However, when she was especially distressed, she would violently bite her forearms. These wounds required many sutures and skin grafts and left deep, half-dollar-sized scars.

Rosa was eventually transferred to a state hospital forensic unit because of her increasingly bizarre behavior. She continued to assault others and to bite and scratch herself. The heart of Rosa's problem was the horrific abuse she had suffered at the hands of her aunt's boyfriend and others. She frequently experienced flashbacks and nightmares that tended to be followed by assaults and major self-injury. Before she could deal with her trauma, Rosa desperately needed some skills to manage her intense rage, shame, guilt, and self-loathing. In group and individual treatment on the forensic unit, Rosa learned a number of breathing skills. She particularly liked a visualization from her childhood when she went to the beach with her aunt. She also used art as a release and found that stroking her arms with a cosmetic brush was a soothing activity. These skills allowed Rosa to reduce her assaults on self and others over time. Her major self-injury (self-biting) stopped, but her cutting episodically continued.

Eventually Rosa made productive use of cognitive therapy. She began to look at her incredibly negative core beliefs, which supported much of her self-loathing, rage, and violence. She has also started working on her body image and developed some strategies whereby she "pampered" her body rather than destroying it. The goal is for Rosa to eventually be ready for exposure treatment. If she can resolve some major aspects of her trauma history, there is still hope for Rosa to have a productive life in the community after her sentence is completed.

CONCLUSION

Major self-injury is among the most challenging behaviors faced by clinicians. Their greatest ally in preventing the behavior is often medication. Ancillary treatments that can be helpful are cognitive therapy, replacement skills training, and exposure therapy (in cases of trauma). Fortunately, cases of major self-injury are rare. When acts of such extreme self-mutilation are encountered, they are often unforgettable. At least in the large majority of cases, the clients survive their extreme acts of self-harm—which provides some small solace to the families and treaters involved.

Conclusion

This book has provided a practical guide to understanding and treating self-injury. It was written for professionals but may be of benefit for self-injuring persons as well. The book began by differentiating self-injury from suicide, the two major forms of direct self-harm. It also placed self-injury in relation to various types of indirect self-harm, such as eating disorders, substance abuse, risk-taking behaviors, and noncompliance with psychotropic medications. The book discussed how self-injury is different from body modification such as professionally obtained tattoos, piercings, brands, etc., and reviewed the emerging problem of self-injury in the general population (such as middle and high schools, colleges, and the community at large), offering some speculations as to why the rate of self-injury is growing so markedly.

The heart of this book focused on the assessment and treatment of self-injury. I provided a format for conducting a detailed assessment of self-injury with an emphasis on the antecedents that trigger self-injury, the myriad details regarding the self-injury itself, and the consequences or aftermath of self-injury. The section on treatment moved from the simplest to the most complex of techniques. Some basic recommendations were provided as to how to respond initially to the behavior. I emphasized the need to employ a "low-key, dispassionate demeanor" and a "respectful curiosity." A series of clinical interventions, including contingency management, replacement skills training, cognitive therapy, body image work, and exposure treatment, were then discussed. I also presented a chapter on family treatment, and Dr. Gordon Harper provided a chapter on the psychopharmacological treatment of self-injury. Some suggestions were also offered as to how to manage the countertransference or therapy-interfering behaviors that often emerge in response to self-injury.

Some clients may require all of the modes of treatment discussed in this book in order to give up self-injury. Others may need only one or two in order to make significant gains. Most clients require some combination of contingency management, replacement skills training, and cognitive therapy. Others, particularly those with histories of trauma, may also need exposure treatment and body image work. Many clients benefit from psychopharmacological treatment. It is important to emphasize that each client is unique and must be assessed and treated individually and idiosyncratically. The key is to select the right treatments from the roster of interventions to match the problems and strengths of each individual.

The third and final section of this book focused on several specialized topics. The first of these was the fascinating problem of self-injury contagion, a phenomenon frequently reported in congregate settings such as schools, group homes, and hospitals. I also presented a protocol for responding to self-injury in educational settings, including middle and high schools and universities. Perhaps the most unpleasant chapter in the book was devoted to the topic of major self-injury, which refers to persons who inflict substantial physical damage on themselves, such as self-enucleation or autocastration.

Although this book has attempted to review current research and to present state-of-the-art treatments, it does not claim to have all, or even most, of the answers. Self-injury remains a challenging clinical problem. Progress has been made in the past 30 years in developing more effective treatments. Nonetheless, therapy still requires the best efforts of clients and therapists, working collaboratively toward the common goal of eliminating self-injury and acquiring healthier forms of self-expression and emotion regulation.

Afterword

Two of the most well-known stories in Zen Buddhism involve extreme self-injury. They both feature Bodhidharma, a monk who is said to have brought Zen from India to China about 526 C.E. This Zen master was so committed to attaining enlightenment that he retreated in solitude to a cave for 9 years to practice meditation. Frustrated by his tendency to doze off and thereby "neglect" his practice, he cut off his eyelids. With such fierce dedication, he eventually obtained his goal of a clear, complete *satori*.

Some years later, a monk named Hui K'o came to Bodhidharma's cave seeking to learn from the master. Bodhidharma turned him away. Again and again this monk appealed for admission as a disciple, and Bodhidharma's answer was always the same: refusal. One day, standing in a blizzard outside Bodhidharma's cave, the monk cut off his arm and presented it to the master as a token of his resolve and conviction. He was then accepted as a disciple and eventually became heir to Bodhidharma's teaching lineage.

Certainly eyelid removal or arm amputation should be imitated by no one. However, there may be a symbolic significance in these mythical actions. Self-injurers can be viewed as pursuing a quest that has a fervor beyond most mortals. Whether the goal is release from pain, the resolution of trauma, or an altered state of consciousness, self-injuring persons are willing to pursue actions that most others eschew. They bring their seeking to a level of conviction that takes on physical proportions. Bodily transformation may have as its goal psychological or even spiritual renewal. We should respect their intensity as indicative of great resolve and promise.

My work with self-injurers has taught me, again and again, that great things are possible from those who are able to transform pain into affirmation. The life stories of self-injurers often move from anguish, isolation, and bodily harm to accomplishment, affiliation, and self-protection. We professionals are fortunate to play some role in assisting these seekers to find a higher ground.

Breathing Manual

This manual presents a number of breathing techniques that can be used to manage distress and eliminate self-injury. The examples come from different traditions, including psychology, psychotherapy, social work, and Buddhist meditation. The first four techniques are simpler; after that, the different types of breathing are listed in no particular order. The suggestion is to find a few that are comfortable and useful and to practice those frequently. None will work without practice; all can be helpful tools in reducing and eliminating self-harm behaviors. For all the techniques, it is best to practice for at least 20 minutes three times a week to achieve a beneficial effect.

As Thich Nhat Hanh said,

> While we practice conscious breathing, our thinking will slow down, and we can give ourselves a real rest. Most of the time, we think too much, and mindful breathing helps us to be calm, relaxed and peaceful. It helps us stop thinking so much and stop being possessed by sorrows of the past and worries about the future. It enables us to be in touch with life, which is wonderful in the present moment. (1991, p. 11)

Nhat Hanh also stated:

> Our breathing is the link between our body and our mind. Sometimes our mind is thinking of one thing and our body is doing another, and mind and body are not unified. By concentrating on our breathing, "In" and "Out," we bring body and mind back together, and become whole again. Conscious breathing is an important bridge. (1991, p. 9)

BREATHING TECHNIQUES

In . . . Out Breathing

As you breathe in, say "in" inside your mind; as you breathe out, say "out" inside your mind. Continue for several minutes.

Comment: This simplest of breathing exercises appeals to many as an introduction to mindful breathing. Its simplicity can also be its weakness, because attention may wander. This technique is especially useful for cognitively limited individuals who have trouble remembering more complex techniques. However, people of all abilities have used this technique effectively.

1 through 10 Exhale Breathing

As you breathe in, say nothing inside your mind; as you breathe out, say "1." Next, as you breathe in, say nothing again, and as you breathe out, say "2." Continue in this manner up to 10, counting only on the exhalations. When you reach 10, return to 1. If you lose count or go beyond 10, return to 1 and start over.

Comment: This is a good alternative introductory exercise to "In . . . Out Breathing." It is more complex and requires more attention; however, it is still quite simple and easily remembered. This technique is 2,500 years old and is often the first taught in various traditions of meditation.

1 through 10 Inhalation and Exhalation Breathing

Start with 1 on the inhalation and continue with 2 on the exhalation, alternating up to 10. Then the breathing continues in reverse: 9 on the inhalation, 8 on the exhalation, back down to 1 and then up again, and so on.

Comment: Many people like this exercise because of its soothing up and down rhythm. It is complicated enough to hold one's attention, but simple enough to support relaxation.

Deeper Breathing

Most of us breathe throughout the day in a fairly shallow way, using only a modest percentage of lung capacity. This exercise involves intentionally deepening the breath. Taking deeper breaths in a calm manner increases relaxation. Alertness is also enhanced as more oxygen reaches the brain. Begin by focusing on your breath. Deliberately slow down the breath and make your "in breath" fuller. Next, as you breathe out, do so more fully; deliberately expel more of the air from your lungs than you normally do. As you practice this exercise, find a comfortable new rhythm for breathing deeply.

Comment: Some people can end up light headed with this type of breathing. Return to normal "shallow" breathing if you start to feel any shortness of breath or other discomfort. With practice, a good rhythm can be found.

Bamboo Breathing

To learn bamboo breathing, see Figure A.1. This breathing technique comes from Sekida (1985). It is called bamboo breathing because bamboo grows in clearly delineated sections, as shown in the figure. The horizontal lines on the chart represent brief pauses in breathing. The long diagonal lines represent long, deep breaths; the short diagonal lines represent short, shallow breaths. More specifically, the breathing begins with two long in-breaths and is followed by two brief out-breaths, then two brief in-breaths. This occurs for five cycles, concluding with four long out-breaths.

Comment: This exercise is complex and requires a good memory and concentration to successfully complete and repeat. People who have persistent trouble with becoming distracted find this exercise quite helpful. When first learning bamboo breathing, it may be necessary to look at the diagram.

This exercise can be too difficult for some. Others initially may find themselves gasping for breath if they are unable to establish a good rhythm. Return to normal, comfortable breathing if you experience shortness of breath or other discomfort. In general, heavy cigarette smokers or asthmatics may have trouble with more complex breathing techniques.

Breathing In, I Calm My Body; Breathing Out, I Smile

This is another breathing exercise from Nhat Hanh (1991). Say the above words recurrently.

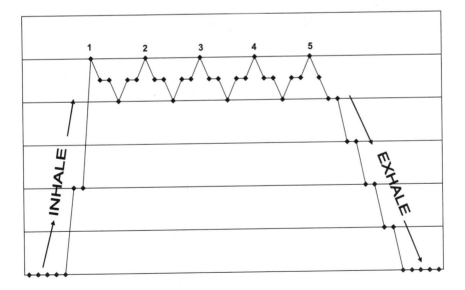

FIGURE A.1. Bamboo breathing.

Comment: He states that smiling relaxes all the muscles in the face and recommends it for this reason.

Letting Go of . . . Breathing

As you breathe in, say: "Mindfully breathing." As you breathe out, say: "Letting go of X . . . " (insert for X whatever you'd like to have less of, such as anxiety, tension, anger, judgments, memories, perfectionism, etc.). You can select one thing to let go of and say that recurrently or you can let go of different emotions with each successive out-breath. The idea is not to "drive out" or forbid any thoughts or feelings, but rather to notice them and then let them go on their way.

Comment: Many individuals identify this exercise as a favorite way to release unwanted, persistent negative thoughts or feelings.

Cultivating . . . Breathing

Same as letting go of . . . breathing, but instead of letting go, you "cultivate" something positive, such as patience, calmness, relaxation, mindfulness, compassion, etc. In this case, breathe out as you say "cultivating," and breathe in as you say "patience," etc. The metaphor is that as you breathe in, the desired state is entering your body and increasing.

Comment: It's usually better to teach this technique after the preceding one, letting go of . . . breathing.

Letting Be, Letting Go, Breathing

This form of breathing comes from Kabat-Zinn (1990). It is designed to assist in dealing with emotions as they emerge. As you become aware of feelings, you say internally:

> On the in-breath: Seeing [insert the relevant feeling, e.g., anger, anxiety].
> On the out-breath: Letting be.
> On the in-breath: Seeing [insert the same feeling name].
> On the out-breath: Letting go.

Comment: This exercise indicates that feelings must be encountered and experienced (letting them be). They cannot just be negated, ignored, or repressed. However, at some point, we also need to let them go.

Wave Breathing

This form of breathing was also inspired by Kabat-Zinn (1990). In his "Guided Mindfulness Meditation" recording he uses the phrase, "riding the wave of the breath." I found this phrase suggestive and used it to create a visualization. As you breathe in, imagine the ocean gently lapping on the beach; as you breathe out, the ocean gently recedes. In imagining the ocean's movement, you can include sight, sound, smell, and touch.

Pleasant Word Breathing

Select a word that appeals to you and repeat it each time you exhale. A colleague of mine, perhaps uniquely, likes the word "onomatopoeia." Others have selected words such as "calm," "ocean," "peaceful," "soothing," "relax," etc.

Breathing with Tapping

Some prefer to make breathing a more active, tactile experience. One way to do this is to gently tap your left finger on your left leg as you breathe in and tap your right finger on your right leg as you breathe out. Decide on a rhythm of tapping that is comfortable for you.

Raised Arm Breathing

A variation of this type of breathing with movement involves sitting with an arm comfortably resting on each leg with the fingertips near the knees. As you inhale, slowly raise both arms up to a comfortable position close to the shoulders; as you exhale return the arms and hands to your legs. Repeat.

Body Scan Breathing

This is a progressive body awareness type of breathing. I learned it from Issho Fujita, a Soto Zen Priest. Begin by bringing your attention gently to the areas of your body that are supported by the chair or floor or cushion. After noticing these sensations, turn your attention to where your feet and legs are supported. After several minutes, shift your attention to focusing on the rise and fall of the abdomen with each in-breath and out-breath. After several more minutes, turn your attention to the rise and fall on the upper chest with each in- and out-breath. After several minutes, bring your attention to the nostrils and become aware of the air going in and out with each breath. You may notice that the air is cooler going in and warmer going out. After several minutes, turn your attention to the full body. Imagine that a single membrane surrounds your body. Imagine that your body is a single cell, a one-celled amoeba. Become aware of the full body. After several minutes of this focusing, the exercise concludes.

Comment: This technique is good for physical grounding and especially helpful for those who are easily distracted, because it provides multiple steps on which to focus.

Pause Breathing

In this exercise you begin by finding a comfortable rhythm of deeper breathing (see above). Once you have this rhythm, concentrate on the gap or pause between the end of the inhalation and the beginning of the exhalation. It is often helpful to deliberately extend the pause beyond its usual length.

Some suggest that this brief moment between breaths symbolizes a break in the constant striving for survival (e.g., taking in oxygen, food, information, expelling carbon dioxide, producing work, speaking to others). It represents an interlude from the effort of balancing inner and outer worlds.

Comment: This type of breathing can produce some unusual thoughts, feelings, insights. However, some find it initially difficult to locate or hold the pause.

Walking Meditation

Nhat Hanh (1975) strongly recommends walking meditation as a complement to meditative breathing in a seated position. Walking meditation involves walking at a slower than normal pace. It also entails focusing on the breath as your body moves through its paces. One way to do walking meditation is to place your right hand on your sternum in a fist with your thumb tucked inside. Then place your left had over the right, covering it (Issho Fujita, personal communication). As you begin walking, extend your left leg very slowly, touching down first on the heel. Focus quite deliberately on the physical sensations in your leg and foot. Continue focusing as you gradually shift your weight first to the instep and then to the ball of the foot and finally to the toes of the left foot. Continue for the right leg, foot and toes. After several moments, a rhythm is established.

As you are walking, it is useful to synchronize your breath with your steps. One way to do this is take one step for each in-breath and out-breath. However, you should discover your own natural synchrony.

Stoplight or Telephone Breathing

Nhat Hanh (1975) suggests using stoplights or ringing phones as meditation bells that signal brief moments of mindful breathing. This is an excellent way to build some self-soothing and mindful concentration into daily activities.

Return to Health Breathing

Psychologist Cindy Sanderson taught this type of breathing at a DBT intensive in 1999. She reported learning it when she was being treated for cancer. She has since died from a recurrence of the disease, making the second half of the mantra all the more meaningful.

In-breath: "Let me be one with the heart."
Out-breath: "Let me be healed."

In-breath: "Let me be free from suffering."
Out-breath: "Let me be at peace."

Comment: Repetitive phrases, sometimes referred to as mantras, are part of many mindful breathing and meditative exercises. They are both relaxing and focusing.

Empty Mind Breathing

This technique is generally for the more advanced mindful breather. As you focus on your breathing, try to think of absolutely nothing. Release all thoughts, feelings, memories, images, anticipations, sensations. Do and think of nothing.

Comment: To get to a point of an empty mind, one may have to breathe mindfully for extended periods of time.

Distress Tolerance Breathing

Derived from Nhat Hanh (1991), this exercise seems very consistent with the concept of "distress tolerance" from DBT (Linehan, 1993b). The instructions are to say to oneself:

Breathing in, I'm aware of my anger [or whatever feeling].
Breathing out, I'm aware of my anger.
Breathing in, I sit with my anger.
Breathing out, I sit with my anger.
Breathing in, I know my anger will pass.
Breathing out, I know my anger will pass.
Breathing in, I will transform my anger into something positive.
Breathing out, I will transform my anger into something positive.

Comment: As with other exercises, this one can be modified to meet the needs of the individual, that is, simplified, shortened, extended, etc.

Breathing Retraining

This technique is used by Foa and colleagues (Foa & Rothbaum, 1998; Meadows & Foa, 1998) in their treatment of trauma survivors.

As you inhale slowly, you count (silently) to 4. As you exhale slowly, you say the word "calm" or "relax" in a long, drawn-out fashion; for example, *caaalllmmmm*. When the breath is fully exhaled, you pause and count to 4 before inhaling again. Then repeat for at least 10 minutes. This technique is designed to help manage anxiety, calm the body physiologically, and teach mastery over unpleasant emotions.

White Light, Black Smoke Breathing

I learned this technique from Lobsang Phuntsok, a Tibetan monk. As you breathe in, imagine a column of white light entering your body and purifying and cleansing your thoughts, feelings, habits, and behaviors. Then as you breathe out, envision black smoke leaving your body. This black smoke carries with it all the toxins, negative thoughts, judgments, feelings, behaviors, and habits. This exercise can be simplified by saying to yourself, as you breathe in, "White light, compassion," and as you breathe out, "Black smoke, anger" or "judgments" or "frustration," etc. Phuntsok emphasizes that it is important to visualize the light entering the body and the black smoke exiting the lungs as vividly as possible.

Comment: The metaphoric images of white light and black smoke are especially evocative and therefore appeal to many.

This Too Shall Pass

As you breathe in, say "This too," and as you breathe out, "shall pass."

Just Breathing

With practice, you may find that you get to the point where you just breathe. There is no need for counting, words, phrases, sentences, images, or other techniques. You focus on the breath and just breathe.

Body Attitudes Scale

This questionnaire concerns body image and satisfaction. Please write the appropriate number on the line next to each question.

1	2	3	4	5
Strongly disagree	Disagree	Neither agree nor disagree	Agree	Strongly agree

____ 1. Most people find me attractive.

____ 2. I try never to do anything that threatens my health.

____ 3. Sometimes I feel disconnected from my body.

____ 4. Most days I feel physically sick.

____ 5. I am good at most sports activities.

____ 6. I often seem to damage my health without meaning to.

____ 7. Everyone deserves to have sexual pleasure.

____ 8. I am not a good-looking individual.

____ 9. I have never had the experience of feeling outside my body.

____ 10. Good health is one of the most important things in my life.

____ 11. Sometimes my body feels out of control.

____ 12. I do not have good physical endurance.

____ 13. I take care of myself when I feel sick.

____ 14. My body is sexually appealing.

____ 15. Sometimes my body feels like an enemy.

____ 16. I hate being touched by others.

____ 17. I am currently at an attractive weight.

____ 18. I like my looks just the way they are.

___ 19. I can imagine having a satisfying sex life in the future.

___ 20. Most of the time when I look in the mirror, I feel ugly.

___ 21. I would prefer to live without a body.

___ 22. I like the idea of having a physically mature body.

___ 23. I enjoy being sexually aroused.

___ 24. I liked my body much better before it matured.

___ 25. I am not a physically coordinated individual.

___ 26. I am presently at a healthy weight.

___ 27. I have to work hard to make myself attractive to others.

___ 28. Sexual experiences give me pleasure.

___ 29. My looks often disgust me.

___ 30. People consider me a very good athlete.

___ 31. I frequently wish I were more sexually attractive.

___ 32. I often feel at war with my body.

___ 33. I am physically ill more often than I am well.

___ 34. I prefer to avoid sexual experiences.

___ 35. I feel that my body is strong.

___ 36. I think of myself as sexually appealing.

Websites Related to Self-Injury

There are scores of websites that focus on self-injury. They fall into two main categories: (1) websites designed by professionals to assist self-injurers, and (2) websites created by self-injurers intended to offer peer support. I have provided brief descriptions of several of the more prominent websites of both types in this appendix. Most of these sites come up on the first two pages of a Google search for the term "self-injury." This review is meant to be representative, not exhaustive.

WEBSITES DESIGNED BY
MENTAL HEALTH PROFESSIONALS

Self-Injury and Related Issues (SIARI)
www.siari.co.uk

The SIARI website is the creation of Jan Sutton, who is based in the United Kingdom. She is the author of *Healing the Hurt Within: Understand and Relieve the Suffering Behind Self-Destructive Behaviour* (1999) and several other books.

The multifaceted website, with its many links, provides many helpful suggestions regarding coping skills and alternatives to self-injury, a self-assessment questionnaire for self-injurers, and first aid information. It also offers information for family and friends, references to many publications regarding self-injury, and a bookstore. An interesting and unusual feature is that the website offers an on-line support group for *professionals* who work with self-injurers. I am not aware of any other website that has this feature.

There is a well-designed *moderated* message board for self-injurers, with guidelines for participants about the dangers of posting triggering information and a request to label it as triggering to forewarn others.

The website presents a "cycle of self-injury" that includes the steps of (1) mental agony, (2) emotional engulfment, (3) panic stations, (4) action stations, (5) feel better, and (6) grief reaction (Sutton, 1999). In all likelihood, Sutton's cycle does not apply to all self-injurers but primarily to trauma survivors and those who tend to dissociate. The SIARI website provides an article by Sutton regarding the link between self-injury, dissociation, and trauma. Although some of the content of the SIARI site may not be relevant for self-injurers from the general population, the suggestions regarding coping skills and alternatives to self-injury are relevant for all.

S.A.F.E. Alternatives
www.selfinjury.com

The S.A.F.E. Alternatives website is the creation of Conterio and Lader, authors of *Bodily Harm* (1998). This website offers concise material about self-injury, a brief summary about the components of successful treatment, a bibliography, and links to purchase Conterio and Lader's book and video. The website also provides a link for admission to their inpatient unit at Linden Oaks Hospital at Edward, in Naperville, Illinois. This program is the only inpatient unit devoted exclusively to the treatment of self-injury in the United States. Optimally, the length of stay for this program is 30 days.

Conterio and Lader also operate the national information line—800-DONT-CUT—which has been an invaluable resource for self-injurers for many years. This line receives about 16,000 calls per year and their e-mail address (wladersafe@aol.com) another 5,000 contacts (Lader, personal communication, 2004). That Conterio personally responds to the phone calls and Lader to the e-mails indicates their heroic level of commitment to help self-injurers.

American Self-Harm Information Clearinghouse
www.selfinjury.org

This website is the creation of Deb Martinson, the author of the notable "Bill of Rights for People Who Self-Harm." It is a strong statement of affirmation for self-injurers that clients and therapists should read. The full text of the Bill of Rights is provided in Appendix D of this volume.

The website carries Favazza's endorsement and offers a brief description of the reasons for self-injury, a discussion of myths regarding self-injury, self-help suggestions, and several links.

There Is No Shame Here
www.palace.net/~llama/psych/injury.html

This is another website by Deb Martinson. It is a complex site that offers information about causes of self-injury, self-help, diagnoses, treatment, and information for families and friends. There is a lengthy list of references and many links. The site offers a monitored message or web board for self-injurers that carefully addresses the issue of triggering content.

The site provides *many* suggestions for replacement behaviors, although some are questionable, such as slashing a plastic bottle or heavy piece of cardboard. Such aggressive modes place a weapon in the hands of self-injurers and may make self-harm more likely. The website takes great pains to be accepting, supportive, and nonjudgmental toward self-injurers.

Self-Injury
www.mirror-mirror.org/selfinj.htm

This simple one-page website presents some basic information about self-injury and concentrates on presenting a long, useful list of alternatives.

WEBSITES CREATED BY SELF-INJURERS OFFERING PEER SUPPORT

LifeSIGNS: Self Injury Guidance and Network Support
www.lifesigns.org.uk

This website is run by a set of directors, "some of whom self-injure, some have beaten self-injury, and some have never self-injured" (quotation from the home page of the site). (I have classified this site under the self-injurer generated category because some of the directors have considerable experience with self-injury.)

This comprehensive site is very professional in appearance. It offers extensive information about self-injury and suggestions for eliminating the behavior. It has a chat room with clearly articulated rules about avoiding triggering content. The authors of the site have written several pamphlets on self-injury, designed for schools and universities, that are available through the site. A monthly electronic newsletter is offered to members. Many links are provided. The site also offers a "Self-Injury Charter," which is similar in some ways to Deb Martinson's Bill of Rights. This appears to be among the best of the peer-generated sites in terms of offering positive, supportive, nontriggering, solution-focused content.

RecoverYourLife.com
www.recoveryourlife.com

This website (formerly RuinYourLife.com) offers a complex combination of benefits and risks. This site is "dedicated to exploring 'self-destruction' in all its forms."

There is no doubt that websites of this type help some self-injurers feel that they are not alone and that their problem can be discussed with others. This multifaceted site offers self-help suggestions, a first aid section (which may be triggering because of its level of detail), and a gift shop selling RYL journals, mouse pads, mugs, teddy bears, and clothing.

Of concern are the poetry and artwork. Some of the art includes graphic color photos of wounds and drawings of lacerations, wounds, and blood. One drawing depicts a person who has died by hanging. In my opinion, the risks that this site takes in terms of triggering cannot be justified. I did consider not drawing attention to it in this appendix, but the site does come up on the first page or two of a Google search of "self-injury."

Self-Injury: A Struggle
www.self-injury.net

This website is said to have been generated by a young adult self-injurer, named Gabrielle. She states she has been self-injuring for 4 years. Although attractively designed, some of the content is alarming—such as the section titled, "Gallery of Pain." This category contains artwork that depicts razor blades, wounds, blood, etc. There is also poetry describing acts of self-injury and at least one short story that culminates in a completed suicide. The site has sections on famous self-injurers and a memorial section for self-injurers who have died. The categories on stopping self-injury, helping family and friends, and finding resources seem less developed than the more negative content areas. There is a message board offered, but I could not find rules or even a statement pertaining to concerns about triggering content.

This is the type of site that provides some support for young self-injurers, but also contains a great deal of triggering material that could do harm. Aspects of this website run the risk of normalizing and even *glamorizing* self-injury. The content is weighted heavily in the direction of describing and depicting self-injury rather than solving the problem of self-injury.

Self-Injury Support
www.sisupport.org

This rather simple peer-generated website is based in California. The mission of the site is "to offer a positive and productive self-injury support site providing alternatives to self-injury, referrals, support groups, affirmations and interactive opportunities" (from the homepage). This site was developed in response to sites such as the two described immediately above. The Self-Injury Support website states, "Much to our dismay we have discovered that many [self-injury websites] . . . are "triggering" and not exactly the type of material we wanted to read about when we were struggling ourselves, usually late at night, with thoughts of self-injury. So, we have decided to focus on positive information regarding self-injury and hope that you will find our site to be both educational and supportive in a positive and reassuring manner to help those in need."

Consistent with these goals, the site emphasizes understanding self-injury and how to recover. There are lists of references and programs that serve self-injurers. There is no chat room.

Bill of Rights for People Who Self-Harm

PREAMBLE

An estimated one percent of Americans use physical self-harm as a way of coping with stress; the rate of self-injury in other industrial nations is probably similar. Still, self-injury remains a taboo subject, a behavior that is considered freakish or outlandish and is highly stigmatized by medical professionals and the lay public alike. Self-harm, also called self-injury, self-inflicted violence, or self-mutilation, can be defined as self-inflicted physical harm severe enough to cause tissue damage or leave visible marks that do not fade within a few hours. Acts done for purposes of suicide or for ritual, sexual, or ornamentation purposes are not considered self-injury. This document refers to what is commonly known as moderate or superficial self-injury, particularly repetitive SI; these guidelines do not hold for cases of major self-mutilation (i.e., castration, eye enucleation, or amputation).

Because of the stigma and lack of readily available information about self-harm, people who resort to this method of coping often receive treatment from physicians (particularly in emergency rooms) and mental-health professionals that can actually make their lives worse instead of better. Based on hundreds of negative experiences reported by people who self-harm, the following Bill of Rights is an attempt to provide information to medical and mental-health personnel. The goal of this project is to enable them to more clearly understand the emotions that underlie self-injury and to respond to self-injurious behavior in a way that protects the patient as well as the practitioner.

THE BILL OF RIGHTS FOR THOSE WHO SELF-HARM

1. **The right to caring, humane medical treatment.** Self-injurers should receive the same level and quality of care that a person presenting with an identical but accidental injury would receive. Procedures should be done as gently as they would be for others. If stitches are required, local anesthesia should be used. Treatment of accidental injury and self-inflicted injury should be identical.

2. **The right to participate fully in decisions about emergency psychiatric treatment (so long as no one's life is in immediate danger).** When a person presents at the emergency room with a self-inflicted injury, his or her opinion about the need for a psychological assessment should be considered. If the person is not in obvious distress and is not suicidal, he or she should not be subjected to an arduous psych evaluation. Doctors should be trained to assess suicidality/homicidality and should realize that although referral for outpatient follow-up may be advisable, hospitalization for self-injurious behavior alone is rarely warranted.

3. **The right to body privacy.** Visual examinations to determine the extent and frequency of self-inflicted injury should be performed only when absolutely necessary and done in a way that maintains the patient's dignity. Many who SI have been abused; the humiliation of a strip-search is likely to increase the amount and intensity of future self-injury while making the person subject to the searches look for better ways to hide the marks.

4. **The right to have the feelings behind the SI validated.** Self-injury doesn't occur in a vacuum. The person who self-injures usually does so in response to distressing feelings, and those feelings should be recognized and validated. Although the care provider might not understand why a particular situation is extremely upsetting, she or he can at least understand that it *is* distressing and respect the self-injurer's right to be upset about it.

5. **The right to disclose to whom they choose only what they choose.** No care provider should disclose to others that injuries are self-inflicted without obtaining the permission of the person involved. Exceptions can be made in the case of team-based hospital treatment or other medical care providers when the information that the injuries were self-inflicted is essential knowledge for proper medical care. Patients should be notified when others are told about their SI and as always, gossiping about any patient is unprofessional.

6. **The right to choose what coping mechanisms they will use.** No person should be forced to choose between self-injury and treatment. Outpatient therapists should never demand that clients sign a no-harm contract; instead, client and provider should develop a plan for dealing with self-injurious impulses and acts during the treatment. No client should feel they must lie about SI or be kicked out of outpatient therapy. Exceptions to this may be made in hospital or ER treatment, when a contract may be required by hospital legal policies.

7. **The right to have care providers who do not allow their feelings about SI to distort the therapy.** Those who work with clients who self-injure should keep their own

fear, revulsion, anger, and anxiety out of the therapeutic setting. This is crucial for basic medical care of self-inflicted wounds but holds for therapists as well. A person who is struggling with self-injury has enough baggage without taking on the prejudices and biases of their care providers.

8. **The right to have the role SI has played as a coping mechanism validated.** No one should be shamed, admonished, or chastised for having self-injured. Self-injury works as a coping mechanism, sometimes for people who have no other way to cope. They may use SI as a last-ditch effort to avoid suicide. The self-injurer should be taught to honor the positive things that self-injury has done for him/her as well as to recognize that the negatives of SI far outweigh those positives and that it is possible to learn methods of coping that aren't as destructive and life-interfering.

9. **The right not to be automatically considered a dangerous person simply because of self-inflicted injury.** No one should be put in restraints or locked in a treatment room in an emergency room solely because his or her injuries are self-inflicted. No one should ever be involuntarily committed simply because of SI; physicians should make the decision to commit based on the presence of psychosis, suicidality, or homicidality.

10. **The right to have self-injury regarded as an attempt to communicate, not manipulate.** Most people who hurt themselves are trying to express things they can say in no other way. Although sometimes these attempts to communicate seem manipulative, treating them as manipulation only makes the situation worse. Providers should respect the communicative function of SI and assume it is not manipulative behavior until there is clear evidence to the contrary.

References

Alderman, T. (1997). *The scarred soul: Understanding and ending self-inflicted violence*. Oakland, CA: New Harbinger.

American Association of Suicidology. (2002). Survivors of suicide fact sheet. Available at *www.suicidology.org/associations/1045/files/SurvivorsFactSheet.pdf*

Arnold, E. L., Vitiello, B., McDougle, C., Scahill, L. M., Shah, B., Gonzalez, N. M., Chuang, S., Davies, M., Hollway, J., Aman, M. G., Cronin, P., Koenig, K., Kohn, A. E., McMahon, D. J., & Tierney, E. (2003). Parent-defined target symptoms respond to risperidone in RUPP autism study: Customer approach to clinical trials. *Journal of American Academy of Child and Adolescent Psychiatry, 42*, 1443–1450.

Ashford, J. B., LeCroy, C. W., & Lortie, K. L. (2001). *Human behavior in the social environment* (2nd ed.). Belmont, CA: Brooks/Cole.

Bandura, A. (1977). *Social learning theory*. Englewood Cliffs, NJ: Prentice-Hall.

Bayda, E. (2002). *Being Zen, bringing meditation to life*. Boston: Shambhala Publications.

Beck, A. T., Freeman, A., Davis, D. D., & Associates. (2003). *Cognitive therapy of personality disorders* (2nd ed.). New York: Guilford Press.

Beck, A. T., Rush, A. J., Shaw, B. F., & Emery, G. (1979). *Cognitive therapy of depression*. New York: Guilford Press.

Beck, J. S. (1995). *Cognitive therapy, basics and beyond*. New York: Guilford Press.

Belsher, G., & Wilkes, T. C. R. (1994). Ten key principles of adolescent cognitive therapy. In T. C. R. Wilkes, G. Belsher, A. J. Rush, & E. Frank (Eds.), *Cognitive therapy for depressed adolescents*. New York: Guilford Press.

Berman, M. E., & Walley, J. C. (2003). Imitation of self-aggressive behavior: An experimental test of the contagion hypothesis. *Journal of Applied Social Psychology, 33*, 1036–1057.

Blew, P., Luiselli, J. K., & Thibadeau, S. (1999). Beneficial effects of clonidine on severe self-injurious behavior in a 9–year-old girl with pervasive developmental disorder. *Journal of Child and Adolescent Psychopharmacology, 9*, 285–291.

Bohus, M., Limberger, M., Ebner, U., Glocker, F. X., Schwarz, B., Wernz, M., & Lieb, K. (2000). Pain perception during self-reported distress and calmness in patients with borderline personality disorder and self-mutilating behavior. *Psychiatry Research, 95,* 251–260.

Boiko, I., & Lester, D. (2000). Deliberate self-injury in female Russian inmates. *Psychological Reports, 87*(3), 789–790.

Brenner, H. D., Roder, V., Hodel, B., Kienzle, N., Reed, D., & Liberman, R. P. (1994). *Integrated psychological therapy for schizophrenic patients.* Cambridge, MA: Hogrefe & Huber.

Briere, J., & Gil, E. (1998). Self-mutilation in clinical and general population samples: Prevalence, correlates, and functions. *American Journal of Orthopsychiatry, 68*(4), 609–620.

Brown, M. (1998). *The behavioral treatment of self-mutilation.* Paper presented at the "self-mutilation, treatment and research symposium," XVI Congress of the World Association for Social Psychiatry, Vancouver, BC, Canada.

Brown, M. (2002). *The impact of negative emotions on the efficacy of treatment for parasuicide in borderline personality disorder.* Unpublished doctoral dissertation, University of Washington, Seattle.

Brown, M., Comtois, K. A., & Linehan, M. M. (2002). Reasons for suicide attempts and nonsuicidal self-injury in women with borderline personality disorder. *Journal of Abnormal Psychology, 111*(1), 198–2002.

Cash, T. F., & Pruzinsky, T. (Eds.). (1990). *Body images: Development, deviance, and change.* New York: Guilford Press.

Cash, T. F., & Pruzinsky, T. (Eds.). (2002). *Body image: A handbook of theory, research, and clinical practice.* New York: Guilford Press.

Cassano, P., Lattanzi, L., Pini, S., Dell'Osso, L., Battistini, G., & Cassano, G. B. (2001). Topiramate for self-mutilation in a patient with borderline personality disorder. *Bipolar Disorders, 3,* 161.

Chengappa, K. N., Ebeling, T., Kang, J. S., Levine, J., & Parepally, H. (1999). Clozapine reduces severe self-mutilation and aggression in psychotic patients with borderline personality disorder. *Journal of Clinical Psychiatry, 60,* 477–484.

Chowanec, G. D., Josephson, A. M., Coleman, B., & Davis, H. (1991). Self-harming behavior in incarcerated male delinquent adolescents. *Journal of American Academy of Child and Adolescent Psychiatry, 30,* 202–207.

Christenson, G. A., Mackenzie, T. B., & Mitchell, J. E. (1991). Characteristics of 60 adult chronic hair-pullers. *American Journal of Psychiatry, 148,* 365–370.

Clark, D. M. (1986). A cognitive approach to panic. *Behavior Research and Therapy, 24,* 461–470.

Clendenin, W. W., & Murphy, G. E. (1971). Wrist cutting. *Archives of General Psychiatry, 25,* 465–469.

Comtois, K. A. (2002). A review of interventions to reduce the prevalence of parasuicide. *Psychiatric Services, 53*(9), 1138–1144.

Connors, R. E. (2000). *Self-injury.* New York: Jason Aronson.

Conterio, K., & Lader, W. (1998). *Bodily harm.* New York: Hyperion Press.

Cookson, M. R. (2003). Pathways to Parkinsonism. *Neuron, 37,* 7–10.

Crabtree, L. H., & Grossman, W. K. (1974). Administrative clarity and redefinition for an open adolescent unit. *Psychiatry, 37*, 350–359.

Cullen, E. (1985). Prediction and treatment of self-injury by female young offenders. In D. Farrington & R. Tarling (Eds.), *Prediction in criminology*. Albany: State University of New York Press.

Darche, M. A. (1990). Psychological factors differentiating self-mutilating and non-self-mutilating adolescent inpatient females. *Psychiatric Hospital, 21*, 31–35.

Davis, M., Eshelman, E. R., & McKay, M. (1982). *The relaxation and stress reduction* workbook (2nd ed.). Oakland, CA: New Harbinger.

Deiter, P. J., Nicholls, S. S., & Pearlman, L. A. (2000). Self-injury and self-capacities: Assisting an individual in crisis. *Journal of Clinical Psychology, 56*(9), 1173–1191.

Denys, D., van Megan, H. J., & Westenberg, H. G. (2003). Emerging skin-picking behavior after serotonin reuptake inhibitor-treatment in patients with obsessive–compulsive disorder: Possible mechanisms and implications for clinical care. *Journal of Psychopharmacology, 17*, 127–129.

Drews, D. R., Allison, C. K., & Probst, J. R. (2000). Behavioral and self-concept differences in tattooed and nontattooed college students. *Psychological Reports, 86*(2), 475–481.

Dulit, R. A., Fyer, M. R., Leon, A. C., Brodsky, B. S., & Frances, A. J. (1994). Clinical correlates of self-mutilation in borderline personality disorder. *American Journal of Psychiatry, 151*, 1305–1311.

Ellis, A. (1962). *Reason and emotion in psychotherapy*. New York: Lyle Stuart.

Farber, S. K. (2000). *When the body is the target: Self-harm, pain, and traumatic attachments*. Northvale, NJ: Jason Aronson.

Farberow, N. L. (Ed.). (1980). *The many faces of suicide: Indirect self-destructive behavior*. NewYork: McGraw-Hill.

Favaro, A., & Santonastaso, P. (1998). Impulsive and compulsive self-injurious behavior in bulimia nervosa: Prevalence and psychological correlates. *Journal of Nervous and Mental Disease, 186*, 157–165.

Favaro, A., & Santonastaso, P. (2000). Self-injurious behavior in anorexia nervosa. *Journal of Nervous and Mental Disease, 188*, 537–542.

Favazza, A. (1987). *Bodies under siege*. Baltimore, MD: Johns Hopkins University Press.

Favazza, A. (1989). Why patients mutilate themselves. *Hospital and Community Psychiatry, 40*, 137–145.

Favazza, A. (1996). *Bodies under siege* (2nd ed.). Baltimore, MD: Johns Hopkins University Press.

Favazza, A. (1998). The coming of age of self-mutilation. *Journal of Nervous and Mental Disease, 186*, 259–268.

Favazza, A., & Conterio, K. (1988). The plight of chronic self-mutilators. *Community Mental Health Journal, 24*(1), 22–30.

Favazza, A., DeRosear, L., & Conterio, K. (1989). Self-mutilation and eating disorders. *Suicide and Life-Threatening Behaviors, 19*(4), 352–361.

Favazza, A., & Rosenthal, R. J. (1990). Varieties of pathological self-mutilation. *Behavioural Neurology, 3*, 77–85.

Fisher, S. (1970). *Body experience in fantasy and behavior.* New York: Appleton-Century-Crofts.

Foa, E. B., Keane, T. M., & Friedman, M. J. (Eds.). (2000). *Effective treatments for PTSD.* New York: Guilford Press.

Foa, E. B., & Rothbaum, B. O. (1998). *Treating the trauma of rape: Cognitive-behavioral therapy for PTSD.* New York: Guilford Press.

Follette, V. M., Ruzek, J. I., & Abueg, F. R. (Eds.). (1998). *Cognitive-behavioral therapies for trauma.* New York: Guilford Press.

Fontana, D. (2001). *Discover Zen: A practical guide to personal serenity.* San Francisco: Chronicle Books.

Freeman, A., & Reinecke, M. A. (1993). *Cognitive therapy of suicidal behavior.* New York: Springer.

Gardner, A. R., & Gardner, A. J. (1975). Self-mutilation: Obsessionality and narcissism. *British Journal of Psychiatry, 127,* 127–132.

Gardner, D. L., & Cowdry, R. W. (1985). Suicidal and parasuicidal behavior in borderline personality disorder. *Psychiatric Clinics of North American, 8,* 389–403.

Gardner, W. I., & Sovner, R. (1994). *Self-injurious behaviors.* Willow Street, PA: VIDA.

Garfield, D. M., & Garfinkel, P. E. (Eds.). (1997). *Handbook of treatment of eating disorders* (2nd ed.). New York: Guilford Press.

Garner, D. M., Vitousek, K. M., & Pike, K. M. (1997). Cogntive-behavioral therapy for anorexia nervosa. In D. M. Garner & P. E. Garfinkel (Eds.), *Handbook of treatment for eating disorders.* New York: Guilford Press.

Geist, R. (1979). Onset of chronic illness in children and adolescents. *American Journal of Orthopsychiatry, 52,* 704–711.

Gerson, J., & Stanley, B. (2002). Suicidal and self-injurious behavior in personality disorder: Controversies and treatment directions. *Current Psychiatry Reports, 4,* 30–38.

Gough, K., & Hawkins, A. (2000). Staff attitudes to self-harm and its management in a forensic psychiatric service. *British Journal of Forensic Practice, 2*(4), 22–28.

Grant, B. F., Harford, T. C., Dawson, D. A., Chou, P., Dufour, M., & Pickering, R. (1994). Epidemiologic Bulletin No. 35: Prevalence of DSM-IV alcohol abuse and dependence, United States, 1992. *Alcohol Health and Research World, 18,* 243–248.

Gratz, K. L., Conrad, S. D., & Roemer, L. (2002). Risk factors for deliberate self-harm among college students. *American Journal of Orthopsychiatry, 72*(1), 128–140.

Green, A. H. (1968). Self-destructive behavior in physically abused schizophrenic children. *Archives of General Psychiatry, 18,* 171–179.

Greilsheimer, H., & Groves, J. E. (1979). Male genital self-mutilation. *Canadian Psychiatric Association Journal, 36,* 441–446.

Grossman, R. (2001). Psychotic self-injurious behaviors: Phenomenology, neurobiology, and treatment. In D. Simeon & E. Hollander (Eds.), *Self-injurious behaviors: Assessment and treatment.* Washington, DC: American Psychiatric Association.

Grossman, R., & Siever, L. (2001). Impulsive self-injurious behaviors, neurobiology and psychopharmacology. In D. Simeon & E. Hollander (Eds.), *Self-injurious behaviors: Assessment and treatment*. Washington, DC: American Psychiatric Association.

Haines, J., & Williams, C. (1997). Coping and problem solving of self-mutilators. *Journal of Clinical Psychology, 53*(2), 177–186.

Hammock, R., Levine, W. R., & Schroeder, S. R. (2001). Brief report: Effects of clozapine on self-injurious behavior of two risperidone nonresponders with mental retardation. *Journal of Autism and Developmental Disorders, 31*, 109–113.

Haw, C., Houston, K., Townsend, E., & Hawton, K. (2002). Deliberate self harm patients with depressive disorders: Treatment and outcome. *Journal of Affective Disorders, 70*, 57–65.

Hawton, K., Townsend, E., Arensman, E., Gunnell, D., Hazell, P., House, A., & van Heeringen, K. (2000). Psychosocial versus pharmacological treatments for deliberate self-harm. *Cochrane Database of Systematic Reviews, 2*, CD001764.

Hayes, S. C. (2004). Acceptance and commitment therapy and the new behavior therapies. In S. C. Hayes, V. M. Follette, & M. M. Linehan (Eds.), *Mindfulness and acceptance: Expanding the cognitive-behavioral tradition*. New York: Guilford Press.

Heinsz, S. V. (2000). Self-mutilation in child and adolescent group home populations. *Dissertation Abstracts International, 2201*, U.S. UMV Microfilms International.

Himber, J. (1994). Blood rituals: Self-cutting in female psychiatric inpatients. *Psychotherapy, 31*, 620–631.

Holdin-Davis, D. (1914). An epidemic of hair-pulling in an orphanage. *British Journal of Dermatology, 26*, 207–210.

Hood, K. K., Baptista-Neto, L., Beasley, P. J., Lobis, R., & Pravdova, I. (2004). Case study: Severe self-injurious behavior in comorbid Tourette's disorder and OCD. *Journal of the American Academy of Child Psychiatry, 43*(10), 1298–1303.

Howard League for Penal Reform. (1999). *Scratching the surface: The hidden problem of self-harm in prison*. London: Author.

Hughes, M. (1982). Chronically ill children in groups: Recurrent issues and adaptations. *American Journal of Orthopsychiatry, 52*, 704–711.

Hyman, J. (1999). *Women living with self-injury*. Philadelphia: Temple University Press.

Ireland, J. L. (2000). A descriptive analysis of self-harm reports among a sample of incarcerated adolescent males. *Journal of Adolescence, 23*, 605–613.

Kabat-Zinn, J. (1990). *Full catastrophe living: Using the wisdom of your body and mind to face stress, pain and illness*. New York: Dell.

Kazdin, A. E. (1994). *Behavior modification in applied settings*. Pacific Grove, CA: Brooks/Cole.

Kennedy, B. L., & Feldman, T. B. (1994). Self-inflicted eye injuries: Case presentations and a literature review. *Hospital and Community Psychiatry, 45*, 470–474.

Kettlewell, C. (1999). *Skin game: A cutter's memoir*. New York: St. Martin's Press.

Keuthen, N. J., Stein, D. J., & Christenson, G. A. (2001). *Help for hair pullers: Understanding and coping with trichotillomania.* Oakland, CA: New Harbinger.

Kingdon, D. G., & Turkington, D. (1994). *Cognitive-behavioral therapy of schizophrenia.* New York: Guilford Press.

Kreitman, N. (Ed.). (1977). *Parasuicide.* Chichester, UK: Wiley.

Kroll, J. C. (1978). Self-destructive behavior on an inpatient ward. *Journal of Nervous Mental Disease, 166,* 429–434.

Kubany, E. S. (1998). Cognitive therapy for trauma-related guilt. In V. M Follette, J. I. Ruzek, & F. R. Abueg, (Eds.), *Cognitive-behavioral therapies for trauma.* New York: Guilford Press.

Langbehn, D. R., & Pfohl, B. (1993). Clinical correlates of self-mutilation among psychiatric inpatients. *Annals of Clinical Psychiatry, 5,* 45–51.

Lester, D. (1972). Self-mutilating behavior. *Psychological Bulletin, 2,* 119–128.

Levenkron, S. (1998). *Cutting: Understanding and overcoming self-mutilation.* New York: Norton.

Levey, J., & Levey, M. (1991). *The fine arts of relaxation, concentration and meditation.* Boston: Wisdom.

Levey, J., & Levey, M. (1999). *Simple meditation and relaxation.* Berkeley, CA: Conari Press.

Liberman, R. (1999). *Social and independent living skills.* UCLA skills training video series. Cambridge, MA: Hogrefe & Huber.

Lightfoot, C. (1997). *The culture of adolescent risk-taking.* New York: Guilford Press.

Linehan, M. M. (1993a). *Cognitive-behavioral treatment of borderline personality disorder.* New York: Guilford Press.

Linehan, M. M. (1993b). *Skills training manual for treating borderline personality disorder.* New York: Guilford Press.

Linehan, M. M., Armstrong, H. E., Suarez, A., Allmon, D., & Heard, H. L. (1991). *Archives of General Psychiatry, 48,* 1060–1064.

Low, G., Jones, D., MacLeod, A., Power, M., & Duggan, C. (2000). Childhood trauma, dissociation and self-harming behaviour: A pilot study. *British Journal of Medical Psychology, 73,* 269–278.

Mace, F. C., Blum, N. J., Sierp, B. J., Delaney, B. A., & Mauk, J. E. (2001). Differential response of operant self-injury to pharmacologic versus behavioral treatment. *Journal of Developmental and Behavioral Pediatrics, 22,* 85–91.

Macy, J. D., Beattie, T. A., Morgenstern, S. E., & Arnsten, A. F. (2000) Use of guanfacine to control self-injurious behavior in two rhesus macaques (*Macaca mulatta*) and one baboon (*Papio anubis*). *Comparative Medicine, 50,* 419–425.

Maltsberger, J. T. (1986). *Suicide risk.* New York: New York University Press.

Markowitz, P. J. (1995). Pharmacotherapy of impulsivity, aggression, and related disorders. In E. Hollander & D. Stein (Eds.), *Impulsivity and aggression.* New York: Wiley.

Marlatt, G. A. (2002). *Harm reduction: Pragmatic strategies for managing high-risk behaviors.* New York: Guilford Press.

Marlatt, G. A., & Vandenbos, G. R. (1997). *Addictive behaviors: Readings on etiology, prevention and treatment.* Washington, DC: American Psychological Association.

Massachusetts Department of Education. (2004). 2003 Youth Risk Behavior Survey Results. Available at www.doe.mass.edu/hssss/program/youthrisk

Matthews, P. C. (1968). Epidemic self-injury in an adolescent unit. *International Journal of Social Psychiatry, 14*, 125–133.

McKay, D., Kulchycky, S., & Dankyo, S. (2000). Borderline personality disorder and obsessive–compulsive symptoms. *Journal of Personality Disorders, 14*(1), 57–63.

McKerracher, D. W., Loughnane, T., & Watson, R. A. (1968). Self-mutilation in female psychopaths. *British Journal of Psychiatry, 114*, 829–832.

Meadows, E. A., & Foa, E. B. (1998). Intrusion, arousal, avoidance: Sexual abuse survivors. In V. M Follette, J. I. Ruzek, & F. R. Abueg (Eds.), *Cognitive-behavioral therapies for trauma*. New York: Guilford Press.

Medinfo.co.uk. (2003). SSRIs. Available at www.medinfo.co.uk/drugs/ssris.html.

Menninger, K. (1966). *Man against himself*. New York: Harcourt, Brace Jovanovich. (Original work published 1938)

Merlo, M., Perris, C., & Brenner, H. (2004). *Cognitive therapy with schizophrenic patients*. Cambridge, MA: Hogrefe & Huber.

Merriam-Webster. (1995). *Merriam-Webster dictionary, home and office edition*. Springfield, MA: Author.

Miller, A. L., & Glinski, J. (2000). Youth suicidal behavior: Assessment and intervention. *Journal of Clinical Psychology, 56*(9), 1131–1152.

Miller, A. L., Rathus, J. H., Linehan, M. M., Wetzler, S., & Leigh, E. (1997). Dialectical behavior therapy for suicidal adolescents. *Journal of Practical Psychiatry and Behavioral Health, 3*(2), 78–86.

Miller, D. (1994). *Women who hurt themselves: A book of hope and understanding*. New York: Basic Books.

Miller, M., & Hemenway, D. (2001). Firearm prevalence and the risk of suicide: A review. *Harvard Health Policy Review, 2*(2), 1–3.

Milnes, D., Owens, D., & Blenkiron, P. (2002). Problems reported by self-harm patients: Perception, hopelessness and suicidal intent. *Journal of Psychosomatic Research, 53*(3), 819–822.

Mitchell, J. E., Boutacoff L. I., & Hatsukami, D. (1986). Laxative abuse as a variant of bulimia. *Journal of Nervous and Mental Disease, 174*, 174–176.

Modesto-Lowe, V., & Van Kirk, J. (2002). Clinical uses of naltrexone: A review of the evidence. *Experimental Clinical Psychopharmacology, 10*,213–227.

Motz, A. (2001). *The psychology of female violence: Crimes against the body*. Hove, UK: Brunner-Routledge.

Murphy, M. (2002). *One bird one stone: 108 American Zen stories*. New York: Renaissance Books.

Nhat Hanh, T. (1975). *The miracle of mindfulness*. Boston: Beacon Press.

Nhat Hanh, T. (1991). *Peace is every step: The path of mindfulness in every day life*. New York: Bantam Books.

Nock, M. K., & Prinstein, M. J. (2004). A functional approach to the assessment of self-mutilative behavior. *Journal of Consulting and Clinical Psychology, 72*, 885–890.

Offer, D. O., & Barglow, P. (1960). Adolescent and young adult self-mutilation incidents in a general psychiatric hospital. *Archives of General Psychiatry, 3*, 194–204.

O'Leary, K. D., & Wilson, G. T. (1987). *Behavior therapy, application and outcome* (2nd ed.). Englewood Cliffs, NJ: Prentice-Hall.

Orbach, I., Lotem-Peleg, M., & Kedem, P. (1995). Attitudes toward the body in suicidal, depressed and normal adolescents. *Suicide and Life-Threatening Behavior, 25*, 211–221.

Orbach, I., Milstein, I., Har-Even, D., Apter, A., Tiano, S., & Elizur, A. (1991). A multi-attitude suicide tendency scale for adolescents. *Psychological Assessment, 3*, 398–404.

Orenstein, P. (1994). *School girls: Young women, self-esteem, and the confidence gap.* New York: Anchor Books.

Osuch, E. A., Noll, J. G., & Putnam, F. W. (1999). The motivations for self-injury in psychiatric inpatients. *Psychiatry, 62*, 334–345.

O'Sullivan, R. L., Phillips, K. A., Keuthen, N. J., & Wilhelm, S. (1999). Near-fatal skin picking from delusional body dysmorphic disorder responsive to fluvoxamine. *Psychosomatics, 40*, 79–81.

Pao, P. E. (1969). The syndrome of delicate self-cutting. *British Journal of Medical Psychology, 42*, 195–206.

Parkin, J. R., & Eagles, J. M. (1993). Bloodletting in bulimia nervosa. *British Journal of Psychiatry, 162*, 246–248.

Patterson, G. (1975). *Professional guide for families and living with children.* Portland, OR: Research Press.

Pattison, E. M., & Kahan, J. (1983). The deliberate self-harm syndrome. *American Journal of Psychiatry, 140*, 867–872.

Paul, T., Schroeter, K., Dahme, B., & Nutzinger, D. O. (2002). Self-injurious behavior in women with eating disorders. *American Journal of Psychiatry, 159*, 408–411.

Phillips, R. H., & Alkan, M. (1961). Some aspects of self-mutilation in the general population of a large psychiatric hospital. *Psychiatric Quarterly, 35*, 421–423.

Pies, R. W., & Popli, A. P. (1995). Self-injurious behavior: Pathophysiology and implications for treatment. *Journal of Clinical Psychiatry, 56*, 580–588.

Pipher, M. (1994). *Reviving Ophelia: Saving the selves of adolescent girls.* New York: Ballantine Books.

Podvoll, E. M. (1969). Self-mutilation within a hospital setting: A study of identity and social compliance. *British Journal of Medical Psychology, 42*, 213–221.

Ponton, L. E. (1997). *The romance of risk: Why teenagers do the things they do.* New York: Basic Books.

Rapaport, J. L., Ryland, D. H., & Kriete, M. (1992). Drug treatment of canine acral lick: An animal model of obsessive–compulsive behavior. *Archives of General Psychiatry, 49*, 517–521.

Rathus, J. H., & Miller, A. L. (2002). Dialectical behavior therapy adapted for suicidal adolescents. *Suicide and Life-Threatening Behavior, 32*(2), 146–157.

Rodham, K., Hawton, K., & Evans, E. (2004). Reasons for deliberate self-harm: Comparison of self-poisoners and self-cutters in a community sample of adolescents. *Journal of the American Academy of Child and Adolescent Psychiatry, 43*, 80–87.

Rodriguez-Srednicki, O. (2001). Childhood sexual abuse, dissociation and adult self-destructive behavior. *Journal of Child Sexual Abuse, 10*(3), 75–90.

Rosen, D. M., & Hoffman, A. (1972). Focal suicide: Self-mutilation in two young psychotic individuals. *American Journal of Psychiatry, 128,* 1367–1368.

Rosen, P., & Walsh, B. (1989). Relationship patterns in episodes of self-mutilative contagion. *American Journal of Psychiatry, 146,* 656–658.

Rosenberg, L. (1998). *Breath by breath, the liberating practice of insight meditation.* Boston: Shambhala.

Ross, R. R., & McKay, H. R. (1979). *Self-mutilation.* Lexington, MA: Lexington Books.

Ross, S., & Heath, N. (2002). A study of the frequency of self-mutilation in a community sample of adolescents. *Journal of Youth and Adolescence, 1,* 67–77.

Rothbaum, B. O., Meadows, E. A., Resick, P., & Foy, D. W. (2000). Cognitive-behavioral therapy. In E. B. Foa, T. M. Keane, & M. J. Friedman (Eds.), *Effective treatments for PTSD.* New York: Guilford Press.

Rothbaum, B. O., & Ninan, P. T. (1999). Manual for the cognitive-behavioral treatment of trichotillomania. In D. J. Stein, G. A. Christenson, & E. Hollander (Eds.), *Trichotillomania.* Washington, DC: American Psychiatric Press.

RUPP (Research Units on Pediatric Psychopharmacology) Autism Network. (2002). Risperidone in children with autism and serious behavioral problems. *New England Journal of Medicine, 347,* 314–321.

Rush, A. J., & Nowels, A. (1994). Adaptation of cognitive therapy for depressed adolescents. In T. C. R. Wilkes, G. Belsher, A. J. Rush, & E. Frank (Eds.), *Cognitive therapy for depressed adolescents.* New York: Guilford Press.

Russ, M. J., Roth, S. D., Kakuma, T., Harrison, K., & Hull, J. W. (1994). Pain perception in self-injurious borderline patients: Naloxone effects. *Biological Psychiatry, 35,* 207–209.

Russ, M. J., Roth, S. D., Lerman, A., Kakuma, T., Harrison, K., Shindledecker, R. D., Hull, J., & Matttis, S. (1992). Pain perception in self-injurious patients with borderline personality disorder. *Biological Psychiatry, 32*(6), 501–511.

Ryckman, R. M., Robbins, M., Thornton, B., & Cantrell, P. (1982). Development and validation of a physical self-efficacy scale. *Journal of Personality and Social Psychology, 42,* 891–900.

Sandman, C. A., & Hetrick, W. P. (1995). Opiate mechanisms in self-injury. *Mental Retardation and Developmental Disabilities Research Reviews, 1,* 130–136.

Sandman, C. A., Hetrick, W., Taylor, D. V., Marion, S. D., Touchette, P., Barron, J. L., Martinezzi, V., Steinberg, R. M., & Crinella, F. M. (2000). Long-term effects of naltrexone on self-injurious behavior. *American Journal of Mental Retardation, 105,* 103–117.

Schilder, P. (1935). *The image and appearance of the human body.* New York: International Universities Press.

Schroeder, S. R., Oster-Granite, M. L., & Thompson, T. (Eds.). (2002). *Self-injurious behavior.* Washington, DC: American Psychological Association.

Schwartz, A. E. (1995). *Guided imagery for groups.* Duluth, MN: Whole Person Associates.

Secord, P. F., & Jourard, S. M. (1953). The appraisal of body cathexis: Body cathexis and the self. *Journal of Consulting Psychology, 17*(5), 343–347.

Segal, Z. V., Williams, J. M. G., & Teasdale, J. D. (2002). *Mindfulness-based cognitive therapy for depressions.* New York: Guilford Press.

Sekida, K. (1985). *Zen training: Methods and philosophy.* New York: Weatherill.

Selekman, M. D. (2002). *Living on the razor's edge: Solution-oriented brief family therapy with self-harming adolescents.* New York: Norton.

Seligman, M. E. P. (1992). *Helplessness: On depression, development, and death.* New York: Freeman.

Shapira, N. A., Lessig, M. C., Murphy, T. K., Driscoll, D. J., & Goodman, W. K. (2002). Topiramate attenuates self-injurious behaviour in Prader-Willi syndrome. *International Journal of Neuropsychopharmacology, 5,* 141–145.

Shapiro, S., & Dominiak, G. M. (1992). *Sexual trauma and psychopathology.* New York: Lexington Books.

Shaw, S. N. (2002). *The complexity and paradox of female self-injury: Historical portrayals, journeys toward stopping, and contemporary interventions.* Unpublished doctoral dissertation, Harvard University Graduate School of Education, Cambridge, MA.

Shea, C. S. (1999). *The practical art of suicide assessment.* New York: Wiley.

Shneidman, E. S. (1985). *Definition of suicide.* New York: Wiley.

Shneidman, E. S. (1993). *Suicide as psychache.* New York: Wiley.

Simeon, D., & Favazza, A. (2001). Self-injurious behaviors, phenomenology and assessment. In D. Simeon & E. Hollander (Eds.), *Self-injurious behaviors, assessment and treatment.* Washington, DC: American Psychiatric Association.

Simeon, D., & Hollander, E. (Eds.). (2001). *Self-injurious behaviors, assessment and treatment.* Washington, DC: American Psychiatric Association.

Simeon, D., Stanley, B., & Frances, A. (1992). Self-mutilation in personality disorders: Psychological and biological correlates. *American Journal of Psychiatry, 148,* 221–226.

Stein, D. J., & Niehaus, D. J. H. (2001). Stereotypic self-injurious behaviors, neurobiology and psychopharmacology. In D. Simeon & E. Hollander (Eds.), *Self-injurious behaviors, assessment and treatment.* Washington, DC: American Psychiatric Association.

Sutton, J. (1999). *Healing the hurt within: Understand and relieve the suffering behind self-destructive behaviour.* Oxford, UK: Pathways.

Symons, F. J., Sutton, K. A., & Bodfish, J. W. (2001). Preliminary study of altered skin temperature at body sites associated with self-injurious behavior in adults who have developmental disabilities. *American Journal of Mental Retardation, 106,* 336–343.

Symons, F. J., & Thompson, T. (1997). Self-injurious behavior and body site preference. *Journal of Intellectual Disabilities Research, 41,* 456–468.

Taiminen, T. J., Kallio-Soukainen, K., Nokso-Koivisto, H., Kaljonen, A., & Helenius, H. (1998). Contagion of deliberate self-harm among adolescent inpatients. *Journal of the American Academy of Child and Adolescent Psychiatry, 37*(2), 211–217.

Thompson, J. K., Berland, N. W., Linton, P. J., & Weinsier, R. L. (1987). Utilization of self-adjusting light beam in the objective assessment of body distortion in seven eating disorder groups. *International Journal of Eating Disorders, 5*(11), 113–120.

Tiefenbacher S., Novak, M. A., Lutz, C. K., & Meyer, J. S. (2005). The physiology and neurochemistry of self-injurious behavior: A nonhuman primate model. *Frontiers in Bioscience, 10*, 1–11.

Tsiouris, J. A., Cohen, I. L., Patti, P. J., & Korosh, W. M. (2003). Treatment of previous undiagnosed psychiatric disorders in persons with developmental disabilities decreased or eliminated self-injurious behavior. *Journal of Clinical Psychiatry, 64*, 1081–1090.

Tucker, L. A. (1981). Internal structure, factor satisfaction, and reliability of the body cathexis scale. *Perceptual and Motor Skills, 53*, 891–896.

Tucker, L. A. (1983). The structure and dimensional satisfaction of the body cathexis construct of males: A factor analytic investigation. *Journal of Human Movement Studies, 9*, 189–194.

Tucker, L. A. (1985). Dimensionalilty and factor satisfaction of the body image construct: A gender comparison. *Sex Roles, 12*(9), 931–937.

Turell, S. C., & Armsworth, M. W. (2000). Differentiating incest survivors who self-mutilate. *Child Abuse and Neglect, 24*, 237–249.

Vale, V., & Juno, A. (1989). *Modern primitives*. San Francisco: Re/Search Publications.

van der Kolk, B. A., McFarlane, A. C., & Wiesaeth, L. (Eds.). (1996). *Traumatic stress*. New York: Guilford Press.

van der Kolk, B. A., Perry, C., & Herman, J. L. (1991). Childhood origins of self-destructive behavior. *American Journal of Psychiatry, 148*, 1665–1671.

Velazquez, L., Ward-Chene, L., & Loosigian, S. R. (2000). Fluoxetine in the treatment of self-mutilating behavior [Letter]. *Journal of the American Academy of Child and Adolescent Psychiatry, 39*, 812–814.

Villalba, R., & Harrington, C. J. (2000). Repetitive self-injurious behavior: A neuropsychiatric perspective and review of pharmacologic treatments. *Seminar in Clinical Neuropsychiatry, 5*, 215–226.

Virkkunen, M. (1976). Self-mutilation in antisocial personality disorder. *Acta Psychiatrica Scandanavica, 54*, 347–352.

Walser, R. D., & Hayes, S. C. (1998). In V. M. Follette, J. I. Ruzek, & F. R. Abueg (Eds.), *Cognitive-behavioral therapies for trauma*. New York: Guilford Press.

Walsh, B. W. (1987). *Adolescent self-mutilation: An empirical study*. Unpublished doctoral dissertation, Boston College Graduate School of Social Work, Chestnut Hill, MA.

Walsh, B. W. (2001). Self-mutilation. In C. D. Bryant (Ed.), *Encyclopedia of criminology and deviant behavior* (Vol. IV). London: Taylor & Francis.

Walsh, B. W., & Frost, A. K. (2005). *Attitudes regarding life, death, and body image in poly-self-destructive adolescents*. Unpublished study.

Walsh, B. W., & Rosen, P. (1985). Self-mutilation and contagion: An empirical test. *American Journal of Psychiatry, 142*, 119–120.

Walsh, B. W., & Rosen, P. (1988). *Self-mutilation: Theory, research and treatment*. New York: Guilford Press.

Warren, F., Dolan, B., & Norton, K. (1998). Bloodletting, bulimia nervosa and borderline personality disorder. *European Eating Disorders Review, 6,* 277–285.

Weintrob, A. (2001). Paxil and self-scratching [Letter to the editor]. *Journal of the American Academy of Child and Adolescent Psychiatry, 40,* 5.

Weissman, M. (1975). Wrist cutting. *Archives of General Psychiatry, 32,* 1166–1171.

Wilson, G. T., Fairburn, C. G., & Agras, W. S. (1997). Cognitive-behavioral therapy for bulimia nervosa. In D. M. Garner & P. E. Garfinkel (Eds.), *Handbook of treatment for eating disorders.* New York: Guilford Press.

Wolpe, J. (1969). *The practice of behavior therapy.* New York: Pergamon Press.

Zweig-Frank, H., Paris, J., & Guzder, J. (1994). Psychological risk factors for dissociation and self-mutilation in female patients with borderline personality disorder. *Canadian Journal of Psychiatry, 39,* 259–264.

Index